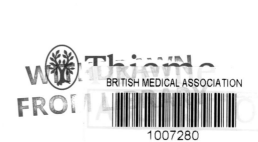

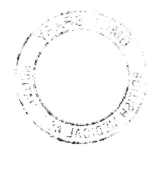

Neurosurgery Oral Board Review

Third Edition

Jonathan S. Citow, MD, FACS
Chief of Neurosurgery
Advocate Condell Medical Center
Libertyville, Illinois;
Assistant Clinical Professor of Neurosurgery
Rosalind Franklin University Medical School
North Chicago, Illinois;
President
American Center for Spine and Neurosurgery
Libertyville, Illinois, USA

Robert J. Spinner, MD
Chair
Department of Neurologic Surgery;
The Burton M. Onofrio, MD Professor of Neurosurgery;
Professor of Orthopaedics and Anatomy
Mayo Clinic
Rochester, Minnesota, USA

Ross C. Puffer, MD
Chief Neurosurgical Resident
Department of Neurosurgery
Mayo Clinic
Rochester, Minnesota, USA

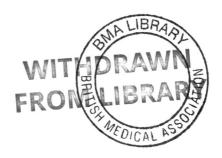

335 illustrations

Thieme
New York • Stuttgart • Delhi • Rio de Janeiro

Acquisitions Editor: Timothy Hiscock
Managing Editor: Madhumita Dey
Director, Editorial Services: Mary Jo Casey
Production Editor: Shivika
International Production Director: Andreas Schabert
Editorial Director: Sue Hodgson
International Marketing Director: Fiona Henderson
International Sales Director: Louisa Turrell
Senior Vice President and Chief Operating
Officer: Sarah Vanderbilt
President: Brian D. Scanlan

Library of Congress Cataloging-in-Publication Data
is available from the Publisher.

Important note: Medicine is an ever-changing science undergoing continual development. Research and clinical experience are continually expanding our knowledge, in particular our knowledge of proper treatment and drug therapy. Insofar as this book mentions any dosage or application, readers may rest assured that the authors, editors, and publishers have made every effort to ensure that such references are in accordance with **the state of knowledge at the time of production of the book.**

Nevertheless, this does not involve, imply, or express any guarantee or responsibility on the part of the publishers in respect to any dosage instructions and forms of applications stated in the book. **Every user is requested to examine carefully** the manufacturers' leaflets accompanying each drug and to check, if necessary in consultation with a physician or specialist, whether the dosage schedules mentioned therein or the contraindications stated by the manufacturers differ from the statements made in the present book. Such examination is particularly important with drugs that are either rarely used or have been newly released on the market. Every dosage schedule or every form of application used is entirely at the user's own risk and responsibility. The authors and publishers request every user to report to the publishers any discrepancies or inaccuracies noticed. If errors in this work are found after publication, errata will be posted at www.thieme.com on the product description page.

Some of the product names, patents, and registered designs referred to in this book are in fact registered trademarks or proprietary names even though specific reference to this fact is not always made in the text. Therefore, the appearance of a name without designation as proprietary is not to be construed as a representation by the publisher that it is in the public domain..

© 2020. Thieme. All rights reserved.
Thieme Publishers New York
333 Seventh Avenue, New York, NY 10001 USA
+1 800 782 3488, customerservice@thieme.com

Thieme Publishers Stuttgart
Rüdigerstrasse 14, 70469 Stuttgart, Germany
+49 [0]711 8931 421, customerservice@thieme.de

Thieme Publishers Delhi
A-12, Second Floor, Sector-2, Noida-201301
Uttar Pradesh, India
+91 120 45 566 00, customerservice@thieme.in

Thieme Publishers Rio de Janeiro,
Thieme Publicações Ltda.
Edifício Rodolpho de Paoli, 25ª andar
Av. Nilo Peçanha, 50 – Sala 2508
Rio de Janeiro 20020-906 Brasil
+55 21 3172 2297

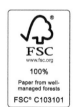

FSC
www.fsc.org
100%
Paper from well-managed forests
FSC® C103101

Cover design: Thieme Publishing Group   5 4 3 2 1
Typesetting by DiTech Process Solutions, India

Printed in USA by King Printing Company, Inc.

ISBN 978-1-68420-126-6

Also available as an e-book:
eISBN 978-1-68420-127-3

I would like to dedicate this book to Mr. Alberto Giorgio Denny Rothschild. He is the distinguished father of my best friend Gary and served as a second father to me after my father passed away in early childhood. His combination of intensity and compassion fit well with my dream of becoming a neurosurgeon. I studied for my medical boards in his suburban basement far from the distractions of my own apartment in the city of Chicago and his entire family has always been an excellent support system for me and my family.

Jonathan S. Citow

Contents

Content

Preface to the Third Edition

Neurosurgery Oral Board Review, Third edition is a substantial update to an already existing excellent resource for preparation of American Board of Neurological Surgery (ABNS) oral examination. Due to recent advances in the field of neurosurgery, the practices of neurosurgery have drastically transformed, and so is the format of the exam. In order to stay up to date and closely mirror the content and style of the exam, we have updated significant portions of the book from the second edition and added 80 new practice cases in oral board format. These cases are self-interactive, that is, they allow you to read the patient presentation/imaging and practice by giving your response to the case. We have also added sample responses to situations that you can refer to if needed. Every operative case will also describe a complication or event and ask you to describe how you would deal with that situation. Again, you can practice your response, or refer to our sample answer if you are stuck. Each case includes a list stating other potential complications (for further practice) and a short list of references should you want to pursue more in-depth literature on the topic from Thieme's MedOne Neurosurgery resource.

We truly hope that this updated version is a valuable resource for quick review and test practice for the real oral board examination. Practicing multiple cases and varying complications should help ease some of the pre-test anxiety and give you the right blend of confidence needed to pass the test and put the neurosurgery oral board examinations behind you for good!

Jonathan S. Citow, MD, FACS
Robert J. Spinner, MD
Ross C. Puffer, MD

Preface to the Second Edition

I wrote this book using the notes that I scribbled down while studying for the neurosurgery oral board examination. This book is not intended to serve as a replacement for classic neurosurgical texts, but as a supplement to the knowledge gained during the long years of residency and in the early stages of practice. I tried to focus on the major aspects of diseases that a neurosurgeon may encounter, both in clinical practice and on the examination. For a more thorough helping of knowledge, consider thumbing through the texts in the reference list. My favorite is *Comprehensive Neurosurgical Board Review (Third Edition)*, but I may be a little biased. That book was geared for the written boards, but the anatomy, pathology/radiology, neurology, and neurosurgery sections provide useful information that is not covered in this text.

I must admit that I was a tad intimidated by the oral examination before I lived through it. I expected to hear "So, Dr. Citow, can you please show me the incision for the hypoglossal-pundendal nerve anastomses used for people who constantly speak out of their asses." But it really was a fair test and a surprisingly pleasant experience. I truly got the sense that the examiners are out to reinforce their preconceived notion that the examinee (you) is indeed competent—not the other way around—and makes reasonable decisions. They are not out to trick you with obscure details. Stay relaxed and suggest exactly what you would do in everyday practice (not in a surreal ivory tower university setting) and all will be fine. The only disheartening aspect of the test is that none of the examiners smile (but this may be their baseline state) or acknowledge that you are correct (but neither do your patients in the hospital, unless they have been on the Internet).

Good luck!

Introduction

Relax, there is little the examiners will ask you that you have not treated successfully numerous times. Remember, this book is only our view of things. There are many ways to skin a nerve root. As long as the patients are well cared for, all will be fine. In this third edition, we have kept true to the major *purpose* of the first successful edition, that is, to serve as a *concise and easy-to-read* review book that can basically be covered in a few days as a *supplement* to additional study. We don't advocate preparing for the boards in one weekend, but the nature of our profession often requires quick reviews. Nevertheless, we have made several changes in this edition that will greatly enhance your preparation. Sections and chapters are reorganized into topics to better follow the format of the real examination. We have added to the end of each chapter some key helpful hints. In addition, we have added a quick reference section, new images, and an expansive case preparation section comprising 80 cases. These cases will allow you to practice individual cases in oral board format and formulate your responses to questions. They also provide basic guidance on safe treatment strategies. There are references for further reading if you want to dive a little deeper into the pathology and treatment strategies for a given pathology.

Because of the nature of the oral board examination, success clearly depends on confidence, which depends on knowing what to expect. Understanding the conditions will help reduce anxiety and improve success. The American Board of Neurological Surgery (ABNS) states that the purpose of the examination is to "determine competency in diagnosis and management;" however, it also explicitly states that the examination "focuses on problems neurosurgeons can expect." We would argue that this latter acknowledgment should receive as much if not more attention than the former during your preparation. Yes, you must know the basics in diagnosing and managing diseases of the nervous system, but the ABNS wants to make sure you are a safe neurosurgeon and that you avoid and appropriately manage complications. Most examinees will have recently completed residency and written board exams, so the basic knowledge of diagnosis and management is there and simply need review. However, many examinees lack extensive practical experience of dealing with complications. Regardless of your experience with complications, you must demonstrate to the ABNS that you have solid complication avoidance skills.

The basic format of the oral examination has not changed for years. It only lasts for three hours. The first hour is based on basic neurosurgery (cranial and spine trauma, basic emergency department evaluation and management, such as subdural hematomas and acute spinal cord injury). The second hour is dedicated to more focused examination in a given specialty field, such as complex spine or vascular neurosurgery. The third hour is dedicated to your submitted case list. During each hour, you will meet two examiners who are mostly leaders in neurosurgery. Do not expect them to ask you questions in their field of expertise, outside of the hour of subspecialty focus. Typically, you will be presented a case history with symptoms and physical exam findings via a PowerPoint slideshow, and then you will be asked how you would proceed. You must formulate a differential diagnosis and then be prepared to discuss how you would work up each diagnosis. As you do this, the examiners will give you results that will guide you to the most likely diagnosis. At this time you must be prepared to discuss in detail your medical and surgical treatment options. There will be paper and cranial and spine models in the room that you can use. Once you demonstrate your knowledge of treatments, the examiners will likely interrupt you to proceed on to something else, for example, postoperative management of a complication.

Time is of essence! It is paramount that you practice the real situation to get used to this very short and fast exam. Being comfortable with the relatively fast format will greatly help you. The exact scoring system is not discussed in detail in the ABNS literature, so we are unsure of the methodology. However, members of the ABNS have reviewed it at the American Association of Neurological Surgeons (AANS) annual meeting sessions devoted to this topic. Basically, each case is scored between 0 to 4 in areas of diagnosis, management, and complications. The "passing" average likely changes each year based on the performances in that year. Achieving a particular score does not appear to be the key; instead, what has been repeatedly emphasized is that you cover at least 6 cases per hour to accumulate enough points to achieve the passing score. This equates to only 10 minutes per case. We have found through our own experiences and teaching review courses that most folks are woefully unsatisfied with how much they discuss a case in 10 minutes. You will likely not say every important fact that the examiner is looking for about a particular case in 10 minutes, but you can let the examiner know that you know a lot about a particular case's diagnosis and management. You achieve that by talking. Think quickly, and then say what's on your mind. You will lose valuable time if you wait for the examiner to ask you a question. Instead, let the examiners interrupt you and redirect the discussion where they want—this is in your best interest.

Most people tackle this examination differently, but over the years we have accumulated some advice that seems to come up consistently from recent examiners:

1. Apply to ABNS to sit for oral exam as soon as you can after accumulating appropriate practice data after residency. The day after completion of your residency may be the smartest day of your life, and it will be helpful to do your oral exam as close to this day as possible. Once you apply, it will take many months for them to schedule your exam.

2. Gather review materials months ahead, but give yourself a dedicated 1 to 2 weeks off work before the exam to really focus on it.

3. Practice the exam, especially with senior colleagues or at review courses. This may be awkward for some, so you need to get over it and practice.

4. Spend the night near the testing site, so you can arrive very early, get familiar with the setup, and relax.

5. Review your submitted practice data and expect questions about it.

6. During the exam, you will be provided with paper and pencil, but taking extensive notes may slow you down, so be judicious if you need notes. We recommend not taking notes.

7. If you know the examiner, forget his or her specialty as you will most likely be asked questions from outside that specialty.

8. Don't guess. If you don't know, say so, but recommend how you might go about getting an answer. If you don't do a certain technique, say so, and tell them what you do in the real world (e.g., send patients to your cerebrovascular neurosurgery colleague). *But,* you will still be expected to discuss the basic craniotomy for clipping a particular aneurysm. Consults are wise, but typically not available during your exam! The assumption is that you should be able to deal with any basic neurosurgery issue if you had to.

9. Be humble. A reasonable assumption is that arrogant and overly self-confident neurosurgeons make deadly mistakes. No matter how well you discuss cases, we suspect this type of attitude will be significantly penalized.

10. Lastly, our knowledge of neurosurgery and educational methods are constantly evolving, as is the field of neurosurgery. We would encourage you to use this book as a broad overview of topics and test prep while using more focused resources for intensive review as you need.

Best of luck!

Suggested Readings

Youmans Neurological Surgery. Winn HR. Philadelphia, PA: Elsevier–Health Sciences Division, 2010.

Handbook of Neurosurgery, 9th Edition. Greenberg MS, New York, NY: Thieme Medical Publishers, 2020.

Adams and Victor's Principles of Neurology, 9th Edition. Ropper A, Samuels M. New York, NY: McGraw-Hill Professional, 2009.

Comprehensive Neurosurgery Board Review, 3rd Edition. Citow JS Macdonald RL, Puffer RC, Khalid SI, Carter BS, Cohen AR, Spinner RJ, Refai D. New York, NY: Thieme Medical Publishers, 2020.

The following journals were referred for information:

Journal of Neurosurgery
Neurosurgery
Surgical Neurology

Part 1

Spinal Disorders

1 Spinal Anatomy and Approaches

I. Spinal Column Anatomy

A. Cervical—should see smooth anterior spinous line, posterior spinous line, spinol-aminar line, and spinous tip line; atlanto-occipital distance should be < 10 mm; C1, odontoid distance should be <5 mm; and facets should look like shingles. Rule of Spence states that C1 (**Fig. 1.1**) lateral masses should not extend more than a total of 7 mm over C2 (on odontoid view).

B. Thoracolumbar (**Fig. 1.2**).

II. Spinal Tracts

A. Upper extremities are medial in the corticospinal tracts and spinothalamic tracts.

B. Lower extremities are medial in the posterior columns (**Fig. 1.3** and **Fig. 1.4**).

III. Arterial Supply to Spinal Cord

A. One anterior spinal artery forms from two vertebral arteries. There are two posterior spinal arteries. Anterior and posterior spinal arteries get radicular artery inputs with a watershed zone in midthoracic.

B. Artery of Adamkiewicz (a radicular artery) usually enters the spinal canal on the left at T9–12 to supply T8 to the conus.

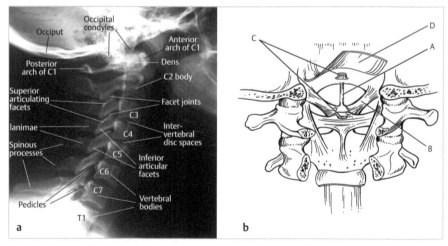

Fig. 1.1 (a) Cervical anatomy. (b) Cervical ligamentous anatomy. A, apical; B, alar; C, cruciform; D, tectorial.

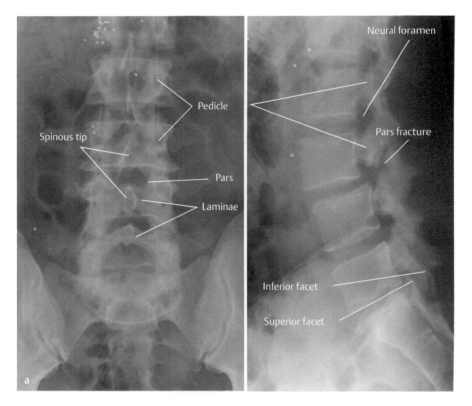

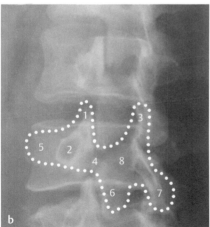

Fig. 1.2 Thoracolumbar anatomy. **(a)** Anteroposterior (AP) view and **(b)** oblique view (to look at pars and down the pedicle axis) "Scotty dog" view: **1.** Ear–superior articular process of facet (left); **2.** Eye–pedicle (left); **3.** Tail–superior articular process of facet (right); **4.** Neck–pars interarticularis, fractured (left); **5.** Snout–transverse process (left); **6.** Inferior articular process of facet (left); **7.** Hind leg–inferior articular process of facet (right); **8.** Body–lamina (left).

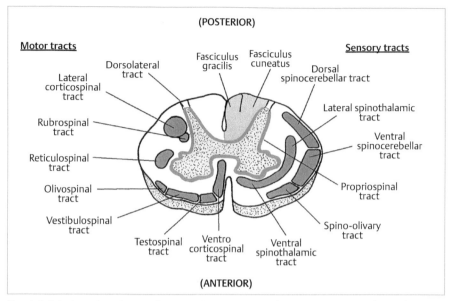

Fig. 1.3 Spinal cord pathways. (Source: Citow JS. Comprehensive Neurosurgical Board Review. New York, NY: Thieme Medical Publishers; 2000: 69, Fig. 1.39.)

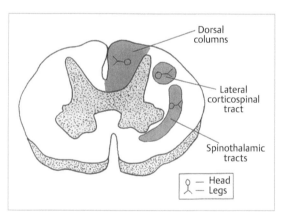

Fig. 1.4 Spinal cord somatotopic organization. (Source: Citow JS. Comprehensive Neurosurgical Board Review. New York, NY: Thieme Medical Publishers; 2000: 70, Fig. 1.40.)

IV. Evaluation

A. Motor examination—deltoid (C5), biceps (C5,6), triceps (C7,8), wrist extension (C6), finger extension (C7), finger flexion (C8), interosseous (T1), hip flexion (L2), knee extension (L4), dorsiflexion (L4), extensor hallucis longus (L5), and plantar flexion (S1).

B. Sensory examination—key levels are C1 (no sensory branch), C2 (posterior head), C6 (thumb), C8 (pinky), T4 (nipples), T10 (umbilicus), L4 (anterior knee), L5 (big toe), and S1 (lateral foot) (**Fig. 1.5**).

C. Deep tendon reflexes—biceps (C5,6), triceps (C7,8), brachioradialis (C6), patellar (L4), and Achilles' (S1).

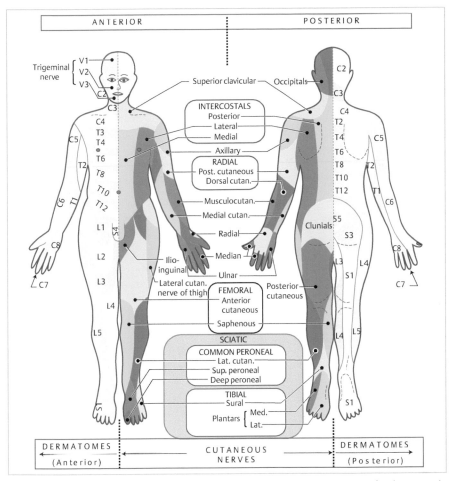

Fig. 1.5 Dermatome chart. (Source: Greenberg MS. Handbook of Neurosurgery. 7th ed. New York, NY: Thieme Medical Publishers; 2010: 94, Fig. 5.13.)

V. Basic Spine Approaches—Accessible Region (Frequent Indications)

A. Transoral (**Fig. 1.6**).

1. Access to lower two-thirds of the clivus, anterior C1, odontoid.

2. Indications—basilar invagination, tumors such as chordoma and chondrosarcoma.

3. Endoscopic approaches can now reliably provide access to lower two-thirds of the clivus, but require advanced training, experience, and assistance from an otorhinolaryngologist (ENT).

4. Risk of infection and swallowing difficulties with standard transoral approach.

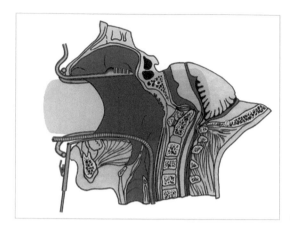

Fig. 1.6 Transoral approach and accessible spine regions.

B. Far lateral transcondylar.
1. Access to foramen magnum.
2. Indications—intradural lesions such as meningioma.

C. Suboccipital with midline posterior cervical.
1. Access from occiput to C2/3.
    a. Indications—unstable conditions such as atlanto-occipital dislocation.
2. May do C2 pedicle or pars screw with C3 pedicle or pars or lateral mass screw based on anatomy (**Fig. 1.7**).

D. Midline high posterior cervical.
1. Access to C1–3 for Brook, Gallie, Sonntag, or C1/2 transarticular screws.
2. Indications—Hangman fracture, dislocation, displaced or unhealed odontoid fracture (**Fig. 1.8**).

E. Anterior odontoid screw.
1. Skin entry at T2, screw enters between C2 and C3 anterior border guided by K wire.
2. Indications—nondisplaced type 2 odontoid fracture (**Fig. 1.7**); can be difficult with large chest; not ideal for comminuted fractures.

F. Posterior cervical.
1. Access to C3–7 for laminectomy or laminoplasty.
2. Indications—cervical spondylotic myelopathy with lordosis, tumor, ossified posterior longitudinal ligament (OPLL), add foraminotomy for foraminal stenosis.
3. Add lateral mass screws (**Fig. 1.7**) for traumatic, degenerative, pathologic spondylolisthesis.

G. Anterior cervical.
1. Access to C3–T1.
2. Indications—corpectomies for trauma, tumor, infection, deformity, OPLL, diskectomy, and fusion for disk bulge (**Fig. 1.9**).
3. Avoid if posterior compression is greater than three levels, prior extensive neck surgery, and severe osteoporosis.

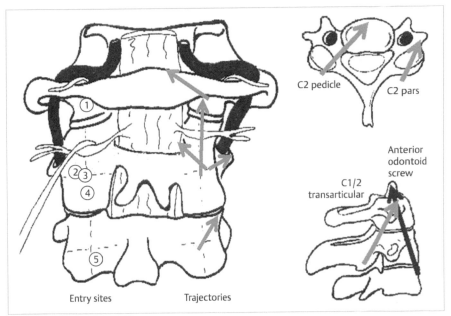

Fig. 1.7 High posterior cervical fusion screw entry sites and trajectories. Use preoperative computed tomography (CT)/CT angiography to check anatomy, vertebral artery, and calculate screw sizes. **1.** C1 lateral mass screw: hold down C2 nerve root, drill notch in inferior C1 arch, palpate medial wall of lateral mass, enter in midline or 5 mm lateral to medial wall of lateral mass, lean your hand 20 degrees lateral and 10 degrees caudal to aim for C1 anterior tubercle, use ~4 × 35 mm screw. **2.** C2 pars screw: enter 3 mm rostral and 3 mm lateral to midpoint, lean your hand 10 degrees medial and 10 degrees caudal, use ~ 4 × 16 mm screw. **3.** C2 pedicle screw: enter 3 mm rostral and 2 mm lateral to midpoint, lean your hand 15 degrees lateral and 20 degrees caudal, use ~4 × 35 mm screw. **4.** C1/2 transarticular screw, enter 3 mm rostral and 3 mm lateral to inferomedial edge of C2/3 facet joint, use K wire as guide, lean hand 5 degrees medial and 45 degrees caudal to aim through joint and into C1 arch, use ~ 4 × 40 mm screw. **5.** C3 through C7 lateral mass screw, enter 1 mm medial and 1 mm caudal to midpoint, lean hand 20 degrees medial and 20 degrees caudal to aim for superolateral corner of lateral mass, use 4 × 16 mm screw.

    4.   May consider cervical arthroplasty for selected patients/indications, such as young patient with single-level disease and preserved lordosis.

H. Median sternotomy (trap-door approach) with cardiothoracic (CT) surgeon.

    1.   Access to T1–4 (stay on right side to avoid heart; use double lumen endotracheal [ET] tube to deflate one lung).

    2.   Indications—corpectomies for trauma, tumor, infection, deformity, and OPLL; diskectomy and foraminotomy for disk bulge.

I. Lower thoracotomy with CT surgeon.

    1.   Access to T5–L2 (stay on left side to avoid great vessels, incise two levels above pathology).

    2.   Indications—anterior pathology such as trauma, infection, fracture, disks.

J. Posterior thoracic.

    1.   Access to posterior T1–12 (only posterior pathology).

    2.   Indications—laminectomy for trauma, tumor, OPLL.

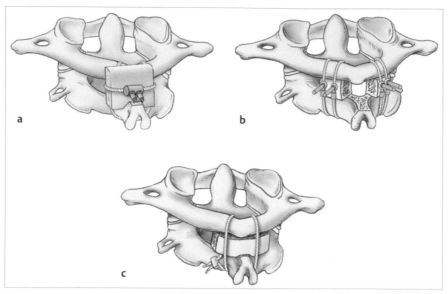

Fig. 1.8 (a) Brook, **(b)** Gallie, and **(c)** Sonntag posterior cervical fusion techniques. (Source: Fessler RG, Sekhar L. Atlas of Neurosurgical Techniques: Spine and Peripheral Nerves. New York, NY: Thieme Medical Publishers; 2006:135–136, Figs. 16.8 and 16.9.)

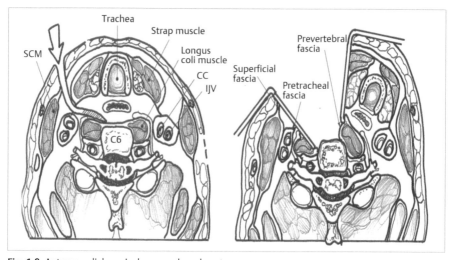

Fig. 1.9 Anteromedial cervical approach and anatomy.

3. Add transpedicular, costotransversectomy, or lateral extracavitary for lateral pathology.
4. Add pedicle screws for instability (**Fig. 1.10a–d**).
   a. Pedicular or extrapedicular (between pedicle and rib head).
   b. Palpate pedicle with Penfield #4 to define its location.

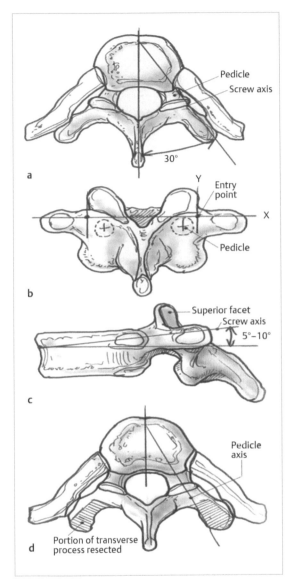

Fig. 1.10 (a–d) Thoracic pedicle screw placement.

    c. Enter 2 mm caudal to superior facet edge and even with superior facet lateral edge.

    d. Lean hand laterally 30 degrees at T1 and only 10 degrees at T12.

K. Retroperitoneal approach.

    1. Access to anterior L1–5 (left side to avoid liver and vena cava).

    2. Incision above umbilicus gets you to L1–4 and below umbilicus for L4–S1.

    3. Divide left anterior abdominal muscles down to preperitoneal fat and dissect laterally cutting latissimus dorsi to expose quadratus lumborum and iliopsoas medially.

4. Sweep sympathetic chain laterally and ureter medially.

5. Clip aortic radicular arteries as needed.

6. Remove pathology leaving contralateral cortex intact.

7. Distract intervertebral space with pins.

8. Place cage filled with bone graft, and secure with anterolateral plates (i.e., Kaneda) (**Fig. 1.11** and **Fig. 1.12**).

9. Indications—tumor, infection, spondylosis, anterior lumbar interbody fusion (ALIF), arthroplasty, trauma.

L. Transabdominal.

1. Access to direct anterior L5–S1 for ALIF or arthroplasty.

M. Posterior lumbosacral.

1. Access to L1–sacrum for laminectomy.

2. Add transforaminal lumbar interbody fusion (TLIF; complete foraminotomy for nerve root decompression) or posterior lumbar interbody fusion (PLIF) if familiar with them.

3. Add pedicle screws for instability.

a. Drill off lateral facet, enter at midpoint of transverse process at facet/transverse process (TP) junction, lean hand laterally 30 degrees (**Fig. 1.13**).

4. Indications—neurogenic claudication from lumbar stenosis, trauma, tumor, infection, recurrent radiculopathy (TLIF).

N. Lateral lumbosacral.

1. Access to L2–4 (e.g., direct lateral interbody fusion and extreme lateral interbody fusion) if you are familiar with them; cannot reach L1 laterally due to ribs or L5 laterally due to iliac crest.

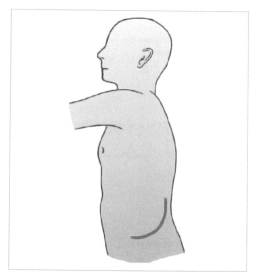

Fig. 1.11 Retroperitoneal approach. (Source: Citow JS. Neurosurgery Oral Board Review. 1st ed. New York, NY: Thieme Medical Publishers; 2003: 139, Fig. 12.13.)

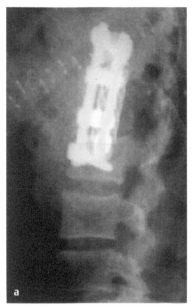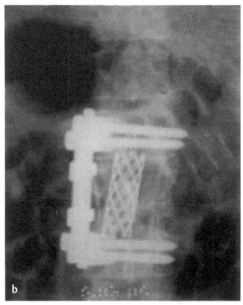

Fig. 1.12 (a) Lateral X-ray of Kaneda plate fusion. (b) Anteroposterior X-ray of Kaneda plate fusion. (Source: Citow JS. Neurosurgery Oral Board Review. 1st ed. New York, NY: Thieme Medical Publishers; 2003: 139, Fig. 12.14.)

O. Sacroiliac joint fusion.

1. Option for patients who have had exhausted conservative therapies and have benefited from several sacroiliac (SI) joint injections; still controversial and under active study.

2. Technique involves lateral to medial placement of often three screws or implants with bone graft.

3. May be performed in minimally invasive fashion.

VI. Common Complications Associated with Basic Approaches (with Prevention/Treatment Strategies)

A. Transoral—cerebrospinal fluid (CSF) leak (lumbar drain), infection (preoperative oral cultures), vascular injury (preoperative computed tomography angiography [CTA]), dysphagia (postoperative percutaneous endoscopic gastrostomy tube [PEG]), respiratory difficulties (postoperative tracheotomy), tongue swelling (relax retractor every hour [q1h]).

B. Anteromedial cervical—wrong level (intraoperative fluoroscopy), paralysis from hyperextension injury in severe stenosis (fiberoptic intubation, examination after positioning, somatosensory evoked potentials [SSEPs]), dysarthria (use left side to avoid the lower coursing left recurrent laryngeal nerve [RLN]), dysphagia (good longus coli release to hold retractor, postoperative barium swallow study for esophageal leak, postoperative steroids), thoracic duct injury (leave drain; low-fat diet), stroke and Horner syndrome (do not dissect lateral to longus coli or around carotid sheath), CSF leak (leave eggshell of bone in OPLL), C5 palsy (don't retract

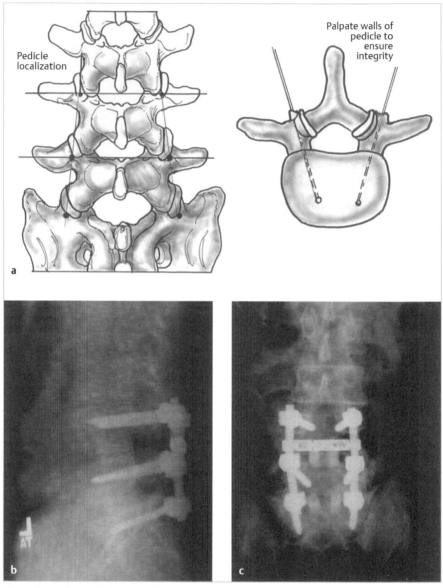

Fig. 1.13 Lumbar pedicle screw placement. **(a)** Pedicle screw placement. **(b)** Lateral X-ray of L4–S1 pedicle screw fusion with tangent bony posterior lumbar interbody fusion (PLIF). **(c)** Anteroposterior X-ray of L4–S1 pedicle screw fusion with tangent bony PLIFs. (Fig. 1.13B, C Source: Citow JS. Neurosurgery Oral Board Review. 1st ed. New York, NY: Thieme Medical Publishers; 2003: 138, Fig. 12.12A, B.)

nerve), vertebral artery injury (don't go beyond lateral annulus), sleep apnea or bradycardia (C3/4 procedures), pneumothorax (check postoperative chest X-ray [CXR] in low cervical cases), CSF leak (treat with fibrin glue and lumbar drain), graft subsidence (too much endplate drilling), pseudoarthrosis (redo, extend fusion, add posterior tension band fusion), worsened myelopathy in 5% (counsel patient preoperative).

C. Posterior cervical—wrong level (intraoperative fluoroscopy), neurologic injury (fluoroscopy, SSEPs, and motor evoked potentials [MEPs]), infection (lavage, Prolene sutures), C5 palsy (1–2 mm Kerrison rongeur during foraminotomy), vertebral artery injury (don't pull out screws that hit artery), instability (fuse if straight or kyphotic).

D. Thoracotomy—pneumothorax (chest tube), chylothorax (try to ligate; leave drain; low-fat diet), vascular (ask CT surgeon), neurologic injury (restrict only to anterior pathology; SSEPs and MEPs), thoracic radiculopathy (avoid neurovascular bundle adhered to inferior rib margin), hypohidrosis or Horner (avoid high thoracic sympathetic chain).

E. Left lateral paramedian incision for anterior lumbar—vascular and visceral injuries (ask general surgeon to expose), infertility (avoid sympathetic plexus, monitor hypogastric plexus), hernia (ask general surgeon to close).

F. Posterior lumbosacral approaches—hematoma (leave drain), infection, misplaced screws (use anteroposterior [AP] and lateral fluoroscopy; intraop navigation; try to stimulate nerve root from within pedicle).

G. Traction with Gardner-Wells or Halo.

1. Epidural hematoma, skull fracture, herniated disk, occipitoatlantal dislocation, infection.

2. Halos can result in swan neck deformity in midcervical (C3–5).

H. Prophylactic surgical antibiotics.

1. Cefazolin—1 g intravenously (IV) 1 hour before incision and 24 hours postsurgery.

2. Vancomycin—if patient is allergic to Cefazolin.

3. For nasal or oral surgery—gentamicin 120 mg IV q8h and clindamycin 300 mg IV q8h for 24 hours.

Helpful Hints

1. Standard spine surgical preoperative—consent with risks; complete blood cell count (CBC), electrolytes, prothrombin time/partial thromboplastin time (PT/PTT), blood available, urinalysis (UA), CXR, electrocardiogram (ECG); antibiotics before incision.

2. Neuromonitor spine cases with SSEP (dorsal cord), MEP (ventral cord), or direct nerve stimulation (when nerve roots exposed).

3. Consider neuronavigation when placing hardware. Preoperative reconstructed CT to ascertain screw location and sizes, preoperative CTA to see vertebral arteries, intraop fluoroscopy or CT to guide screw placement.

4. During spine procedure, localize with intraop fluoroscopy before incision, upon bony exposure, before placing hardware, and after placing hardware.

5. C5 takes a dive. C5 is most common nerve root injury after surgery, likely retraction injury due to larger nerve in smaller foraminal canal.

Case 1

A 61-year-old male presents with difficulty with fine motor control in hands and frequent tripping. Past medical history is significant for degenerative joint disease. Examination revealed symmetric hyperreflexia in arms and legs, positive Hoffman and clonus, and up going Babinski (**Fig. 1.14**).

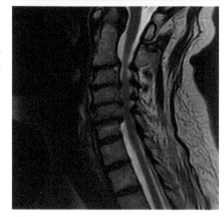

Fig. 1.14

Case 2

A 30-year-old plumber presents with new onset of pain in neck radiating down left lateral arm and into thumb and index finger for past 2 weeks; no other symptoms. Past medical history is significant for diabetes and recent pneumonia. Examination was normal. Axial T2-weighted magnetic resonance image taken through C4/5 disk (**Fig. 1.15**).

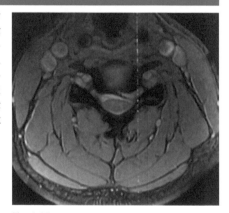

Fig. 1.15

Case 3

A 48-year-old construction worker presents with new onset of sharp shooting pain around his left torso and difficulty walking. Past medical history is significant for degenerative spine disease, smoking, and hypertension. Examination revealed thoracic dermatomal loss of pinprick, motor strength four-fifth throughout legs, hyperreflexia in his legs, three beats of bilateral clonus, and upgoing Babinski (**Fig. 1.16**).

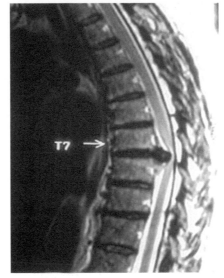

Fig. 1.16

2 Spine Trauma

I. Spinal Shock

A. Loss of sympathetic tone and muscle paralysis cause venous pooling with hypotension (usually occur with injuries above T7).

B. Loss of voluntary and reflex movements as well as sensation after a spinal cord injury; may last as long as 2 weeks; priapism is a bad sign.

C. Spinal shock may make accurate American Spinal Injury Association (ASIA) diagnosis incorrect. Must wait for spinal shock to wear off (indicated by the return of the bulbocavernosus reflex) before accurate ASIA examination.

II. Hypotension

A. Causes—hypovolemia, myocardial dysfunction, or loss of sympathetic tone.

B. Treatment:
   1. Loss of sympathetic tone—levophed (norepinephrine), phenylephrine (may cause reflex bradycardia), or dopamine to maintain systolic blood pressure (SBP) to greater than 90 mm Hg.
   2. Prevent pulmonary edema from overhydration.
   3. Use atropine for bradycardia.

III. Initial Management

A. Immobilize patient with cervical collar and backboard.

B. Address airway, breathing, circulation (ABC); consider nasotracheal intubation if no suspected cribriform plate trauma.

C. Insert nasogastric (NG) tube (ileus common), Foley catheter, and A-line.

D. Initiate deep vein thrombosis (DVT) prophylaxis with thrombo-embolic deterrent (TED) hose, sequential compression devices (SCDs), and subcutaneous (SQ) heparin or Lovenox.

E. Watch for hypothermia and electrolyte abnormalities.

F. Consider initiating mean arterial pressure target of greater than 85 mm Hg, using pressors if necessary.

IV. Radiologic Evaluation

A. Cervical, thoracic, and lumbar spine X-rays; chest X-ray (CXR); kidney, ureter, bladder (KUB); and pelvic X-ray.

B. No need to perform flexion–extension X-rays if greater than 3.5 mm subluxation because there is almost certainly instability.

C. Children of less than 4 years-age may have pseudospread of the atlas on anteroposterior (AP) view of 2–8 mm (a fracture must be determined by computed tomography [CT]).

D. Children may also have 3 mm of subluxation at C2–3 up to 10 years.

V. Solumedrol (Methylprednisolone) Protocol

A. Traumatic spinal cord dysfunction—Medication must be started within 8 hours of injury.

B. Dose—30 mg/kg over 45 minutes, wait 15 minutes, then 5.4 mg/kg/h over 23 hours.

C. Third NASCAS study suggests that if steroids are started within 3 hours of injury, they should be continued for 24 hours; if started from 3–8 hours after injury, they should be continued for 48 hours.

D. Controversial protocol, so know the risks (acute corticosteroid myopathy, pneumonia, hyperglycemia, sepsis) and exclusion criteria (cauda equina syndrome, gunshot wounds, pregnancy, age <13 years) if using it.

E. Steroid side effects—avascular necrosis, mood changes, hypertension, glucose intolerance.

F. In 2013, Congress of Neurological Surgeons did not recommend the use of high-dose methylprednisolone because of high rates of complications and limited efficacy in studies conducted during that time. Some providers still use methylprednisolone in incomplete cervical spinal cord injuries, hoping to achieve better recovery, although evidence is lacking.

VI. Traction

A. Avoid in cases of atlanto-occipital dislocation, type 2 or 3 Hangman fractures, or children less than 3 years age.

B. Consider magnetic resonance imaging (MRI) before initiating traction to make sure there is not a herniated disk that may be pulled into the spinal cord (rare occurrence). Not necessary if patient is awake and has an examination that can be followed.

C. Place Gardner-Wells tongs with pins 2.5 fingerbreadths above the pinna; for neutral position above the external acoustic meatus (EAM), for flexion 2 cm posterior, and for extension 2 cm anterior.

  1. Tighten pins daily for 3 days to 60 lbs (pin indicator 1 cm beyond surface).

  2. Avoid using traction weight more than 40–50 lbs.

  3. Obtain frequent X-rays to evaluate alignment and make sure that the disk spaces do not exceed 10 mm and the occipital condyle–C1 lateral mass spaces do not exceed 5 mm.

  4. Halo pins should be placed while the eyes are closed to 8 lb/inch and the bars tightened to 30 lb/inch.

  5. Dislocation reduction is best performed with fluoroscopy to save time.

6. Avoid raising the head, preventing the patient from seeing the ground, but avoid overflexion, preventing the patient from swallowing.
7. Use pin care with half-strength hydrogen peroxide and bacitracin ointment three times daily.

VII. Spinal Cord Levels

A. To determine the location of a spinal cord level in relation to the vertebral level, subtract 2 from T2–10 to be at the spinal cord level.
B. Bones of T11–L1 are over the spinal cord levels L1–5, S1–5, and C x 1 (**Fig. 2.1**).

VIII. Complete Injury (May Repair Nonurgently)

A. No voluntary movement, sensation, or sphincter control below injured spinal cord level.
B. Priapism may occur from lack of sympathetic input.
C. Watch for hypotension and bradycardia.
D. Autonomic dysreflexia may occur with an injury above T6; includes an exaggerated sympathetic response with hypertension, sweating, and flushing.
   1. May be stimulated by bowel or bladder emptying.
   2. Treatment—head of bed (HOB) elevation, Nipride or phentolamine, Diazepam, and maintaining an empty bladder and bowel.

IX. Incomplete Injuries

A. Central cord syndrome—the most frequent incomplete injury.
   1. Cause—hyperextension, usually with preexisting cervical stenosis.
   2. Signs/symptoms—weakness (more in the upper extremity [UE] than the lower extremity [LE] because the UE fibers are medial in the corticospinal and spinothalamic tracts), and various sensory and sphincter dysfunction.
   3. Treatment:
      a. Spinal cord compression with incomplete cord injury should be decompressed and repaired as soon as safely possible. Within 24 hours is preferable, but studies have failed to demonstrate benefit from emergent repair in the middle of the night.
      b. Supportive care until the procedure can be performed safely under ideal circumstances.
B. Anterior cord syndrome.
   1. Cause—anterior spinal artery cardiovascular accident (CVA) causing decreased motor function and loss of pain and temperature sensation, with sparing of proprioception.
      a. Frequently associated with aortic dissection.
   2. Prognosis—poor.

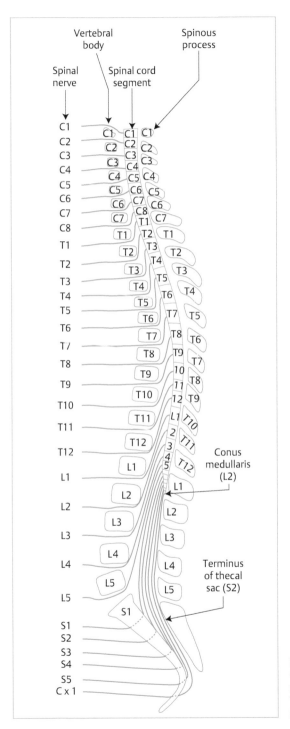

Fig. 2.1 Spinal cord levels. (Source: Greenberg MS. Handbook of Neurosurgery. 7th ed. New York, NY: Thieme Medical Publishers; 2010: 944, Fig. 28-1.)

C.   Brown–Séquard syndrome—hemicord injury with ipsilateral motor and light touch/proprioception deficit with contralateral pain/temperature deficit:
   1.   Cause—usually a penetrating injury.
   2.   Prognosis if the deficit is partial—relatively good.
D.   Posterior cord injury—causes only paresthesias and rarely occurs.

X. Spinal Cord Injury without Radiographic Abnormality (Sciwora Syndrome)

A.   Cause—usually occurs in children due to ligamentous flexibility.
B.   Evaluation—in patient with MRI and flexion–extension X-rays.
C.   Treatment—collar should be worn for 3 weeks and sports avoided for 3 months.

XI. Cervical Fracture Stability (See Quick Reference Guide for SLIC Grading System)

A.   Nondisplaced fracture—assess stability with flexion–extension X-rays:
   1.   Unstable—place in collar (or other orthosis) for 6–12 weeks and assess fusion at that point with another flexion–extension X-rays (various injury types are discussed in this chapter).
   2.   No instability on the dynamic X-rays—no collar needed; however, study may be insufficient because cervical muscle spasm may prevent adequate motion to demonstrate instability.
   3.   Study questionable—keep patient in collar and repeat study in 2 weeks.
   4.   Ligamentous instability—present if >3.5 mm of subluxation or >11 degrees of angulation:
      a.   These injuries usually require surgical stabilization because only 10–15% heal with immobilization.

XII. Atlanto-Occipital Dislocation

A.   Joint stabilized mainly by tectorial membrane (posterior longitudinal ligament [PLL] from C2 to occiput) and alar ligaments (from dens to C1 and occiput) (see **Fig. 2.1**)
B.   Distance from occipital condyle to superior facet of atlas should be <5 mm.
C.   Distance from basion to tip of dens should be <5 mm in adults and <10 mm in children.
D.   Power's ratio—(anterior basion to posterior arch of C1)/(opisthion to anterior arch) >1 suggests anterior dislocation (most frequent injury).
E.   Type 1 injury is anterior subluxation, type 2 is distraction, and type 3 is posterior subluxation (very rare).

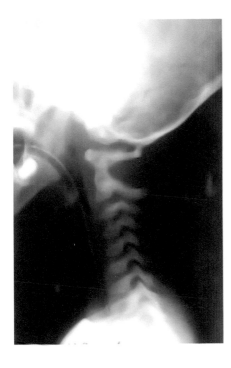

Fig. 2.2 Atlanto-occipital and atlantoaxial dislocations. Lateral cervical spine X-rays film demonstrates increased distance from the occiput to the atlas and the atlas to the axis. (Source: Citow JS. Neuropathology and Neuroradiology: A Review. New York, NY: Thieme Medical Publishers; 2001: 211, Fig. 295.)

F. Treatment:

1. Place patient in a halo immediately.

2. Stabilize with occiput–C3 fusion (using combination of occipital plating, C1 lateral mass screws, C2 pars/pedicle screws, and subaxial lateral mass screw techniques).

3. Lateral mass plates with occipital extension may also be used.

4. If a condylar fracture presses on brainstem, the patient should be placed in a halo position and treated with transoral decompression followed by posterior fusion.

5. Evaluate for associated vertebral artery dissection with magnetic resonance angiography (MRA); if present treat with heparin/Warfarin for 3 months (**Fig. 2.2**).

XIII. Atlantoaxial Dislocation

A. Anterior dislocation.

1. Cause—transverse ligament injury or dens fracture.

2. Treatment:

a. C1–2 fusion using C1 lateral mass screws and C2 pars or pedicle screws. Older techniques include sublaminar wires (i.e., Brooks', Gallie, or Sonntag) or transarticular screws: (**1**) C1 lateral mass screws.

Starting point is the midpoint of the C1 lateral mass. Trajectory is 5–10 degrees medial and parallel to the arch of C1. Fluoroscopy or image guidance should be considered during placement (**Fig. 2.3**); (**2**) C2 fixation techniques include C2 pedicle screws, C2 pars screws, C1/2 transarticular screws, and C2 translaminar screws (**Fig. 2.4**); (**3**) Subaxial lateral mass screws. Starting point is approximately 1 mm medial to the center point of the lateral mass. Should be directed 30 degrees lateral and 15–20 degrees superior (**Fig. 2.5**); (**4**) Subaxial pedicle screws are now being used. More lateral starting point and medial trajectory. Image guidance recommended (**Fig. 2.6** and **Fig. 2.7**).

   b.   Brooks' technique—sublaminar wires under both C1 and 2 with two cubes of bone between the laminas.

   c.   Gallie technique—H-shaped bone graft over C1 and 2 held by a wire sublaminar at C1 and around the spinous process of C2.

   d.   Dickman and Sonntag technique—similar to Gallie techniquewith the wire sublaminar under C1 only, but the bone graft is U-shaped and lodged between the laminas of C1 and 2 as well as around the spinous process of C2.

   e.   Songer titanium cables should be tightened to 30 lb/inch (see **Fig. 2.8**).

B.   Rotatory subluxation—occurs in children (often after an upper respiratory infection) or rheumatoid patients.

   1.   Signs/symptoms—head tilt, flexion, and rotation.

   2.   Evaluation—CT.

   3.   Treatment—attempt reduction with 7–15 lbs of traction.

      a.   If reduced—immobilize for 6 weeks and reassess with dynamic studies.

      b.   Fuse early at C1–2 if there is anterior subluxation or the transverse atlantal ligament is disrupted (see **Fig. 2.9a–d**).

XIV. C1 Fracture

A.   Jefferson fracture—4-, 3-, or 2-point fractures from axial loading.

B.   Usually unstable.

C.   Evaluation—evaluate with open-mouth-view X-rays and CT.

   1.   According to the rule of Spence, >7 mm of C1–2 combined over hang on open-mouth X-rays suggests disruption of the transverse atlantal ligament.

   2.   Ligament can usually be visualized on axial MRI and a disruption determined.

D.   Treatment.

   1.   Fracture of the tubercle connecting the transverse ligament usually heals well with immobilization.

   2.   If ligament intact—halo or sternal occipital mandibular immobilizer (SOMI) brace.

   3.   If ligament disrupted—perform occiput–C3 posterior fusion or possibly a C1–2 posterior fusion if arch is stable (see **Fig. 2.10a–c**).

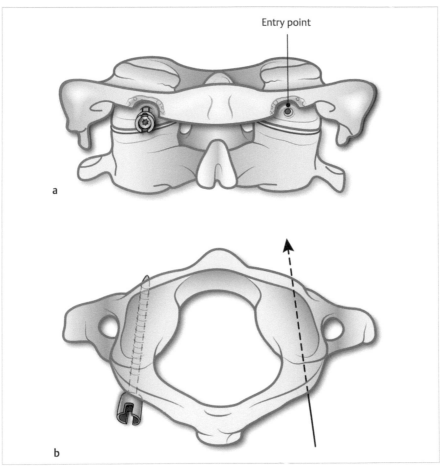

Entry point

a

b

Fig. 2.3 After posterior approach to the arch of C1, use blunt dissection to expose the posterior arch of C1 and C2. Use the bipolar and hemostatic agents to control bleeding from the atlantoaxial periver-tebral venous plexus. Using a Penfield no. 4, retract the C2 nerve root caudally in order to expose the C1 lateral mass and the C1–2 joint space just inferior to its arch. Find the medial and lateral borders of the C1 lateral mass by palpation. The inferior aspect of the posterior arch of C1 often needs to be drilled down to gain further access to this region and to allow the screw to sit flush with the proper angulation. **(a)** For the screw entry point, make a small hole with a drill at the center of C1 lateral mass. **(b)** With the aid of a fluoroscopic lateral view of the high cervical spine, aim the drill toward the anterior tubercle of C1 and medialize the trajectory by 5 to 10 degrees, depending on the anatomy of the lateral mass of C1. Stop drilling when the drill tip is just short of posterior margin of the anterior tubercle or you feel that you have gone through the anterior cortical margin of the lateral mass of C1. Tap the hole and insert a partially threaded screw so that the shaft of the screw in contact with the C2 nerve root does not have any threads. The screw length is typically 34 to 36 mm. For particularly unstable or immature spines, bicortical screw fixation is paramount and requires controlled tapping to penetrate the anterior cortical surface without risking vascular injury. A probe is helpful in determining depth and length of screw. (Source: Ullman J, Raksin P, Hrsg. Atlas of Emergency Neurosurgery. New York, NY: Thieme Medical Publishers; 2015, Fig. 29.8.)

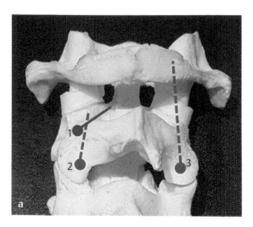
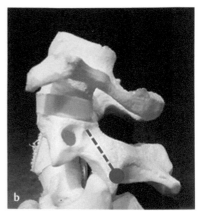
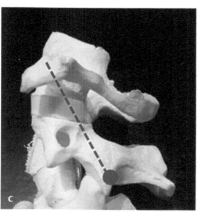
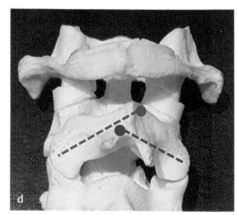

Fig. 2.4 (a) Posterior view of C1–2–3. 1—Illustrated perspective of the trajectory of the C2 pedicle screw and entry point: we start in line with the cranial edge of the C2 lamina and just lateral to the midpoint of the C2 pars; the more caudal the starting point, the harder it is to get into the pedicle and the easier it is to hit the artery. 2—Trajectory of the C2 pars screw and entry point, just superior and slightly lateral to the medial junction of the C2–3 joint (approx. 3 to 5 mm above the junction, as medial as possible but without violating the spinal canal and the medial portion of the pars). 3—Trajectory of the C2 transarticular screw, with the same entry point of C2 pars screw. **(b)** Lateral View of C1–2–3. Lateral perspective of the trajectory of the C2 pars screw. **(c)** Lateral View of C1–2–3. Lateral perspective of the trajectory of the C2 transarticular screw. **(d)** Posterior view of C1–2–3. Illustrated perspective of the trajectory of bilateral C2 laminar screws and their respective entry points, in the junction of the lamina and the spinous process. (Source: Joaquim A, Riew K. Axis Screw Fixation: A Step-by-Step Review of the Surgical Techniques. Arquivos Brasileiros de Neurocirurgia: Brazilian Neurosurgery 2017; 36(02):101–107, Fig. 2.)

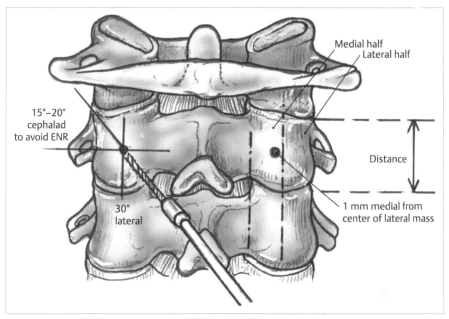

Fig. 2.5 Posterior view of the cervical spinal bony elements. The entry point for a lateral mass screw is 1 mm medial to the center of the lateral mass. ENR, exiting nerve root. (Source: Nader R, Berta SC, Gragnaniello C, Sabbagh AJ, Levy ML. Neurosurgery Tricks of the Trade. Spine and Peripheral Nerves. New York, NY: Thieme Medical Publishers; 2014, Fig. 13.1.)

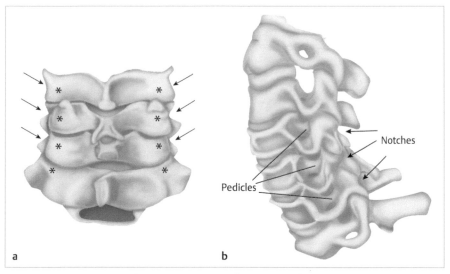

Fig. 2.6 (a) Starting points of C3–7 pedicle screw placement. Each arrow indicates a notch on the lateral margin of the lateral mass. Asterisks show the screw starting points. **(b)** Lateral view of notches and pedicles. (Source: Cervical Pedicle Screw Placement. In: Vaccaro A, Albert T, Spine Surgery. Tricks of the Trade. 3rd Edition. New York, NY: Thieme Medical Publishers; 2016, Fig. 12.4.)

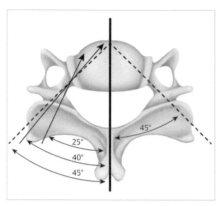

Fig. 2.7 C3–7 screw direction in the horizontal plane. (Source: Cervical Pedicle Screw Placement. In: Vaccaro A, Albert T, Spine Surgery. Tricks of the Trade. 3rd Edition. New York, NY: Thieme Medical Publishers; 2016, Fig. 12.5.)

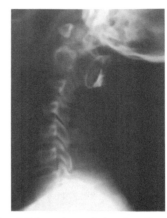

Fig. 2.8 Lateral cervical spine X-rays of Brooks' fusion. (Source: Citow JS Neurosurgery Oral Board Review. 1st ed. New York, NY: Thieme Medical Publishers; 128, Fig. 12.4.)

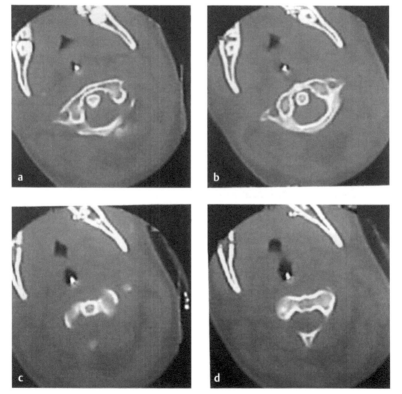

Fig. 2.9 Atlantoaxial rotatory subluxation. (a–d) Axial computed tomography demonstrates the 45-degree rotation of the atlas on the axis. (Source: Citow JS. Neuropathology and Neuroradiology: A Review. New York, NY: Thieme Medical Publishers; 2001:212, Fig. 297.)

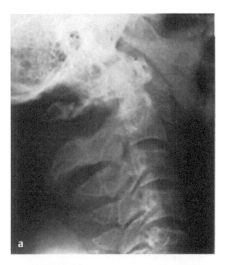
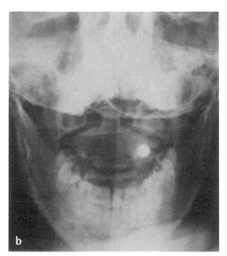
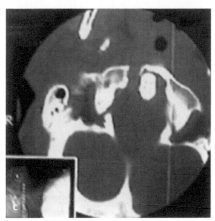

Fig. 2.10 Jefferson fracture. (a) Lateral and (b) open-mouth X-rays films. (c) Axial computed tomography demonstrates anterior and posterior arch fractures with prominent right-sided overhang seen in (b). (Source: Citow JS. Neuropathology and Neuroradiology: A Review. New York, NY: Thieme Medical Publishers; 2001:211, Fig. 296.)

E. C1 and C2 fractures:

1. Treatment—according to C2 injury:

a. Hangman fracture—likely C1–2 posterior fusion using C1 lateral mass and whatever C2 fixation can be adequately placed depending on fracture. Halo is possible if approximation is good.

b. Type 2 dens fracture with <6 mm displacement—halo and >6 mm displacement (occiput–C2 fusion or C1–2 transarticular screws).

c. Type 3 dens fracture—often considered stable, but should still be treated with rigid collar or halo and follow-up imaging.

XV. C2 Fracture

A. Hangman fracture—pars fracture (spondylolisthesis) between the superior facet process (anterior, in line with the occiput–C1 joint) and inferior facet process (posterior, in line with the other cervical facet joints).

    1. Cause—usually from hyperextension and axial loading (not distraction as with judicial hangings of the past).

    2. Usually stable and rarely presents with a deficit (see **Fig. 2.11**).

    3. Effendi classification (by C2–3 subluxation at the PLL line):

        a. Type 1—<3 mm of C2–3 subluxation; treat with SOMI brace for 3 months.

        b. Type 2—>4 mm subluxation or >11 degrees angulation; reduce with traction then place in a halo or Minerva brace (surgery only if unable to maintain reduction).

        c. Type 3—C2–3 locked facets with 50% subluxation; treat with an anterior C2–3 fusion or a posterior C1–3 fusion (or C1–2 fusion).

B. Dens fracture—C1–2 joint provides 50% of the motion of the cervical spine.

    1. Steele's rule of thirds—at the level of the dens, the spinal canal is filled by thirds of spinal cord, cerebrospinal fluid (CSF), and dens.

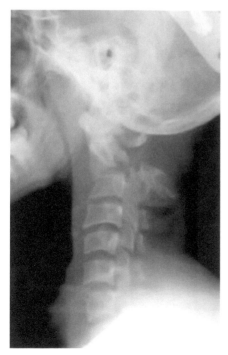

Fig. 2.11 Hangman fracture. Lateral cervical spine X-rays film demonstrates the C2 traumatic spondylolisthesis with anterior angulation. (Source: Citow JS. Neuropathology and Neuroradiology: A Review. New York, NY: Thieme Medical Publishers; 2001:213, Fig. 300.)

2. Anderson and D'Alonzo classification:

   a. Type 1—oblique fracture through the tip of the dens (rare); treat often nonoperatively with halo or rigid collar; may develop instability requiring fusion.

   b. Type 2—fracture at base of dens; may treat nonoperatively if <6 mm displacement or if <7 years: (1) Perform fusion if unable to maintain reduction in cervical collar/halo; (2) 30% nonunion rate in a collar/halo, but only 10% if <6 mm displacement; (3) Treatment—surgical options include anterior odontoid screw (maintains range of motion, requires intact transverse ligament, avoid if fracture >2 weeks old or if patient has barrel chest), posterior transarticular C1–2 screw (need a CT to determine if screws can be placed without vertebral artery injury), or posterior screw/rod fusion (as described earlier using C1–2 techniques) (see **Fig. 2.12a–c**).

   c. Type 3—fracture through body of axis; stable; treat with a SOMI brace.

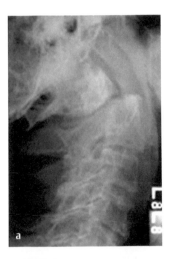
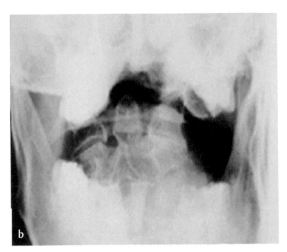
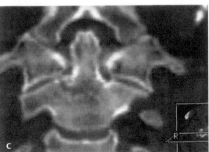

Fig. 2.12 Odontoid fracture (type 2). **(a)** Lateral and **(b)** open-mouth cervical spine X-rays films demonstrate the fracture through the base of the dens with posterior dislocation. **(c)** Coronal tomography of type 3 dens fracture. (Source: Citow JS. Neuropathology and Neuroradiology: A Review. New York, NY: Thieme Medical Publishers; 2001:212, Fig. 298.)

XVI. Clay-Shoveler Fracture—Involves Spinous Process of C7, C6, or T1

A. Stable if no associated ligamentous injury.
B. No collar needed.

XVII. Tear Drop Fracture

A. Cause—major flexion/compression injury. Classic "dive into shallow pool" injury.
B. Produces wedge-shaped fracture on anteroinferior aspect of vertebral body.
C. Usually severe ligamentous injury and instability.
D. Should be differentiated from a stable compression fracture.
E. Treatment—anterior and posterior fusion (with lateral mass plates or interspinous wiring), though a single approach may be sufficient.

XVIII. Locked Facets—May Be Unilateral or Bilateral (With >50% Subluxation)

A. Treatment:
    1. Reduction with traction starting at 3 lb/level and increasing the weight by 5 lbs every 10 minutes while obtaining X-rays to determine alignment and rule out distraction injury (stop if occipitoatlantal dislocation >5 mm or disk space >10 mm).
    2. Avoid >5 lbs per level.
    3. Muscle relaxants may help achieve reduction, but keep patient alert and examinable.
    4. MRI prior to traction to rule out disk herniation in the comatose patient. If awake with an examination that can be followed, repeat examination after each addition of weight.
    5. Once patient is reduced, lower the weight to 10 lbs.
    6. Bilateral facet injury—all patients should be stabilized surgically.
    7. Unilateral facet dislocation—many patients will heal in a brace, but surgery should be performed in the presence of radiculopathy or failure to maintain reduction.
    8. Stabilization can be performed anteriorly (with a plate), but the posterior approach (with lateral mass screws rods) is preferred:
        a. Lateral mass screws inserted into middle of lateral mass and angled 10–30 degrees laterally and rostrally per X-rays and 14–20 mm deep per X-rays to be bicortical with 3.5 mm screws.
        b. Remember to prepare patient for iliac bone graft if not using allograft.
        c. After stabilization, patient is placed in a brace for 6–12 weeks.
    9. There is often vertebral artery occlusion with facet dislocation (**Fig. 2.13a, b**).

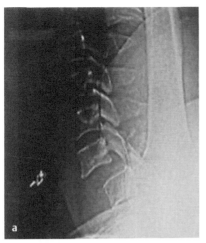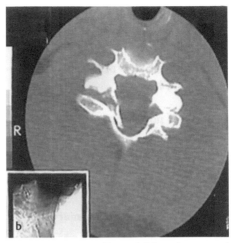

Fig. 2.13 Bilateral interfacetal dislocation. (a) Lateral cervical X-rays film and (b) axial computed tomography demonstrates the C6–7 injury with bilateral jumped facets. (Source: Citow JS. Neuropathology and Neuroradiology: A Review. New York, NY: Thieme Medical Publishers; 2001:214, Fig. 302.)

XIX. Flexion Ligamentous Injury with Posterior Instability

A. Reduce and fuse posteriorly with standard posterolateral cervical fusion with screw technique depending on bony integrity and injury type (**Fig. 2.14**).

XX. Extension Ligamentous Injury or Anterior Compression Fracture

A. Fix anteriorly with cervical diskectomy, fusion, and plating.

XXI. Cervical Orthotics

A. Philadelphia collar—most effective for decreasing motion in the lower cervical spine (C5–T1).
B. SOMI brace—most effective for reducing flexion in the upper cervical spine.
C. Minerva brace—most effective for midcervical instability.
D. Halo vest—most effective for instability at C1–2 or C5–T1.

XXII. Thoracolumbar Fractures (See Quick Reference Guide for TLIC Grading Scale)

A. Denis' three-column model:
    1. Anterior column—anterior longitudinal ligament (ALL) and half disk.

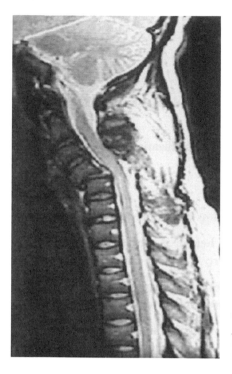

Fig. 2.14 Flexion dislocation. Sagittal T2-weighted magnetic resonance imaging demonstrates the C4–5 subluxation and angulation. (Source: Citow JS. Neuropathology and Neuroradiology: A Review. New York, NY: Thieme Medical Publishers; 2001:214, Fig. 303.)

    2. Middle column—PLL and half disk.

    3. Posterior column—facets, laminas, spinous processes, and associated ligaments.

B. Two-column injury considered unstable.

C. Compression fracture:

    1. Only anterior column is injured.

    2. Considered unstable if vertebral height is decreased >50% or there is >30 degrees angulation.

    3. Treatment—thoracolumbosacral orthosis (TLSO) brace or surgical stabilization (anterior or posterior approach).

D. Burst fracture:

    1. Both the anterior and middle columns are injured.

    2. Considered unstable if vertebral height is decreased <50%, the angulation is >20 degrees, or there is >50% canal compromise.

    3. Treatment—TLSO brace (3–6 months) or surgical decompression and stabilization (anterior and/or posterior approaches may be used as long as decompression and fusion are achieved). Some studies show evidence that burst fractures without neurological deficit can be treated nonoperatively and without bracing, however, this isstill under active study. Concern for treatment without brace revolves around risk for long-term kyphosis above the injured level.

    4. L5 burst fracture is difficult to instrument anteriorly; consider L4–S1 posterior fusion and TLSO brace with thigh cuff in 10 degrees flexion (**Fig. 2.15a, b**).

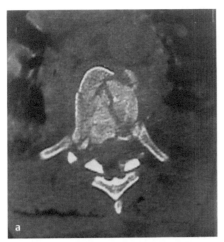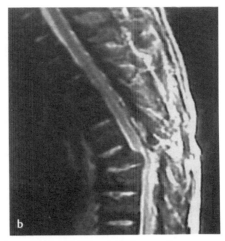

Fig. 2.15 Burst fracture. (a) Axial computed tomography and (b) sagittal T2-weighted magnetic resonance imaging scans demonstrate angulation with retropulsion at T9. (Source: Citow JS. Neuropathology and Neuroradiology: A Review. New York, NY: Thieme Medical Publishers; 2001:215, Fig. 305.)

E. Seat-belt fracture:

1. Both the middle and posterior columns are injured.

2. Evaluation—sagittal CT reconstructions.

3. Treatment—posterior instrumented fusion.

4. Chance fracture—through vertebral bodies.

F. Fracture-dislocation—three-column injury requiring anterior and posterior stabilization.

G. Instrumentation:

1. Pedicle screws may be placed from C2 through the sacrum. C1 fixation is via lateral mass screws.

2. Exposure—must extend to tip of transverse processes to allow decortication of transverse processes and lateral facets.

3. Entrance site—junction of medial transverse process and superior articulating process. Intraoperative fluoroscopy or image guidance/navigation can be used to help guide starting point and trajectory of screw placement.

4. Awl is used to open into the pedicle.

5. Fluoroscopy is used to place screws (5.5 or 6.5 mm) parallel to end plates and ending 80% into vertebral body.

6. Intraoperative monitoring is used to stimulate screws to make sure there is no violation of cortex with pressure on a nerve root.

7. Rod–hook systems may be connected to pedicle screws, but these are rarely used anymore.

8. Instrumentation should extend three levels above and two levels below the injury.

9. Construct may need to be extended to avoid ending at a transition level (cervicothoracic, thoracolumbar, or lumbosacral) or at a thoracic kyphosis.

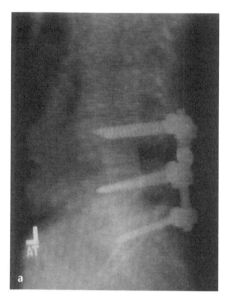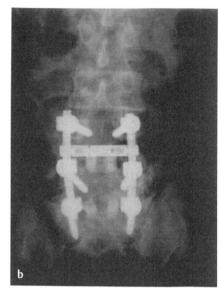

Fig. 2.16 (a) Lateral X-rays of L4–S1 pedicle screw fusion with tangent bony posterior lumbar interbody fusion (PLIF). **(b)** Anteroposterior X-rays of L4–S1 pedicle screw fusion with tangent bony PLIF. (Source: Citow JS. Neurosurgery Oral Board Review. 1st ed. New York, NY: Thieme Medical Publishers; 2003: 138, Fig. 12.12.)

10. Space lateral to facets should be packed with morselized bone.
11. Anterior instrumentation with plates or rods involves bicortical screws (**Fig. 2.16a, b**).

H. Pathological fractures:
   1. If mechanism not severe enough to explain the bony destruction, consider a tumor, infection, or osteoporosis.
   2. Evaluation—MRI, inflammatory markers (erythrocyte sedimentation rate [ESR], C-reactive protein [CRP], white blood cell [WBC], cultures), bone scan, and CXR.

XXIII. Osteoporosis

A. Evaluation—bone mineral density and dual-energy X-rays absorptiometry (DXA) scan of proximal femur and lumbosacral spine.
   1. Rule out hyperthyroidism, increased parathyroid hormone (PTH), steroids, and tumor.

B. Treatment:
   1. Exercise.
   2. Calcium.

3. Estrogen:

    a. Increases DVT risk, possibly increases breast cancer risk, and decreases coronary artery disease.

    b. Add progesterone to decrease endometrial carcinoma risk.

4. Vitamin D.

5. Calcitonin.

6. Fosamax—decreases bone resorption.

C. Compression fractures:

    1. Treatment:

        a. Bracing, kyphoplasty, or vertebroplasty—methylmethacrylate injected to decrease pain; also used for pathological fractures and hemangiomas.

        b. Surgery—rarely needed.

XXIV. Gunshot Wounds

A. Treatment:

    1. Surgery—useful only for incomplete spinal cord injury, CSF leak, instability (rare), or copper bullets.

    2. Colon perforation with CSF leak—explore to clean and pack the defect (80% infection rate).

    3. Gastric and small bowel injuries are less contaminated.

        a. Use antibiotics but not steroids.

    4. Lead from the bullet may rarely cause lead poisoning with neuropathy, encephalopathy, anemia, abdominal pain, and renal dysfunction.

Helpful Hints

1. ABCs first!
2. All trauma patients should be immobilized on a board with a cervical collar.
3. Denis' three-column classification is essential for ascertaining stability and guiding therapy.
4. Spine trauma cases are often great for percutaneous or minimally invasive procedures, but do not propose unless you are quite familiar with technique, instrumentation, imaging, and complications.

Case 4

A 55-year-old man presents with acute neck pain after a minor motor vehicle accident when he hit his head on the dashboard. Past medical history is significant for bladder cancer, degenerative disk disease, painful large nodules on finger joints, and diabetes mellitus. Examination was normal (**Fig. 2.17**).

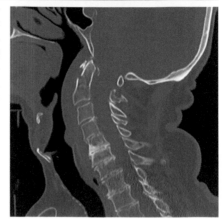

Fig. 2.17

Case 5

A 19-year-old presents in the emergency department after an all-terrain vehicle (ATV) rollover accident. Past medical history is significant for alcohol abuse. Examination was normal except for low back pain (**Fig. 2.18**).

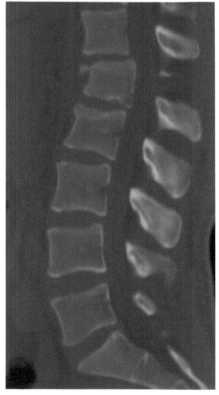

Fig. 2.18

Case 6

A 65-year-old man presents with new-onset back pain after a fall from a 20-foot ladder where he landed on his feet (short T1-inversion recovery magnetic resonance image [STIR MRI] shown). Past medical history is significant for prostatic hypertrophy, 40-year smoking history, oxygen-dependent chronic obstructive pulmonary disease, and recent headaches. Examination was normal, except for focal pain to palpation over upper midlumbar region (**Fig. 2.19**).

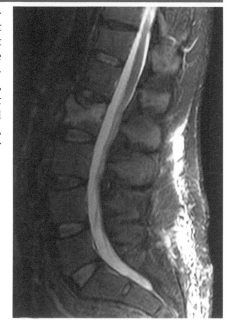

Fig. 2.19

3 Spinal Degenerative Disease

I. Cervical Disk Disease

A. Signs/symptoms:
1. Radiculopathy—neck and interscapular pain, radicular arm pain, numbness and paresthesias, a sensory level and incontinence may be present, and lower motor neuron weakness; C8 and T1 radiculopathies may cause a partial Horner's syndrome.
2. Myelopathy—upper motor neuron weakness, hyperreflexia, Hoffman's sign, clonus, Babinski, a sensory level, and incontinence.

B. Evaluation:
1. Magnetic resonance imaging (MRI).
2. Nerve conduction study—occasionally useful to differentiate radiculopathy from neuropathy.
3. Lhermitte's sign—neck flexion causes caudal electrical shocks; often seen with multiple sclerosis and subacute combined system disease (SCSD); consider awake intubation if present.
4. Spurling's sign—pressing the vertex of the head with the head extended and tilted to the symptomatic side reproduces radicular pain.

C. Treatment:
1. Most of patients (90%) with acute cervical radiculopathy improve by 6 weeks with nonspecific conservative management.
2. Useful medical therapy—oral steroids (Medrol dose pack), nonsteroidal anti-inflammatory drugs (NSAIDs), antispasmodics (for neck spasm), and narcotics.
3. Physical therapy for range of motion and traction exercises may be helpful.
4. Epidural steroids—not of clear benefit.
5. Anterior cervical diskectomy and fusion—consider for patients who have significant weakness, long tract signs (bladder dysfunction), or debilitating pain, or who have failed conservative management.
6. Posterior keyhole laminotomy with partial diskectomy for soft lateral disks—avoids the need for a fusion (consider with professional singers).
7. Plating—probably useful for two- and three-level procedures, though not proven for one-level fusions, however, still commonly used (**Fig. 3.1**).
8. Hard cervical collar—often used postoperative for 6 weeks.

II. Cervical Spondylitic Myelopathy

A. Signs/symptoms—same as cervical disk disease but more often myelopathy (usually when the canal is <12 mm and rarely when it is >16 mm).

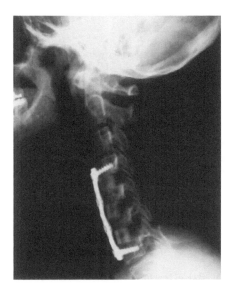

Fig. 3.1 Lateral X-ray of C4–5, 5–6, and 6–7 cervical diskectomy and fusion. (Source: Citow JS. Neurosurgery Oral Board Review. 1st ed. New York, NY: Thieme Medical Publishers; 2003: 144, Fig. 13.2.)

  1. Caused by direct neural compression, ischemia, and microtrauma.

  2. There may be a central cord syndrome.

 B. Evaluation:

  1. MRI and computed tomography (CT) (better bony detail).

  2. Myelography—may be helpful, use Omnipaque 180 (lumbar) or 300 (cervical).

  3. Avoid these medications if the patient is taking Metformin (also stop it 3 days preop), due to elevated risk of lactic acidosis.

  4. Rule out—amyotrophic lateral sclerosis (ALS; no sensory deficit, tongue fasciculations, distal fasciculations, or neck pain), multiple sclerosis, and SCSD.

 C. Treatment:

  1. Anterior cervical diskectomy and removal of osteophytes around canal and foramen.

  2. Less often—full corpectomies.

  3. Posterior decompression if more than three levels are symptomatic or the pathology is mainly posterior.

  4. Add lateral mass fusion to posterior decompression if no lordoses.

  5. Posterior decompression—precipitates swan-neck deformity in 30% of cases (try to avoid by leaving the soft tissue on the facets) and does not stop progression of osteophytes.

  6. If both anterior and posterior approaches are needed, perform the anterior decompression and fusion first and follow with the posterior procedure in 8 weeks (consider supplemental fusion with lateral mass plates).

  7. Success rate of surgery—improved 60%, unchanged 25%, worse 15%.

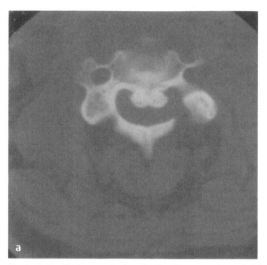 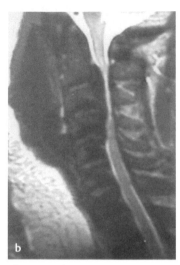

Fig. 3.2 Ossified posterior longitudinal ligament (OPLL). **(a)** Axial computed tomgraphic bone window and **(b)** sagittal T2-weighted magnetic resonance imaging demonstrate C2–5. PLL calcification with cord compression. (Source: Citow JS. Neuropathology and Neuroradiology: A Review. New York, NY: Thieme Medical Publishers; 2001: 208, Fig. 292.)

D. Ossified posterior longitudinal ligament (OPLL).
    1. Treatment:
        a. Decompress with anterior corpectomy followed by fusion, or posterior laminectomy or laminoplasty. (Laminoplasty contraindicated with cervical kyphosis.)
        b. Postsurgery—use a collar for 3 months.
        c. Complication rate includes increased deficit 10%, failure to fuse 10%, and dural tear 25% (leave eggshell of floating bone on dura) for anterior approaches; risk of C5 palsy with posterior decompression.
        d. Cerebrospinal fluid (CSF) leaks—common and should be treated with fibrin glue and lumbar drainage (usually temporary) (**Fig. 3.2a, b**).

III. Upper Cervical Spine Diseases

A. Ankylosing spondylitis:
    1. Most often occurs in young boys.
    2. Associated with rheumatoid arthritis and HLA-B27.
    3. Many spinal levels may fuse, but it spares the occipito-atlas and atlantoaxial joints.
    4. Joints may be unstable.
    5. Frequent cause of lower back pain with sacroiliac erosion.
B. Trisomy 21—patients often develop atlantoaxial dislocation and cervical stenosis.

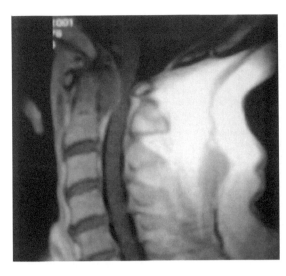

Fig. 3.3 Sagittal T1-weighted magnetic resonance image with a large pannus posterior to the dens. (Source: Citow JS. Neurosurgery Oral Board Review. 1st ed. New York, NY: Thieme Medical Publishers; 2003: 149, Fig. 13.4.)

C. Morquio syndrome—patients often develop atlantoaxial subluxation by hypoplasia of the dens and ligamentous laxity.

D. Rheumatoid arthritis:

1. Most (80%) of the patients have cervical spine involvement.

2. Causes synovial proliferation with destruction of bone and ligaments.

3. Atlantoaxial subluxation—occurs in 25% of patients:

a. Transverse ligament attachment becomes loose and symptoms are produced by a compressive pannus and instability (**Fig. 3.3**).

b. Atlantodental interval (ADI) should be <4 mm if the transverse ligament is not lax.

c. Treatment—C1–2 fusion if ADI >6 mm or patient is symptomatic (a Brook's fusion with sublaminar wires and possible transarticular screws to add stability).

d. Dislocation may need to be reduced before surgery, with up to 7 days of traction with 5–15 lbs.

e. Occiput–C2 fusion may be needed if C1 laminectomy is required for decompression or if the injury is unstable (there are frequent C1 arch fractures).

f. May be necessary to perform a dens resection before or after stabilization.

g. Failure of fusion—up to 50% of cases.

h. Use a halo until the level is fused, around 12 weeks.

i. Before removing the halo ring, check a flexion–extension X-ray: (**1**) Operative mortality—15%, mainly due to cardiac and pulmonary issues, should be cleared with preanesthetic medical evaluation.

4. Basilar impression:

a. Degenerative condition with ventral compression of the spinal cord or lower brainstem by skull settling over the dens.

    b. Signs/symptoms—headache and cranial nerve dysfunction.

    c. Treatment—reduction with 7–15 lbs followed by transoral or endoscopic-assisted odontoidectomy and then occiput–C2 fusion.

    d. If reducible—usually no need for anterior decompression.

    e. Basilar invagination—congenital condition with a fusion of C1 to the occiput: Not reducible with traction, but occasionally requires decompression.

    f. Treatment—transoral odontoidectomy: (**1**) Performed supine with head in neutral position; (**2**) Place the Crockard retractor to move tongue caudally, soft palate rostrally, and endotracheal tube laterally; (**3**) Clean mouth with betadine; (**4**) Palpate anterior tubercle of C1, inject posterior pharyngeal wall with lidocaine and epinephrine, and make longitudinal incision from above arch to base of C2; (**5**) Retract pharyngeal tissue as one layer after subperiosteal dissection with Bovie; (**6**) Remove anterior arch of C1 and dens with a drill and pituitary forceps; (**7**) Underlying soft tissue pannus may be carefully dissected off dura, but be careful to avoid a dural tear; (**8**) Close incision in one layer; (**9**) Most patients will require a fusion.

IV. Thoracic Disk Disease

A. Posterolateral transpedicular approach—may be adequate exposure for some thoracic disks, but central disk removal is performed blindly with angled instruments (Woodson elevator):

    1. Remove hemilamina above and below disk space as well as the facet joint.

    2. Drill off pedicle from level below and clear out lateral and inferior disk space.

    3. Use Woodson elevator to push disk material down into the created trough.

B. Costotransversectomy—allows direct line of vision to extend more medially:

    1. Initiate dissection; then remove transverse process and 4 cm of proximal adjacent rib.

    2. Complications—pneumothorax and radicular artery injury.

C. Lateral extracavitary approach—allows better view of midline, but not as good as transthoracic approach.

D. Transthoracic approach—best view for anterior pathology such as disk disease, burst fractures, or tumors:

    1. Upper T-spine—use transsternal approach.

    2. Middle T-spine—use right thoracotomy (avoid the heart).

    3. Lower T-spine—use left thoracotomy (**Fig. 3.4**).

    4. Thoracolumbar junction—use left retroperitoneal approach (avoid the liver).

    5. Complications—radicular artery injury, pulmonary injury, and CSF-pleura fistula.

    6. Thoracoscopic approaches are gaining in popularity.

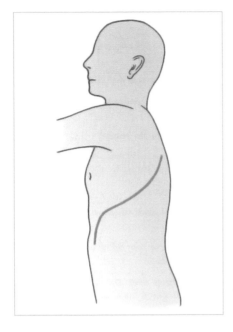

Fig. 3.4 Transthoracic approach. (Source: Citow JS. Neurosurgery Oral Board Review. 1st ed. New York, NY: Thieme Medical Publishers; 2003: 151, Fig. 13.6.)

V. Lumbar Disk Disease

A. Signs/symptoms—lower back and radicular leg pain, numbness, paresthesias, lower motor neuron weakness, and rarely incontinence.

1. Cauda equina syndrome—saddle anesthesia and bladder and bowel incontinence or retention, usually due to a massive L5–S1 disk herniation.

B. Evaluation:

1. Straight leg raise (SLR; Lasègue's sign)—performed supine with leg straight to test lower lumbar roots (L5–S1).

2. Reverse straight leg raise—performed prone with flexed knees to test upper lumbar roots (L2–4).

3. MRI—most useful test.

4. CT-myelography—reserved for more subtle pathology.

5. Nerve conduction velocity (NCV) test—needed (though rarely) to distinguish radiculopathy from neuropathy.

C. Treatment:

1. Most (90%) of the patients with acute lumbar radiculopathy improve by 6 weeks with nonspecific conservative management.

2. Useful medical therapy—same as for cervical disk disease.

3. Physical therapy—strengthening of abdominal and back muscles will help prevent future back problems.

4. Lumbar epidural steroid injections—may be helpful for treatment of pain, but also localization of pain generator with multilevel spondylosis.

5. Indications for early surgery—significant weakness, bowel or bladder dysfunction, or debilitating pain not controlled by narcotics.

6. Gold standard procedure—microdiskectomy.

7. For an extraforaminal (lateral) lumbar disk, there are two standard approaches:

   a. Hemilaminotomy to identify the nerve root followed by a complete facetectomy until the disk is identified (consider fusion if taking entire facet).

   b. Extrafacet approach with dissection over the lateral facets and transverse processes to find the nerve root and disk under the intertransverse ligament.

   c. Iliac crest may need to be drilled down to reach the extruded disk.

D. Complications:

   1. Infection—5%.

   2. Disk reherniation—5%.

   3. Increased deficit—1–5%.

   4. Dural tear—10% (20% on reoperations).

   5. Positioning pressure sore.

   6. Arachnoiditis—central adhesive nerve root cords or roots adherent to the dura seen on MRI.

   7. Deep vein thrombosis (DVT).

   8. Pulmonary embolism.

   9. Reflex sympathetic dystrophy 1%—occurs 4 days to 20 weeks after surgery and treated with physical therapy, steroids, and sympathetic blocks.

   10. Vessel injury (rarely)—aorta and vena cava bifurcate into iliac vessels at L4.

   11. Superficial infection—treat with antibiotics.

   12. Deep infection—usually requires debridement with closure over a drain:

       a. Evaluate the infection with complete blood count (CBC), erythrocyte sedimentation rate (ESR), cultures, and contrasted MR.

VI. Lumbar Stenosis

A. Signs/symptoms:

   1. Similar to lumbar disk disease symptoms but usually with a more insidious onset.

   2. Typically, neurogenic claudication with leg pain and weakness exacerbated by ambulation and relieved over minutes by sitting, lying down, or leaning forward on a grocery cart.

      a. This may be confused with vascular claudication that improves immediately with rest and is evaluated with lower extremity arterial Doppler studies and an ankle/brachial blood pressure <0.6.

   3. Thigh pain—can be caused by trochanteric bursitis or hip arthritis, but the pain should not extend past the knee and there should be no sensory loss.

   4. Lateral recess syndrome—compression of the nerve root adjacent to the pedicle by an enlarged superior facet process (<4 mm of anterior-posterior space).

B. Evaluation—MRI and CT myelography if needed.

C. Treatment:

1. Conservative management as with disk disease, though some will eventually require laminectomy with medial facetectomies, foraminotomies, and lateral recess decompression.

2. Try to leave as much of the facet as possible because 1–5% of patients become unstable after lumbar decompression.

3. Vertically aligned facets—more likely to become unstable.

4. Fusion—not needed if 50% of facet is left intact and disk is untouched.

5. Lumbar fusion—best performed with pedicle screws augmenting a bony lateral fusion over decorticated transverse processes.

6. Posterior lumbar interbody fusion (PLIF) cages—may be placed to augment a posterior fusion with a tall disk space, but have not been proven to be an effective stand-alone device (this is an area of controversy).

7. Open or laparoscopic anterior lumbar interbody fusion (ALIF) cages may also be used in place of a PLIF. ALIF is typically reserved for discogenic back pain confirmed by discogram. Some surgeons use ALIF in deformity surgery to allow for significant correction of lordosis and improvement in interbody fusion rates.

8. Incision for ALIF placement is at the lateral edge of the rectus abdominis with a retroperitoneal dissection and great vessel mobilization.

9. Pedicle screws—usually 5.5 or 6.5 mm in diameter and 40–55 mm in length:

    a. Should be aimed 20 degrees medial at L5, 30 degrees medial at S1, and sink 80% into the body (as guided by fluoroscopy or an image-guided system) (see the "Lumbar Trauma" section for more information).

10. Most (80%) of the patients are improved with surgery.

D. Complications—same as lumbar disk disease complications:

1. Few (10–20%) of postfusion patients develop adjacent stenosis over 10 years.

VII. Spondylolisthesis—Subluxation; May Have a Pars Defect

A. Spondylolysis refers to the defect without subluxation.

B. Spondylolisthesis varieties:

1. Isthmic—little degenerative changes, possibly traumatic, usually at L5–S1.

2. Dysplastic.

3. Degenerative—90% at L4–5 and most others at L3–4.

4. Traumatic.

5. Pathologic.

C. Evaluation—same as lumbar stenosis with flexion–extension X-rays to rule out instability and oblique films to evaluate pars.

D. Treatment—as with lumbar stenosis with the addition of pedicle screws (though some reports suggest fusion not needed because most cases of degenerative spondylolisthesis do not slip more after decompression) (**Fig. 2.16a, b**).

E. Symptomatic spondylolysis (back pain):
1. Evaluation—dynamic studies and local injections into the pars (to determine if this is indeed the pain source).
2. Treatment—consider repairing the pars directly with a screw (avoiding a fusion) or performing the traditional fusion (most common treatment).

VIII. Facet-Mediated Back Pain (Typically Facet Arthropathy)

A. Signs/symptoms—pain is mainly in the paraspinal lower back but can be referred to upper thigh in nonradicular pattern.
B. Evaluation—MRI (rule out tumor or infection) and dynamic X-ray (rule out instability) and may be tender to palpation over facets.
C. Treatment—physical therapy and NSAIDs:
1. Refractory cases may be treated with radiofrequency facet denervation, facet injections, or fusion.

IX. Coccydyni A

A. Signs/symptoms—local tenderness over the coccyx.
B. Evaluation—MRI.
C. Treatment—NSAIDs, doughnut cushion, injections, and possibly resection (low success rates).

X. Myelopathy Differential Diagnosis (See Neurology Section)

A. Spinal cord compression—disk, bone, tumor, abscess.
B. Spinal cord tumor.
C. ALS—tongue fasciculations, normal sensation.
D. Transverse myelitis.
E. Spinal cord cerebrovascular accident (CVA)—aortic dissection.
F. Syphilis—tabes dorsalis.
G. SCSD.

XI. Femoral Neuropathy

A. The femoral nerve arises from L2, 3, and 4 to supply sensation to the anterior thigh and innervate the iliopsoas and quadriceps muscles.
B. Thigh adductors—not weak with a femoral neuropathy; innervated by the obturator nerve (L2, 3).

C. L4 radiculopathy should have sensory loss from knee to medial malleolus (not anterior thigh), normal iliopsoas strength, and weakness of quadriceps, ankle dorsiflexion, and thigh adductors.

XII. Foot Drop

A. Usually from an L4 or 5 radiculopathy (painful) or a common peroneal nerve palsy (painless, normal gluteus medius strength with internal rotation of flexed hip and normal foot inversion); parasagittal meningioma may also present with footdrop.

B. Superficial peroneal nerve (L4, 5)—foot eversion and sensation to the dorsum of the foot.

C. Deep peroneal nerve (L4, 5)—dorsiflexion and a small area of sensation at the big toe web space.

D. Tibial nerve (L5, S1)—foot inversion and plantar flexion with sensation to the sole of the foot.

E. L5 proximal branches—gluteus medius (L4, 5) for internal thigh rotation and gluteus maximus (L5–S1) to resist SLR.

F. Sciatic nerve injury proximal to the peroneal division produces flail foot (no plantar- or dorsiflexion).

XIII. Adult Deformity

A. Characterized by abnormal coronal and sagittal curvature of the spine.

B. Most common presenting symptom is progressively worsening back pain, often with coexisting leg pain from muscle strain (patients with positive sagittal balance).

C. Radiographic parameters are important:

1. Sagittal balance—distance between a plumb line drawn from midpoint of C7 to the posterior superior corner of the sacral endplate. Normal is <5 cm; anything >5 cm is considered pathologically increased.

2. Pelvic incidence/lumbar lordosis—the measurements of pelvic incidence and lumbar lordosis should be matched within approximately 10 degrees.

3. If either of these two measurements is abnormal, consideration should be given to a deformity focused procedure, as a limited procedure may lead to poor long-term outcomes.

4. If a PI/LL mismatch is present, consider obtaining standing, 36-in long cassette X-rays to evaluate for global spine alignment.

D. Multiple techniques can be used to correct global spine malalignment, including anterior interbody approaches, extensive posterior decompression with long segment fusion and osteotomies, such as Smith-Peterson, pedicle subtraction, and vertebral column resection.

E. Deformity correction procedures are often very invasive and have high rates of postoperative medical comorbidity. Patients should undergo extensive preoperative workup to ensure the procedural risk is acceptable.

Helpful Hints

1. Most degenerative spine disorders improve with medical therapy first!
2. Postoperative leg pain should prompt search for DVT.
3. Positional back pain may suggest instability (check flex/ex films and oblique films for pars defect).
4. Be careful while operating an ankylosing spondylitis—prepare for poor bone quality and significant bleeding.
5. There are various interspinous devices on the market for treating lumbar stenosis and instability, but none are standard of care.

Case 7

A 35-year-old man presents with progressive low back pain (LBP) after a fall 2 days ago. Past medical history is significant for cervical fracture 2 years prior. Examination found intact, focal LBP at the L4 level (**Fig. 3.5**).

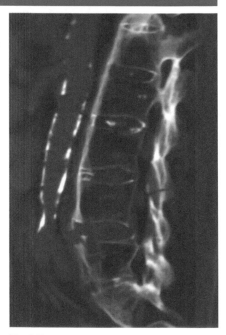

Fig. 3.5

Case 8

A 60-year-old man presents with new-onset leg numbness for the past 3 months. Legs get weak after walking and improve with leaning forward; LBP improves with sitting down. Past medical history is significant for obesity, high blood pressure, and peripheral vascular disease. Examination was normal **(Fig. 3.6)**.

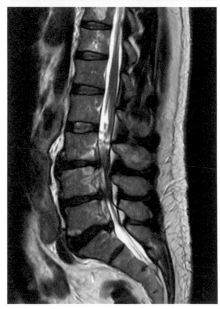

Fig. 3.6

Case 9

A 53-year-old man presents with progressive LBP, intractable to medication, physical therapy, and cortisol injections. Past medical history is significant for obesity, osteoarthritis, renal carcinoma status post nephrectomy, severe peripheral vascular disease (PVD) and coronary artery disease (CAD), and intravenous drug use (IVDU). Examination was negative **(Fig. 3.7)**.

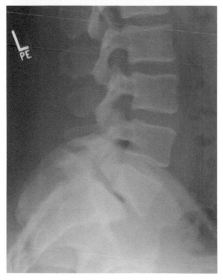

Fig. 3.7

4 Spinal Tumors

I. Primary Spinal Tumors

A. Ependymoma—the most frequent tumor in the lower spinal cord:
    1. Treatment—surgical resection; use intraoperative nerve root monitoring (avoid paralytics).
    2. Lesions of the cauda equina—section the upper filum first to prevent retraction (**Fig. 4.1**).
B. Astrocytoma—more common in children and in the upper spinal cord; usually low grade:
    1. Treatment—surgery (using somatosensory-evoked potential [SSEP] monitoring) and radiation (XRT; only if not low grade) (**Fig. 4.2a, b**).
C. Hemangioblastoma—usually cystic with a vascular mural nodule and located near the cord surface:
    1. Treatment—surgical resection.
D. Vertebral hemangioma:
    1. Treatment (only if symptomatic)—XRT, embolization, vertebroplasty, and rarely surgical resection.

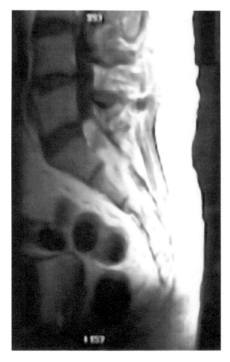

Fig. 4.1 Myxopapillary ependymoma. Sagittal-infused, T1-weighted magnetic resonance image demonstrates enhancing nodular mass filling the distal spinal cord. (Source: Citow JS. Neurosurgery Oral Board Review. 1st ed. New York, NY: Thieme Medical Publishers; 2003: 74, Fig. 9.5.)

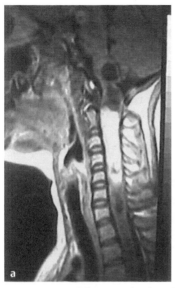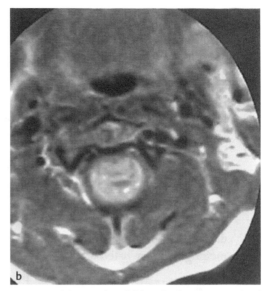

Fig. 4.2 Intramedullary juvenile pilocytic astrocytoma. **(a)** Sagittal- and **(b)** axial-infused, T1-weighted magnetic resonance images demonstrate the enhancing tumor with the associated syrinx extending into the brainstem. (Source: Citow JS. Neuropathology and Neuroradiology: A Review. New York, NY: Thieme Medical Publishers; 2001: 195, Fig. 268.)

E.   Multiple myeloma (an isolated lesion is called a plasmacytoma):

   1.   Evaluation—urinalysis (Bence Jones protein), complete blood count (CBC; anemia), blood serum electrophoresis (immunoglobulin G [IgG] kappa chains), and skeletal bone survey.

   2.   Treatment—XRT and chemotherapy.

II. Secondary Spinal Tumors

A.   Metastatic tumors.

   1.   Treatment:

      a.   Surgery—depends on several factors, including operability. (Can the lesion be safely accessed for adequate resection and subsequent stabilization?)

      b.   Radiosensitivity—if the lesion is radiosensitive, surgical decompression may not be appropriate. (Resistant tumor types include renal cell, sarcoma, primary colon cancer, and specific lung carcinomas.)

      c.   Life expectancy—patient should be expected to survive for at least 3 months, and ideally 6 months after substantial resection and fusion, otherwise the patient may not benefit from the procedure given the length of time for recovery.

   2.   Length of neurological deficit:

      a.   If a patient has a complete spinal cord injury for >24 hours, there is very little chance of recovery after resection of the offending lesion.

Helpful Hints

1. Neuromonitor all cases with SSEPs, motor evoked potentials (MEPs), and/or use Ojemann stimulator when working around individual nerve roots.

2. Extramedullary tumors are typically benign.

3. Intramedullary ependymomas typically have a good resection plane.

4. Embolize large metastatic tumors preop, prepare for transfusions and fusions; consider XRT for poor surgical candidates (reduces pain, stabilizes).

Case 10

A 30-year-old man presents with a new onset neurogenic claudication and urinary incontinence. Previous medical history is unremarkable. Examination was positive for bilateral L1 sensory loss (**Fig. 4.3**).

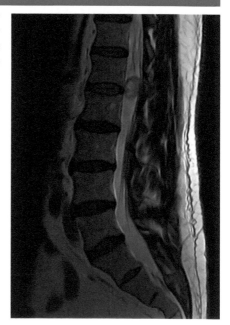

Fig. 4.3

Case 11

A 37-year-old man presents with acute foot drop and incontinence. Previous medical history is significant for obesity, diabetes mellitus, and a recent minor motor vehicle accident with minor lacerations. Examination revealed two-fifth motor strength in right tibialis anterior (TA) and extensor hallucis longus (EHL), an L1 sensory level, increased deep tension reflexes (DTRs) in legs with clonus (**Fig. 4.4**).

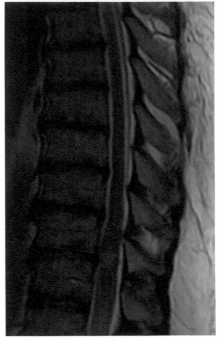

Fig. 4.4

Case 12

A 75-year-old man presents with difficulty walking and urinary incontinence. Previous medical history is significant for hypertension, kidney transplant, osteoarthritis, and diabetes mellitus. Examination revealed a T5 sensory level, spasticity in both legs, and ataxic gait (**Fig. 4.5**).

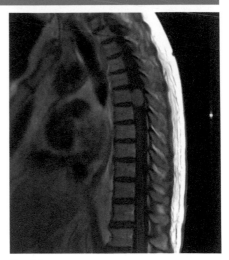

Fig. 4.5

5 Other Spinal Disorders

I. Spinal Arteriovenous Malformations (AVMs)

A. Type I—dural artery to a spinal vein in a foramina:
   1. Most frequent type (70%).
   2. Usually occurs in older men.
   3. Causes progressive myelopathy.
   4. Foix-Alajouanine syndrome—subacute necrotizing myelitis due to venous hypertension.
B. Type II—glomus AVM is intramedullary.
C. Type III—juvenile AVM is intra- and extramedullary:
   1. Carries a worse prognosis.
D. Type IV—intradural perimedullary arteriovenous fistula (AVF):
   1. Occurs in younger patients.
   2. Frequently hemorrhages.
E. Evaluation—magnetic resonance imaging (MRI) and angiography:
   1. Type I and IV AVMs—usually in adults; present with progressive weakness by venous hypertension.
   2. Type II and III AVMs—usually in children.
F. Treatment—endovascular embolization of feeding vessel or open coagulation and division of feeding vessels:
   1. Type I AVMs—radicular artery can be divided or clipped on the foramen.

II. Syringomyelia

A. Communicating—central canal is patent (i.e., Chiari malformation).
B. Noncommunicating—trauma or tumor.
C. Signs/symptoms—cape-like, suspended, dissociated sensory loss (of pain and temperature); pain; Charcot joint; upper motor neuron findings in the lower extremities and lower motor neuron findings in the upper extremities.
D. Evaluation—MRI and possibly cine-MRI.
E. Treatment—occipitocervical decompression with duraplasty in the presence of a Chiari malformation (over 80% of these syrinxes will resolve without shunting):
   1. Other types of syrinxes—treat by local decompression if possible or syringo-peritoneal shunting (midline or dorsal root entry zone incision with 26-gauge tubing).
   2. Syringosubarachnoid shunting—less successful.

III. Paget Disease

A. Cause—increased resorption of bone and replacement with irregular weak bone.

B. Signs/symptoms—bone pain, fractures, back pain, and deafness:

    1. Occurs in the skull, axial, and long bones.

    2. Rarely develops into a sarcoma.

C. Evaluation—increased serum alkaline phosphatase, normal calcium, increased urine hydroxyproline from cartilage, bone scan, and X-ray (thickened bones and lytic skull).

D. Treatment—calcitonin, bisphosphonates, and surgical decompression (there is frequently much blood loss).

IV. Laminectomy Infection

A. Cause—usually *Staphylococcus aureus;* increased risk in the obese, elderly, ill, diabetic, or immunosuppressed.

B. Treatment:

    1. Culture-guided antibiotics—14 days for superficial infection.

    2. Surgical debridement.

    3. Closing over a drain or packing.

    4. Plastic surgery closure—consider for infection extending down to the bone.

V. Spinal Epidural Abscess

A. Causes—usually due to staph rather than strep; most often seen in intravenous drug abusers and diabetics.

B. Signs/symptoms—pain, tenderness, fever, and focal symptoms related to pressure or thrombophlebitis.

C. Evaluation—MRI, complete blood cell count (CBC), and erythrocyte sedimentation rate (ESR).

D. Treatment—antibiotics, immobilization, and decompression.

VI. Vertebral Osteomyelitis

A. Causes—usually staph, strep, or tuberculosis (TB).

B. Treatment—antibiotics and immobilization (**Fig. 5.1**).

VII. Diskitis

A. Causes—staph and strep.

B. Treatment—antibiotics and immobilization.

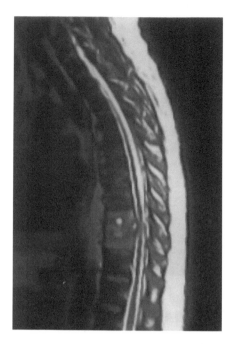

Fig. 5.1 Osteomyelitis. T2-weighted magnetic resonance image of the thoracic spine demonstrating Pott disease with diskitis and osteomyelitis at T7 and 8. (Source: Citow JS. Neuropa- thology and Neuroradiology: A Review. New York, NY: Thieme Medical Publishers; 2001: 199, Fig. 272d.)

Helpful Hint

1. For infection, follow X-ray and serum markers for treatment response. Consider repeating biopsies.

Case 13

A 25-year-old presents with progressively worsening back pain. Previous medical history is significant for uncomplicated lumbar diskectomy 2 months before presentation and diabetes mellitus. Examination revealed new right foot drop (**Fig. 5.2**).

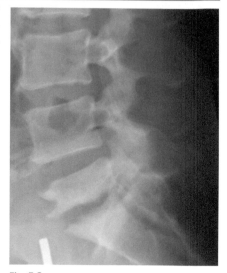

Fig. 5.2

Case 14

A 22-year-old man presents with progressive difficulty running track at college. There is no previous medical history. Examination was remarkable for increased reflexes in his legs, clonus, and upgoing Babinski (**Fig. 5.3**).

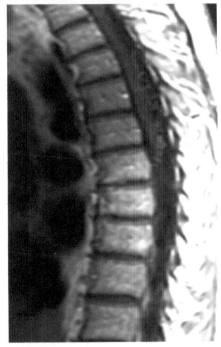

Fig. 5.3

Case 15

A 57-year-old man presents with new bladder incontinence, leg weakness, and gait difficulty. Previous medical history is significant for a motor vehicle accident 10 years ago with temporary leg weakness, diabetes mellitus, peripheral vascular disease, and alcoholism. Examination revealed cape-like loss of pain temperature from T1 to T9, motor strength ⅘ throughout legs, reflexes 1+ in arms and 2+ in legs (**Fig. 5.4**).

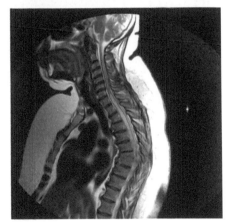

Fig. 5.4

Part 2

Cranial Disorders

6 Cranial Anatomy and Approaches

I. Pterion

A. Junction of frontal, parietal, temporal, and greater wing of sphenoid bones.

B. Located two fingerbreadths above the zygomatic arch and two fingerwidths behind the frontal process of zygoma (**Fig. 6.1**).

II. Asterion

A. Junction of lambdoid, parietomastoid, and occipitomastoid sutures.

B. Located over the transverse–sigmoid junction.

III. Bregma

A. Junction of coronal–sagittal suture.

IV. Frankfort Plane

A. From inferior orbit to top of external acoustic meatus (EAM).

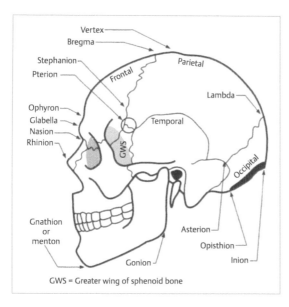

Fig. 6.1 Craniometric points. (Source: Greenberg MS. Handbook of Neurosurgery. 7th ed. New York, NY: Thieme Medical Publishers; 2010: 86, Fig. 5.4.)

V. Posterior Earline

A. Midmastoid up rostrally perpendicular to baseline (Frankfort plane).

VI. Sylvian Fissure

A. Lateral canthus to three-fourth of nasion–inion line and ending at posterior ear line.

VII. Motor Strip

A. 4–5 cm behind coronal suture; top is at posterior ear line and direction is 45 degrees from Frankfort baseline.

VIII. Central Sulcus

A. Top is 2 cm behind nasion–inion line (3–4 cm behind coronal suture); bottom is 5 cm above EAM.

IX. Angular Gyrus

A. Located just above the pinna; caps the superior temporal sulcus.
B. The Wernicke receptive speech area also includes the supramarginal gyrus that caps the sylvian fissure.

X. Broca Area

A. Expressive speech center located in inferior frontal gyrus pars opercularis (behind the pars orbitalis and triangularis).

XI. Superior Orbital Fissure Contents

A. Cranial nerves (CNs) III, IV, VI (all three branches: nasociliary, frontal, and lacrimal).
B. Sympathetic fibers from the internal carotid artery (ICA) plexus.
C. Superior orbital vein
D. Orbital branch of the middle meningeal artery.
E. Recurrent meningeal branch of the lacrimal artery.

XII. Inferior Orbital Fissure

A. CN V2.
B. Zygomatic nerve.

C.   Pterygopalatine branch of the maxillary nerve.

D.   Infraorbital artery and vein.

E.   Inferior ophthalmic vein.

XIII. Orbital Tendinous Ring (Annulus of Zinn)

A.   Structures passing above it include the lacrimal nerve, the frontal nerve, and CN IV.

B.   Structures passing through it include the superior and inferior divisions of CN III, the nasociliary nerve, and CN VI.

C.   Mnemonic—*l*uscious (lacrimal) *F*rench (frontal) *t*arts (trochlear) *s*tand (superior division III) *n*aked (nasociliary) *in* (inferior division III) *a*nticipation (abducens) (**Fig. 6.2**).

XIV. Circle of Willis

A.   Complete in only 20% of the population.

XV. Fetal Circulation

A.   ICA supplies the posterior circulation (occurs in 25% of the population, do not perform Wada test in these patients).

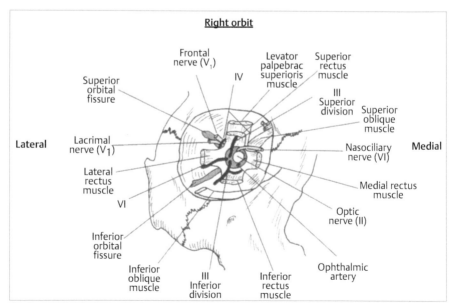

Fig. 6.2 Tendinous ring. (Source: Citow JS. Comprehensive Neurosurgical Board Review. New York, NY: Thieme Medical Publishers; 2000: 76, Fig. 1.41.)

XVI. Vertebral Artery

A. Enters the foramen transversarium at C6.

B. Distal to the C1 foramina transversarium, it curves posteromedially toward the lamina of C1 and then pierces the dura to move anterosuperomedially toward the anterior brainstem.

XVII. Surgical Approaches

A. Temporal lobe lesions.

1. Key points:

    a. Consider a lateral or supine patient position.

    b. Skin incision may be horseshoe anterior and posterior to the ear, question mark extending posterior to the ear (gives widest exposure), or linear (for anterior lesions) (**Fig. 6.3**).

    c. Enter through the inferior or middle temporal gyrus and spare the superior temporal gyrus.

    d. Safe to remove 5 cm of the dominant side and 7 cm of nondominant side (larger resection into optic radiation causes "pie in the sky" visual field cut).

    e. Be careful with the uncus (preserve medial arachnoidal plane near tentorium to avoid CN III, posterior cerebral artery (PCA), and anterior choroidal artery) and middle cerebral artery (MCA) branches in the sylvian fissure (stay in a subpial plane).

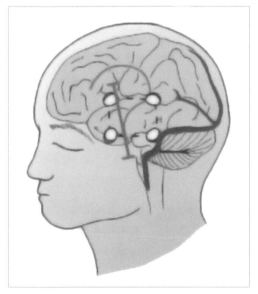

Fig. 6.3 Temporal lobe exposure. (Source: Citow JS. Neurosurgery Oral Board Review. 1st ed. New York, NY: Thieme Medical Publishers; 2003: 78,Fig. 9.7.)

B. Lateral ventricle atrium (trigone)—patient in lateral position; enter through the middle temporal gyrus, lateral temporoparietal cortex, or the superior parieto-occipital region.

C. Frontal horn of lateral ventricle—patient in supine position; enter through the middle frontal gyrus.

D. Body of lateral ventricle—patient in supine position; transcallosal approach.

E. Third ventricle—patient in supine position; transcallosal approach (less seizure risk than with transcortical approach, but may cause contralateral leg weakness due to retraction):

1. We prefer a linear incision to a horseshoe incision in this and most procedures.

2. Be careful with superior sagittal sinus retraction, the surrounding veins, and the fornix.

3. Incise only 2.5 cm of the anterior corpus callosum.

4. Disconnection syndrome more likely with posterior incision through the splenium.

5. Fenestrate the lateral ventricle and then proceed into the third ventricle via an interforniceal approach or extend the foramen of Monro posteriorly by opening the choroidal fissure, but avoid anteriorly through fornix.

6. Prepare both sides of the head in case interhemispheric veins are prohibitive for interhemispheric approach (craniotomy is positioned one-third behind coronal suture and one-third over midline; perform strip craniotomy over sinus separately (**Fig. 6.4** and **Fig. 6.5**).

F. Anterior fossa skull base—for olfactory groove meningiomas, etc.

1. Patient in supine position.

2. Bicoronal incision is made connecting the two zygomatic arches (Soutor incision allows easier skin closure).

3. The scalp flap should be dissected forward above the pericranium to provide a vascularized flap for closure.

4. Dissection over the temporalis muscles should be in the interfascial plane or below the fascia when the fat pads are reached to avoid injuring the frontalis branch of the facial nerve.

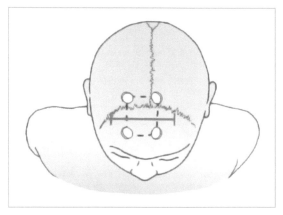

Fig. 6.4 Transcallosal exposure. (Source: Citow JS. Neurosurgery Oral Board Review. 1st ed. New York, NY: Thieme Medical Publishers; 2003: 80, Fig. 9.8.)

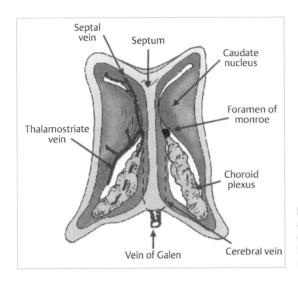

Fig. 6.5 View inside the lateral ventricles. (Source: Citow JS. Neurosurgery Oral Board Review. 1st ed. New York, NY: Thieme Medical Publishers; 2003: 80, Fig. 9.9.)

5. Burr holes are placed at the keyholes and around the anterior superior sagittal sinus; bone flap is turned.

6. Anterior one-third of the sinus may usually be sacrificed when needed.

7. Frontal sinus should be cranialized by removing the posterior wall and removing the mucosa.

8. Frontal ostium should be plugged with muscle.

9. Blood supply is usually under the lesion; try to ligate as early as possible (preop embolization for meningiomas!).

10. At closure, the pericranial flap should be placed over the base of the anterior fossa and sutured to the planum sphenoidale dura.

11. Outer dura should then be closed in a water-tight fashion.

12. Cerebrospinal fluid leak (CSF) should be treated with a lumbar drain and intermittent skull X-rays to watch for pneumocephalus.

13. Complications—Injury to CNs I (almost always) and II, brain injury (cognitive impairment and seizures), anterior cerebral artery injury, and infection (**Fig. 6.6**).

G. Transpetrosal approach—Used to expose anterior or lateral lesions from the midbrain to the lower pons (i.e., cavernous malformation, clivus chordoma, and petroclival meningioma) (**Fig. 6.7**):

1. Patient positioned with falx parallel to floor (usually lateral).

2. Horseshoe incision is fashioned from the base of the mastoid, around the pinna, to the zygoma.

3. Zygoma, mastoid, and external auditory canal are identified.

4. Locate the asterion (junction of the parietomastoid, occipitomastoid, and lambdoid sutures) that overlies the junction of the transverse and sigmoid sinuses.

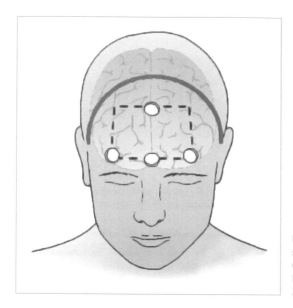

Fig. 6.6 Bicoronal craniotomy incision. (Source: Citow JS. Neurosurgery Oral Board Review. 1st ed. New York, NY: Thieme Medical Publishers; 2003: 81, Fig. 9.10.)

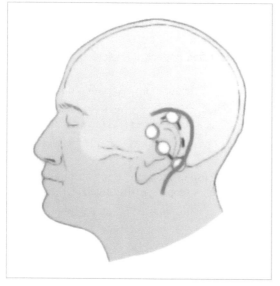

Fig. 6.7 Transpetrosal craniotomy. (Source: Citow JS. Neurosurgery Oral Board Review. 1st ed. New York, NY: Thieme Medical Publishers; 2003: 82, Fig. 9.11.)

5. Transverse sinus is usually under the superior nuchal line.

6. Burr holes are placed on both sides of the transverse and sigmoid sinuses.

7. Do not dissect across the sinus with a Penfield #3; instead use a kerasin punch or eggshell the bone with a diamond drill.

8. Remove the boomerang-shaped bone flap.

9. Drill off the mastoid bone to expose the semicircular canals and the superior petrosal sinus (in the dura at the junction of the tentorium, middle, and posterior fossa).

10. Maximize bony removal to minimize brain retraction.

11. Open the presigmoid dura and divide the superior petrosal sinus.

12. Locate the trochlear nerve under the tentorium.

13. Operative window is between CNs V/VII and VII/IX.

14. The exposure will not reach lesions below the jugular foramen.

15. Close with a fat graft, fibrin glue, and a lumbar drain to prevent CSF leak (as high as 20%).

16. Complications—Injury to the CNs, hearing loss by damage to the semicircular canals with loss of endolymph (be sure to obtain a preop contralateral audiogram), and sinus injury.

H. Anterior foramen magnum lesions—consider transoral approach, far lateral (transcondylar), or posterior approaches.

I. Far lateral (transcondylar) approach—For lesions involving the lower ⅓ of clivus to the upper cervical spine (contralateral vertebrobasilar junction aneurysm):

1. Patient positioned supine, head laterally flexed, vertex down, with ipsilateral mastoid as highest point.

2. Incision is made over the spinous processes of C1–3 and curved laterally over the mastoid bone, or S-shaped incision 2 cm behind mastoid for small lesions.

3. Vertebral artery is identified at the superior C1 transverse arch as it pierces the dura to move up the foramen magnum.

4. Greater occipital nerve may be identified under sternocleidomastoid muscle and followed down to the C2 nerve root.

5. C1 hemilaminectomy is performed and the foramen magnum is opened.

6. Lateral mass of C1 and posteromedial occipital condyle are drilled off to the hypoglossal canal (if more is removed, an occipitocervical fusion is needed).

7. Vertebral artery is mobilized from the C2 arch to the foramen magnum and retracted medially (**Fig. 6.8**).

8. Complications—Injury to lower CNs (use intraoperative monitoring and consider preop trach and percutaneous endoscopic gastrostomy [PEG]).

J. Perforate methylmethacrylate if used as a skull replacement to decrease the fluid accumulation under the bone flap.

K. Intraoperative brain swelling—consider edema, blood clot, hydrocephalus, internal jugular vein occlusion, or hypercapnia.

1. Evaluation—intraoperative ultrasound.

2. Treatment—mannitol, Lasix, hyperventilation, and ventricular drainage:

a. Always consider placement of an occipital Frazier burr hole with posterior fossa surgery.

L. White matter tracts and "zero footprint" approaches to intraparenchymal tumors.

1. Supratentorial fibers can be assigned to three categories:

a. Association fibers (green on DTI)–cingulum, superior longitudinal fasiculus, inferior longitudinal fasiculus. Fibers are intrahemispheric, connecting cortical areas within ipsilateral hemisphere.

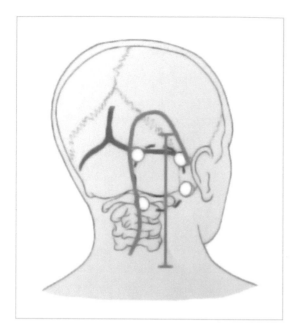

Fig. 6.8 Far-lateral (transcondylar) incision. (Source: Citow JS. Neurosurgery Oral Board Review. 1st ed. New York, NY: Thieme Medical Publishers; 2003: 83, Fig. 9.12.)

    b. Commisural fibers (red on DTI)—corpus callosum and anterior commissure. Fibers are interhemispheric, connecting hemispheres of the brain.

    c. Projection fibers (blue on DTI)—corticospinal tract, optic radiations. Connect cortex to subcortical and distant structures, often for motor control or sensory perception.

2. Association fibers:

    a. Cingulum—connects limbic and neocortical centers. Provides situational inhibition of limbic drives (**Fig. 6.9**).

    b. Superior longitudinal fasiculus—large associative bundle, connects frontal, parietal, occipital and temporal lobes in an ipsilateral hemisphere. Wide ranging effects on sensory processing and motor regulation (**Fig. 6.10**).

    c. Inferior longitudinal fasiculus—connects occipital lobe to temporal lobe in an ipsilateral hemisphere. Functions in visual object identification and classification (**Fig. 6.11**).

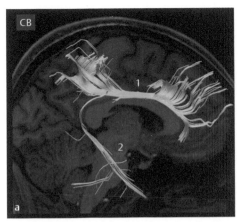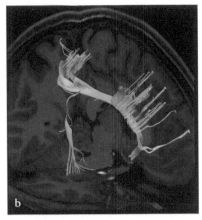

Fig. 6.9 (a) Sagittal and (b) oblique images showing tractography of the cingulum bundle (CB), depicting the anterior arm (1) of the tract extending posteriorly around the corpus callosum (the retrosplenial cingulum) to enter the ipsilateral temporal lobe (2) as the parahippocampal cingulum. Note the dense contributions to this tract from the anterior frontal and parietal white matter. (Source: Leite C, Castillo M, ed. Diffusion Weighted and Diffusion Tensor Imaging. A Clinical Guide. 1st edition. Thieme; 2015: 40, Fig. 3.3.)

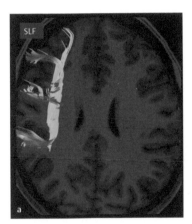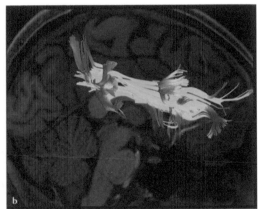

Fig. 6.10 (a) Axial and (b) sagittal depictions of the large superior longitudinal fasciculus (SLF), which connects the anterior hemisphere to the posterior hemisphere through the centrum semiovale and frontal operculum. (Source: Leite C, Castillo M, ed. Diffusion Weighted and Diffusion Tensor Imaging. A Clinical Guide. 1st edition. Thieme; 2015: 41, Fig. 3.4.)

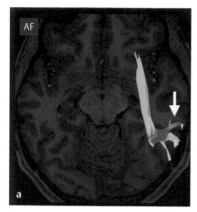
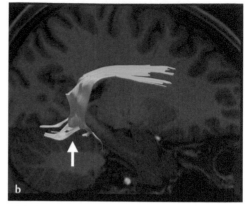

Fig. 6.11 **(a)** Axial and **(b)** sagittal illustrations of the left arcuate fasciculus (AF), a major pathway for normal language function that connects the superior temporal gyrus (*arrows*) to the ipsilateral frontal lobe. (Source: Leite C, Castillo M, ed. Diffusion Weighted and Diffusion Tensor Imaging. A Clinical Guide. 1st edition. Thieme; 2015: 41, Fig. 3.5.)

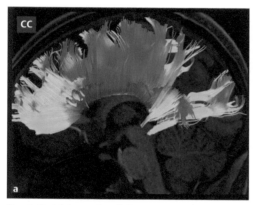
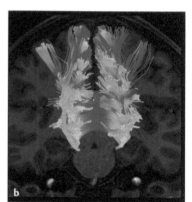

Fig. 6.12 **(a)** Sagittal and **(b)** coronal projections of the massive corpus callosum (CC) show how branches of this bundle follow a topographic arrangement from anterior to posterior, connecting many homologous areas of the cortex across the hemispheres. (Source: Leite C, Castillo M, ed. Diffusion Weighted and Diffusion Tensor Imaging. A Clinical Guide. 1st edition. Thieme; 2015: 44, Fig. 3.10.)

3. Commisural fibers:

    a. Corpus callosum—connects homologus regions of each hemisphere. Coordinates function between hemispheres. Injury can cause disconnection syndromes (**Fig. 6.12**).

    b. Anterior commissure—connects orbitofrontal cortex with temporal and occipital lobes to process olfactory, auditory and visual information.

4. Projection fibers:

    a. Pyramidal tracts (corticospinal and corticobulbar tracts)—primary descending motor fibers involved in voluntary motor control (**Fig. 6.13**).

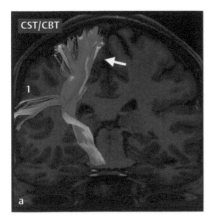
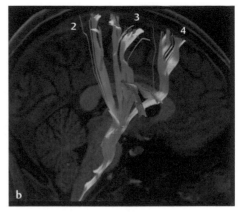

Fig. 6.13 Best seen on (a) coronal images, the lateral branches of the pyramidal tract (1) project to the lateral precentral gyrus, and are more difficult to identify than the dominant medial branches (*white arrow*). These branches are not depicted well with diffusion tensor imaging (DTI) tractography, and require high angular resolution diffusion imaging (HARDI) or diffusion spectrum imaging (DSI) to be visualized. (b) Note on sagittal projection that the pyramidal tract extends not only to the precentral gyrus (3), but also to the parietal lobe (2) and the supplementary motor area (4). CST, corticospinal tract; CBT, corticobulbar tract. (Source: Leite C, Castillo M, ed. Diffusion Weighted and Diffusion Tensor Imaging. A Clinical Guide. 1st edition. Thieme; 2015: 46, Fig. 3.12.)

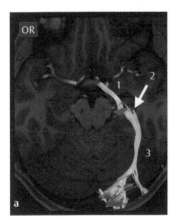
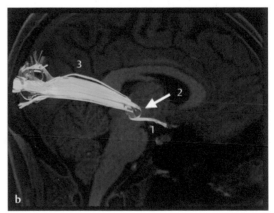

Fig. 6.14 (a) Axial and (b) sagittal images of the left optic tract (1) and optic radiation (OR) (3), carrying topographically organized information from the right visual field to the occipital cortex. From the lateral geniculate nucleus, anterior fibers from this pathway extend a variable length into the ipsilateral temporal lobe (2) before sweeping back into the occipital lobe within the sagittal striatum (*arrow*). Disruption of this segment, the Meyer loop of the optic radiations, gives rise to superior quadrantanopia. (Source: Leite C, Castillo M, ed. Diffusion Weighted and Diffusion Tensor Imaging. A Clinical Guide. 1st edition. Thieme; 2015: 47, Fig. 3.13.)

     b.   Optic radiations—carries visual information from the optic pathways to the occipital lobes. Damage causes visual field deficits (**Fig. 6.14**).

5.   Zero footprint strategies include use of image-guided tube approaches or minimal retraction through a trans-sulcal access corridor planned to avoid disrupting these eloquent white matter tracts as much as safely possible.

Helpful Hints

1. Standard craniotomy preop—consent with risks, complete blood cell count (CBC), electrolytes, prothrombin time/partial thromboplastin time (PT/PTT), blood available, urinalysis (UA), chest X-ray (CXR), electrocardiogram (ECG), antibiotics before incision, antiepileptics, dexamethasone 20 mg/kg every 4 hours (q4h); mannitol 1 gm/kg bolused at drilling; hydrocortisone 100 mg q8h if pituitary surgery.

2. Consider what neural structures should be monitored or localized, e.g., brainstem auditory-evoked responses (BAERs) and CNs V, VII, and VIII during vestibular schwannoma tumor resection; must do awake craniotomy to map speech areas.

3. Consider how to neuronavigate.

4. Plan dural closure for skull base approaches (e.g., periosteal flap).

These cases have a broad differential and multiple approaches, they will help you to practice working up various diagnoses and consider various approaches and anatomic considerations.

Case 16

A 35-year-old woman presents with a mild, chronic headache after a fall. Past medical history and examination were unremarkable (**Fig. 6.15**).

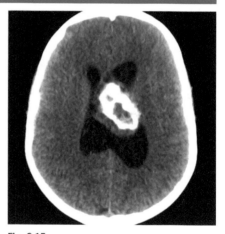

Fig. 6.15

Case 17

An 18-year-old man presents with episodic headaches, worse in the morning and during Valsalva maneuvers. Past medical history is significant for posterior fossa tumor resection 5 years earlier. Examination revealed some balance difficulty (**Fig. 6.16**).

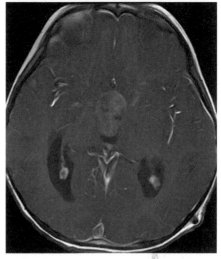

Fig. 6.16

Case 18

A 55-year-old man presents with progressive frontal headaches. Past medical history is significant for smoking history, nonsmall cell cancer after resection and adjuvant therapies. Examination revealed bitemporal heteronymous hemianopsia (**Fig. 6.17**).

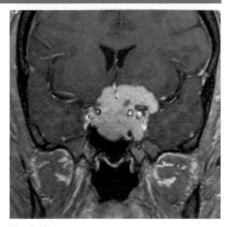

Fig. 6.17

7 Head Trauma

I. Glasgow Coma Scale (GCS)

A. Eye opening—none (1), to pain (2), to voice (3), spontaneously (4).

B. Verbal output—none (1), sounds (2), words (3), disoriented (4), oriented (5).

C. Motor function—none (1), extensor posturing (2), flexor posturing (3), withdrawal from pain (4), localizing (5), following commands (6).

II. Head Trauma Grading

A. Severe (GCS 3–8), moderate (GCS 9–12), mild (GCS 13–15).

III. Good Outcomes

A. GCS 3–6 (8%), 7–8 (41%), 9–12 (81%).

B. Outcome worse if systolic blood pressure (SBP) <90 mm Hg or pO_2 <60 mm Hg.

IV. Intracranial Pressure (ICP) Monitor

A. Place if examination does not correlate with findings on computed tomography (CT) scan (concern for intracranial pressure (ICP)- related examination changes) or in patients with GCS 8 or less who are not immediately postictal.

V. Cerebral Perfusion Pressure (MAP–ICP)

Maintain >70; try to keep ICP <20 mm Hg.

VI. ICP Control

A. Cerebrospinal fluid (CSF) drainage.

B. Mannitol—1 g/kg bolus and 0.25 g/kg every 6 hours (q6h):
   1. Check serum osmolarity q6h and hold mannitol if <320 to avoid acute tubular necrosis.
   2. Maintain euvolemia and normokalemia.
   3. Avoid mannitol with congestive heart failure or renal failure.

C. Sedation and paralytics.

D. Pentobarbital coma:
   1. Lowers ICP and cerebral metabolic rate of oxygen ($CMRO_2$).
   2. Decreases free radicals.

3. Produces hypotension by decreasing sympathetic tone and causing myocardial depression.

4. Increase dose until burst suppression achieved on electroencephalogram (EEG).

5. Insert Swan-Ganz catheter and nasogastric (NG) tube (for hyperalimentation).

6. Dose—thiopental 5 mg/kg intravenously (IV) over 10 minutes, 5 mg/kg/h × 24 hours, and 2.5 mg/kg/h to control ICP/EEG (level 6–8.5 mg/dL).

7. Consider propofol 10 µg/kg/min up to 170 µg/kg/min in place of barbiturates.

VII. Other Measures

A. Fever control—cooling blanket and rectal paracetamol.

B. Sucralfate or Famotidine.

C. Deep vein thrombosis (DVT) prophylaxis—Thromboembolic deterrent (TED) hose, sequential compression device (SCD), and heparin subcutaneously (SQ).

D. Tube feeds after 3 days (may need up to 140% of standard daily caloric intake).

VIII. Skull Fracture

A. Surgical repair if open (also needs antibiotics), CSF leak, an underlying clot causing significant mass effect, or a fragment depressed more than the thickness of the skull.

IX. Sinus Wall Fracture

A. Treat with 10 days of antibiotic and surgical repair.

X. Epidural Hematoma (EDH)

A. EDH <15 mm thickness or <30 cm^3 total volume with <5 mm of midline shift and good GCS can be observed, but repeat imaging and regular neurologic examinations are indicated.

B. Use question mark or linear incision but be sure to expose low enough to reach foramen spinosum (middle meningeal artery).

C. Consider placement of ICP monitor if there is also cerebral edema.

D. Have blood available.

XI. Gunshot Wound

A. Monitor airway, breathing, circulation (ABCs) and address other injuries.

B. Shave around the wound, irrigate and debride, and finally staple the wound closed.

C. Use antiepileptic (e.g., keppra), Cefazolin, and tetanus toxoid.

D. Consider an angiogram to rule out vessel injury for lesions crossing the sylvian fissure or interhemispheric fissure.

E. Don't operate if GCS 3–6 without a mass lesion.

XII. Facial Palsy

A. If partial or worsening, consider ear, nose, and throat (ENT) decompression; surgery rarely needed.

XIII. Tension Pneumocephalus

A. When nitrous oxide not stopped before dural closure; burr hole for subdural drain if symptomatic.

XIV. Post-Traumatic Leptomeningeal Cyst (Growing Skull Fracture)

A. Fix with craniotomy around lesion and dural repair.

XV. Benign Subdural Collections of Infancy

A. Most resolve spontaneously.

XVI. Cephalohematoma

A. Subgaleal hematoma—does not calcify, resolves spontaneously.

B. Subperiosteal hematoma:
    1. Occurs mainly in newborns and is limited by sutures.
    2. 80% resorb spontaneously.
    3. May calcify.
    4. Surgical evacuation for cosmesis is performed after 6 weeks.

XVII. Concussion

A. Transient altered mentation or loss of consciousness following head trauma.

B. For management guidelines for sports-related concussions, see **Table 7.1**, **Table 7.2**, **Table 7.3**, and **Table 7.4**.

Table 7.1 Concussion grading

Grade	Cantu system	AAN system
Mild	A. PTA <30 min B. No LOC	A. Transient confusion B. No LOC C. Symptoms resolve in <15 min
Moderate	A. LOC >5 min, or As above, but symptoms B. PTA >30 min last >15 min (still no LOC) (PTA is common)	
Severe	A. LOC ≥5 min, or Any LOC, whether brief B. PTA ≥24 h (seconds) or prolonged	

Abbreviations: AAN, American Academy of Neurology; LOC, loss of consciousness; PTA, posttraumatic amnesia.

Table 7.2 Cerebral contraindications for return to contact sports

A. Persistent postconcussion symptoms

B. Permanent CNS sequelae from head injury (e.g., organic dementia, hemiplegia, homonymous hemianopsia)

C. Hydrocephalus

D. Spontaneous SAH from any cause

E. Symptomatic (neurologic or pain-producing) abnormalities about the foramen magnum (e.g., Chiari malformation)

Abbreviations: CNS, central nervous system; SAH, subarachnoid hemorrhage.

Table 7.3 Recommendations for multiple sports-related concussions in the same season

Concussion No.	Severity	Guidelines to be met before return to Competition
2	Mild	1 Week[a]
	Moderate or severe	1 Month[a] + normal CT or MRI[b]
3	Mild	Most consider this a season ending injury and recommend CT or MRI[b]
	Moderate	Season-ending injury, consideration for ending all participation in contact sports
2	Severe	Season-ending injury, consideration for ending all participation in contact sports

Abbreviations: CT, computed tomography; MRI, magnetic resonance imaging.

[a]Without symptoms at rest and with exertion (see text).

[b]If any acute abnormalities on CT/MRI: Terminate season. Consider ending all participation in contact sports.

Table 7.4 Management options following concussion

AAN grade management options[a]

1. Mild
   A. Remove from contest.
   B. Examine every 5 min for amnesia or postconcussive symptoms[a].
   C. May return to contest if symptoms clear within 15 min.

2. Moderate
   A. Remove from contest.
   B. Disallow return that day.
   C. Examine on-site frequently for signs of evolving intracranial pathology.
   D. Re-examination the next day by a trained individual.
   E. CT or MRI if H/A or other symptoms worsen or last >1 week[b].
   F. Return to practice after 1 full week without symptoms[a].

3. Severe
   A. Ambulance transport from field to ER if still unconscious or for concerning signs (C-spine precautions if indicated).
   B. Emergent neuro examination; neuroimaging as appropriate.
   C. May go home with head-injury instructions if normal findings at time of initial neuro examination.
   D. Admit to hospital for any signs of pathology or for continued abnormal mental status.
   E. Assess neuro status daily until all symptoms have stabilized or resolved.
   F. Prolonged unconsciousness, persistent mental status alterations, worsening postconcussion symptoms, or abnormalities on neuro examination → urgent neurosurgical evaluation or transfer to a trauma center.
   G. After brief (<1 min) grade 3 concussion, do not return to practice until asymptomatic for 1 full week[a].
   H. After prolonged (>1 minute) grade 3 concussion, return to practice only after 2 full weeks without symptoms[a][c].
   I. CT or MRI if H/A or other symptoms worsen or last >1 week[b].

Abbreviations: AAN, American Academy of Neurology; CT, computed tomography; ER, emergency room; H/A, headache; MRI, magnetic resonance imaging.

[a]Evaluation at rest and with exertion.

[b]Season is terminated for that player if CT/MRI shows edema, contusion, or other acute intracranial pathology. Return to play in any contact sports in the future should be seriously discouraged.

[c]Some experts also require a normal CT scan.

XVIII. CSF Leak

A. Increased risk of infection, mainly from *Streptococcus* and *Staphylococcus*, and a mortality rate <10%.

B. Rhinorrhea—CSF may travel from middle ear through eustachian tube to nasopharynx or directly through cribriform plate to nasopharynx.

C. Otorrhea—CSF leak requires perforated tympanic membrane.

D. Evaluation:
   1. CSF fluid glucose—should be >30 (with tears and mucus it should be <5).
   2. B2-transferrin—found only in CSF.

3. Leak site—localize with coronal thin-cut CT of anterior fossa to sella or with CT cisternography with iohexol lumbar puncture (LP) injection followed by Trendelenburg position prone.

E. Treatment:

1. Bed rest, stool softeners, acetazolamide (decreases CSF production), and fluid restriction (1500 mL/d).

2. Prophylactic antibiotics—not proven helpful.

3. Leak persists >3 days—place lumbar drain with head of bed (HOB) elevated 10 degrees and drip chamber at shoulder:

   a. Avoid tension pneumocephalus—treat by bedrest flat with 100% O_2 and rarely aspiration.

4. Leak persists >2 weeks or patient develops meningitis—consider surgical intradural repair.

Helpful Hints

1. ABCs first.

2. Make sure spine is evaluated.

3. Rule out nonsurgical causes of depressed consciousness, e.g., illicit drugs, narcotics, hypoglycemia, hypoxia, hypotension, seizure.

4. Be aggressive with temporal (prepare for middle meningeal artery bleeding) and posterior fossa hematomas (prepare for sinus involvement).

Case 19

A 25-year-old presents in the emergency department (ED) after a motor vehicle accident (MVA). Past medical history is significant for cocaine abuse. Examination was consistent with GCS = 8 and no movement in right leg (**Fig. 7.1**).

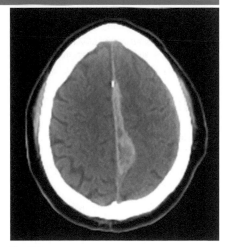

Fig. 7.1

Case 20

A 24-year-old man presents in the ED with a self-inflicted gunshot wound (GSW). Past medical history is significant for bipolar disorder, suicidal ideation, and drug abuse. Examination in ED revealed GSW entrance through hard palate and exit wound at right frontal skull; GCS = 12 and decreased to GCS = 8 an hour after initial examination (**Fig. 7.2**).

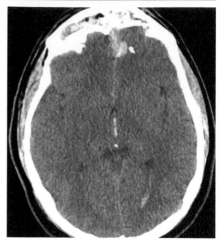

Fig. 7.2

Case 21

An infant is ejected from a car during an MVA. Past medical history is unremarkable. Examination revealed GCS = 5, intact brainstem reflexes (**Fig. 7.3**).

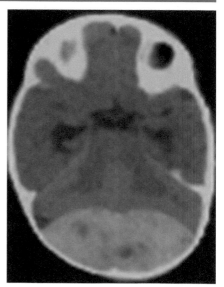

Fig. 7.3

8 Brain Tumors

I. Low-Grade Astrocytoma (WHO Grade 1 or 2)

A. Treatment:
   1. Usually with surgery alone (curative if juvenile pilocytic astrocytoma).
   2. Radiation dose, if used—45 Gy to the tumor with a 2-cm margin; hold off if young due to long-term side effects.
   3. Chemotherapy—procarbazine, lomustine (CCNU), and vincristine (PCV).

II. High-Grade Astrocytoma (WHO Grade 3 or 4)

A. Prognosis—Depends on age (younger is better), Karnofsky score, and histology.
B. Treatment:
   1. Cytoreductive surgery—image-guided surgery suggested.
   2. External beam radiation—typically 60 Gy at 2 Gy fractions 5 days a week, and may add boost to resection cavity.
   3. Temodar—an oral alkylating agent that increases median survival—from 12 to 14 months when given concurrently with radiation therapy.
   4. Gliadel (carmustine [BCNU]) wafers—increase survival minimally by 8 weeks.
   5. Avastin—an anti-vascular endothelial growth factor (VEGF) agent may increase survival minimally.
   6. PCV chemotherapy.
   7. Surgery—avoid if tumor is bilateral, or in patients with low Karnofsky score.
C. Survival:
   1. Per grade—1 (10 years), 2 (8 years), 3 (2 years), and 4 (1.5 year).
   2. Average—17 weeks with biopsy, 30 weeks with surgery alone for grade 4.

III. Oligodendroglioma

A. Treatment—surgery, chemotherapy (PCV helps significantly), radiation therapy (XRT; for the anaplastic variety).
B. Survival—30% at 10 years; 1p19q loss predicts better chemotherapy response and longer survival.

IV. Ependymoma

A. Evaluation—evaluate for drop metastasis (mets) with lumbar puncture (LP) and spinal magnetic resonance imaging (MRI).

B. Treatment:
1. Surgery.
2. XRT—50 Gy to the tumor bed, and spinal XRT if drop mets are seen or cells detected in the cerebrospinal fluid (CSF).
C. Survival—tumor is usually very radiosensitive; survival is 40% at 5 years in children, 80% at 5 years in adults.

V. Choroid Plexus Tumors

A. Treatment—surgery only; consider preoperative embolization.

VI. Primitive Neuroectodermal Tumor (PNET)

A. Evaluation—evaluate for drop mets with spinal MRI and LP.
B. Treatment:
1. Surgery.
2. XRT—radiate craniospinal axis after resection; in children older than 3 years.
3. Surgical resection for medulloblastoma:
    a. Craniospinal XRT—40 Gy with 15 Gy to the tumor bed and drop mets over 6 weeks.
    b. Chemotherapy—CCNU and vincristine.
4. Shunt—required in 30% of cases.
C. Survival—tumor is usually very radiosensitive; survival depends on molecular subtyping, with Wnt-type tumors having the best long-term survival, and Group 3/4 tumors having poor long-term survival. Overall survival may be 43% at 10 years.

VII. Ganglioglioma

A. Treatment—surgery alone.

VIII. Pineal Tumors—Pineal Region Borders are the Tectum, Vermis, Splenium of the Corpus Callosum (Posteriorly), Third Ventricle (Superiorly), and Thalami (Laterally)

A. Evaluation:
1. Evaluate for drop mets with all varieties.
2. Tumor varieties:
    a. Germ cell—most common; most often germinoma
    b. Pineocytoma/pineoblastoma, astrocytoma, embryonal carcinoma, choriocarcinoma, and teratoma.

3. CSF for alpha fetal protein (AFP)—in embryonal carcinoma, endodermal sinus tumor, and teratoma.

4. Beta HCG—choriocarcinoma and germinoma.

B. Treatment:

1. If tumor resection does not relieve hydrocephalus—place ventriculoperitoneal (VP) shunt or perform third ventriculostomy (penetrate floor of third ventricle anterior to mamillary bodies).

2. Avoid performing a stereotactic biopsy due to the hazard of adjacent vessels unless you are comfortable with third ventricular biopsy.

3. Germinoma may be treated with biopsy followed by radiation and chemotherapy.

4. Resection carries 10% mortality.

C. Operative approaches.

1. Infratentorial/supracerebellar:

   a. Not as easy with a steep tentorium.

   b. Usually safe to divide the precentral cerebellar vein.

   c. Operative window—between the two basal veins of Rosenthal (**Fig. 8.1**).

2. Suboccipital/transtentorial:

   a. Risk of visual loss.

   b. Best for tumors above the tentorial edge and vein of Galen (**Fig. 8.2a, b**).

   c. Incise the tentorium 1 cm lateral to the straight sinus.

   d. Operative window—between internal cerebral vein and basal vein of Rosenthal.

3. Transcallosal—minimalize to avoid disconnection syndrome.

4. Transventricular—through the nondominant superior temporal gyrus.

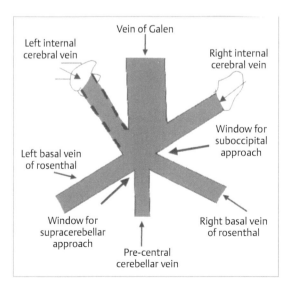

Vein of Galen

Left internal cerebral vein

Right internal cerebral vein

Window for suboccipital approach

Left basal vein of rosenthal

Window for supracerebellar approach

Right basal vein of rosenthal

Pre-central cerebellar vein

Fig. 8.1 Surgical windows around the deep venous anatomy for pineal region lesions. (Source: Citow JS. Neurosurgery Oral Board Review. New York, NY: Thieme Medical Publishers; 2003: 60, Fig. 9.1.)

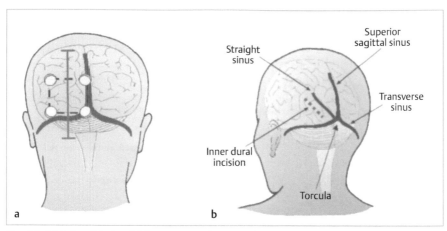

Fig. 8.2 (a) Suboccipital and **(b)** transtentorial incision. (Source: Citow JS. Neurosurgery Oral Board Review. 1st ed. New York, NY: Thieme Medical Publishers; 2003: 61, Fig. 9.2A, 9.2B.)

IX. Pituitary Adenoma

A. Apoplexy:

    1. Signs/symptoms—typically presents with headache and ophthalmoplegia due to tumor infarction or hemorrhage.

    2. One-third of prolactin-secreting adenomas will hemorrhage.

    3. Not an emergency if asymptomatic.

    4. Treatment in cases with mass effect—steroids and surgical decompression.

B. Signs/symptoms:

    1. Bitemporal hemianopsia.

    2. Cavernous sinus invasion—impaired cranial nerves (CNs), chemosis, proptosis, and rarely cerebrovascular accident (CVA).

    3. Hypo- or hyperpituitarism:

        a. Increased prolactin (rule out Hook effect): (1) Amenorrhea, galactorrhea, and impotence; (2) May also be seen with hepatic or renal disease, phenothiazines, verapamil, cimetidine, and pregnancy.

        b. Increased adrenocorticotropic hormone (ACTH)—increased serum and urine cortisol, hyperpigmentation (Nelson syndrome), hypertension, hyperglycemia, abdominal stria, moon face, truncal obesity, extremity wasting, bruising, osteoporosis, amenorrhea, peripheral neuropathy, and depression.

        c. Decreased ACTH—orthostatic hypotension and fatigue.

        d. Increased growth hormone (GH): (1) Increased somatomedin C—synthesized in the liver and produces insulin-like growth factor (IGF)-1; (2) Acromegaly—coarse facial features, enlarging head, hands, and feet; (3) Peripheral neuropathy, cardiomyopathy, hypertension, glucose intolerance (diabetes), upper airway obstruction, perspiration, colon cancer, and giantism (if occurs before growth plate closes); (4) Somatostatin decreases GH release.

        e. Decreased GH—dwarfism.

f. Decreased thyroid stimulating hormone (TSH)—cold intolerance, fatigue, coarse hair, peripheral neuropathy, and myxedema coma.

g. Decreased follicle-stimulating hormone/luteinizing hormone (FSH/LH)—amenorrhea, decreased libido, and infertility (hypogonadism).

h. Decreased antidiuretic hormone (ADH)—diabetes insipidus (very rare with a sellar mass).

C. Evaluation:

1. Endocrine history (as above), visual fields, extraocular movements.

2. Prolactin—mild elevation to 25–150 is usually by stalk effect from decreased dopamine that normally inhibits prolactin.

3. Morning cortisol, 24-hour urine cortisol.

4. ACTH—decreased with adrenal tumor, increased with pituitary adenoma or ectopic lung mass.

5. Dexamethasone suppression test:

a. Low dose of 1 mg—normally decreases ACTH.

b. High dose of 8 mg—decreases ACTH with Cushing disease (pituitary adenoma).

c. There is no suppression with an ectopic tumor.

6. TSH, T4, GH, somatomedin C, FSH/LH, estrogen, testosterone.

7. MRI:

a. May be normal in 50% of cases.

b. Enlarged pituitary gland on MRI: (1) May be caused by pregnancy (also with amenorrhea and increased prolactin); (2) May be caused by primary hypothyroidism (elevated TSH, treat with Levothyroxine).

8. Petrosal sinus sampling—has been used to evaluate the location of an ACTH-secreting tumor; however, normal people have different amounts of ACTH on each side.

9. Rapid-sequence infused MRI—may demonstrate location of a small adenoma.

D. Treatment.

1. Prolactinoma:

a. Bromocriptine (Parlodel)—dopamine agonist that decreases tumor size 75% by 8 weeks.

b. Lifelong therapy needed to control tumor growth.

c. Starting dose—2.5 mg orally three times daily (PO three times a day).

d. Initial bothersome side effects—emesis and postural hypotension; normally resolve over several weeks.

e. Watch for low estrogen—May cause osteoporosis.

f. Safe to take oral contraceptives (OCP) with bromocriptine and safe to take bromocriptine while pregnant.

g. If tumor enlarges during pregnancy, surgically resect it or increase the bromocriptine.

h. Follow patient with visual field examinations.

i. Dostinex is another medical option.

j. Consider transsphenoidal or subfrontal resection if medical therapy fails.

2. Acromegaly:
   a. Surgical resection—best option, followed by therapy with bromocriptine or octreotide, and finally XRT if GH levels do not normalize.
   b. Postoperative steroid withdrawal is a good sign.
   c. IGF-1 levels usually drop 4 weeks after surgery.
   d. Tumors with GH levels > 40 are difficult to cure.
3. Cushing disease:
   a. Surgical resection—best option.
   b. Ketoconazole may be used to temporarily lower cortisol levels.
   c. Bilateral adrenalectomy—last resort (patient may develop Nelson syndrome).
4. Hyperthyroidism—surgical resection favored over octreotide.
5. Radiation:
   a. 50 Gy over 6 weeks.
   b. 50% decrease in ACTH, FSH/LH, and TSH in 10 years.
   c. Visual loss may occur.
   d. Consider only if unable to reoperate.
6. Surgery—subfrontal or transsphenoidal:
   a. Transnasal transsphenoidal—most common approach: (1) Insert a throat pack, prep the thigh or abdomen for a fat graft, inject the nasal mucosa with epinephrine, enter the right nostril; (2) In a submucosal plane, dissect the left side of the nasal cartilage and bilateral nasal bone to the sphenoid bone (find the sphenoid ostium posterior to middle/superior turbinates); (3) Insert the Cushing speculum and finally the Hardy speculum, assess the midline (sphenoid ridge may be off-center), chisel off the anterior wall of the sphenoid sinus, remove the mucosa; (4) Chisel off the anterior wall of the sella, incise the dura in cruciate fashion, and curette out the soft tumor; (5) A newer approach is to insert the speculum directly to the floor of the sphenoid sinus, open the speculum to displace the nasal bone, and open the mucosa over the sinus wall and proceed from there; (6) A lumbar drain may be inserted and air injected to help push the tumor down during resection; (7) Postop MRI should be done at 3 months.

E. Complications:
   1. Diabetes insipidus (DI), injuries to CNs II–VI, carotid artery injury, hypopituitarism, and CSF leak.
   2. Antibiotics—use until the packs are removed at 3 days (chloramphenicol and ampicillin) as well as a hydrocortisone stress dose followed by a replacement dose (100 mg intravenously every 8 hours [IV q8h] × 3 then 20 mg PO every morning and 10 mg every bedtime [qHs]).
   3. Hydrocortisone—stop 2 days after surgery and send a urine cortisol (<9 needs steroid replacement).
   4. Diabetes insipidus—diagnosed as a urine output (UOP) > 250 mL/h × 3 hours with specific gravity (SG) < 1.005.
   5. Lost fluid—replace with half normal saline and use 0.1 μg desmopressin acetate (DDAVP) IV q6h or intranasal 10–40 μg twice a day for long-term maintenance.

6. CSF leak—treat initially with a lumbar drain and if this is unsuccessful, consider exploration and packing.

7. Carotid injury with pulsatile bleeding—should be treated with packing followed by an angiogram to determine if bypass or endovascular treatment (occlusion, stenting, etc.) is needed.

X. Craniopharyngioma

A. Treatment:

1. Perform preop and postop endocrine evaluation.

2. Steroids—consider after surgery to avoid adrenal crisis.

3. Subtotal resection—appears to be the best treatment (unless complete removal can be safely achieved), followed by XRT.

4. Surgical approach—multiple approaches can be used, subfrontal, pterional, endoscopic endonasal. Depends on tumor characteristics and surgeon preference.

5. Surgical mortality—10%; morbidity includes hyperthermia, lethargy, impaired thirst mechanism, and endocrine deficiencies.

B. Survival—5-year rate is 75%.

XI. Colloid Cyst

A. Treatment:

1. If<7 mm and without hydrocephalus, consider conservative management with follow-up MRI at 6 months.

2. Surgical management—stereotactic aspiration or open transcallosal resection (remember to fenestrate the septum pellucidum).

3. Surgical pitfalls—damage to anterior cerebral artery, cingulate gyrus, fornix, internal cerebral veins; enter wrong ventricle; intraventrical hemorrhage.

XII. Meningioma

A. Treatment:

1. Surgical resection—consider if symptomatic.

   a. Preoperative—remember to consider dural patch material (autograft or synthetic), dural sinus patency, and possibility of embolization (may cause distant strokes).

   b. Recurrence with partial resection—60% at 10 years without XRT; 30% with XRT.

B. Survival—91% at 5 years.

XIII. Vestibular Schwannoma

A. Evaluation—should include pure tone audiogram and speech discrimination test (50/50 is considered serviceable hearing with 50 Db pure tone hearing and 50% speech discrimination).

B. Treatment—if asymptomatic, consider following with MRI evaluation every 6 months (**Fig. 8.3a, b**):

1. Suboccipital retrosigmoid resection.

2. Middle fossa approach—for small intracanalicular tumors distal in the canal.

3. Translabyrinthine approach—sacrifices hearing.

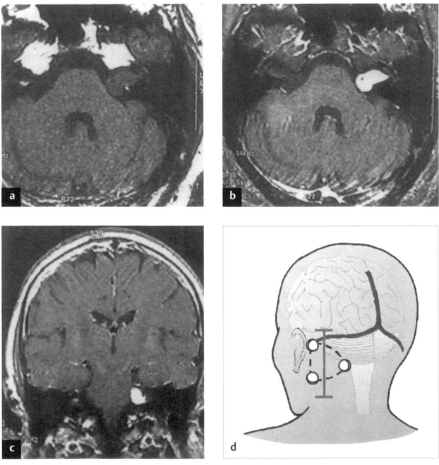

Fig. 8.3 (a) Vestibular schwannoma, noninfused, (b) infused, and (c) axial and infused coronal T1-weighted magnetic resonance images demonstrating an enhancing mass emanating from the left internal acoustic meatus. (d) Vestibular schwannoma exposure via suboccipital–retrosigmoid craniotomy. (Source: Citow JS. Neuropathology and Neuroradiology: A Review. New York, NY: Thieme Medical Publishers; 2001: 105, Fig. 147.)

4. XRT/stereotactic radiosurgery—12–13 Gy dose to the tumor margin undetermined indication with primary or recurrent tumors, and associated with higher hearing preservation and decreased risk of facial palsy.

5. Use intraop 8th (brainstem auditory evoked response [BAER]), 7th, and 5th nerve monitoring.

6. Suboccipital retrosigmoid craniotomy:

   a. Place the patient semiprone (45 degrees) or lateral with the falx parallel to the floor.

   b. Incision is the length of the pinna and located 2 cm posterior to the mastoid notch.

   c. A burr hole is made at the asterion and a small craniotomy fashioned after eggshelling edge of transverse and sigmoid sinuses.

   d. Dura is opened with triangular flaps based on the transverse and sigmoid sinuses.

   e. Cerebellum is gently and slowly retracted medially to expose the CNs.

   f. Water-tight dural closure is essential.

   g. Complications: (1) Facial palsy—if unable to close eyes, use natural tears q2h, Lacri-Lube, and tape eyes shut qHs; (2) Tarsorrhaphy—if after 1 year the weakness hasn't improved, perform a XII–VII anastomosis (or even after only 2 months if the nerves were directly cut); (3) CSF leak—treat with a lumbar drain, shunt, or ENT (ear, nose, and throat) packing; (4) Vertigo—resolves with rehab.

C. Preservation of function:

   1. Seventh nerve—95% (< 1 cm), 80% (1–2 cm), 50% (> 2 cm).

   2. Eighth nerve—57% (< 1 cm), 33% (1–2 cm), 6% (> 2 cm).

XIV. Trigeminal Schwannoma—less common than vestibular schwannoma

A. Tumor limited to the Meckel cave in the middle fossa—pterional craniotomy should provide sufficient exposure.

B. Dumbbell-shaped tumor with extension into the posterior fossa—more aggressive approach such as the transpetrosal.

C. Dissection may be epidural (find V2 and V3 and trace to the tumor) or intradural (**Fig. 8.4**).

XV. Hemangioblastoma—Usually Located in the Posterior Fossa near the Sigmoid–Transverse Junction

A. Evaluation—evaluate for pheochromocytoma and renal cell carcinoma.

B. Treatment—surgical resection after embolization is performed similar to arteriovenous malformation (AVM) surgery by dissecting around the lesion and initially avoiding the veins.

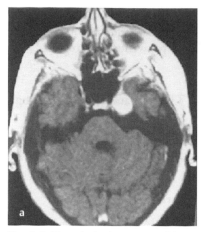 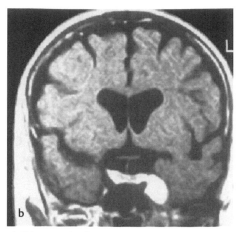

Fig. 8.4 Trigeminal schwannoma. **(a)** Axial and **(b)** coronal infused T1-weighted magnetic resonance images demonstrating a smooth, circumscribed, enhancing mass in the Meckel cave. (Source: Citow JS. Neuropathology and Neuroradiology: A Review. New York, NY: Thieme Medical Publishers; 2001: 105, Fig. 148.)

C.   Only 20% are associated with Von Hippel-Lindau syndrome (CNS hemangioblastomas, retinal hemangiomas, renal cell carcinoma, pheochromocytoma, and cysts of the liver, pancreas, and kidney).

XVI. Chordoma—usually located in the sacrum or clivus

A.   Treatment—Wide en bloc surgical resection and proton beam XRT; prognosis usually poor with median 10-year survival of 20–30%.

XVII. Epidermoid and Dermoid Tumors

A.   Treatment:
   1.   Symptomatic—Treat with surgical resection.
   2.   Steroids—Mollaret meningitis (inflammation by leakage of cholesterol crystals) so avoid spillage during resection.

XVIII. Lymphoma—Metastatic Lesions are Usually Meningeal, whereas Primary Intracranial Lymphoma (Usually in the Immunocompromised) is Usually Located in the Deep Frontal or Paraventricular Region

A.   Evaluation:
   1.   Hyperdense on computed tomography (CT), hyperintense on T1-weighted MRI, and enhances strongly like a meningioma.

2. Examination of lymph nodes, chest X-ray (CXR), CT of the chest and abdomen, bone marrow biopsy, testicular ultrasound, and eye examination for uveitis.

B. Treatment—tumors may disappear with steroids.

1. Biopsy.

2. XRT—50 Gy fractionated.

3. Chemotherapy—intrathecal methotrexate in ventricular access device 12 mg twice a week × 6 with IV leucovorin rescue.

C. Survival—3 months without treatment, 10 months with XRT.

XIX. Paragangliomas

A. Carotid body tumor:

1. Signs/symptoms—usually presents as a neck mass with CN X or XII palsy and internal carotid artery (ICA) insufficiency.

2. Evaluation—MRI and angiogram (external carotid artery feeders and a splayed bifurcation). The tumors may release catecholamines and 5% are bilateral.

3. Treatment—(frequent CN X and XII injury 40%, stroke 10%, and death 10%) and XRT.

B. Glomus jugulare or tympanicum:

1. Signs/symptoms—usually presents with CN IX–XII palsies (jugulare) or CN VII and VIII palsy and bruit (tympanicum).

2. Evaluation:

   a. Evaluate with otoscope—pulsatile red/blue mass behind eardrum.

   b. Urine vanillylmandelic acid (VMA)—tumors may release catecholamines, serotonin, or histamine.

   c. MRI and CT.

3. Treatment—surgical resection (with preoperative embolization) and XRT.

   a. Histamine release at surgery may cause hypotension or bronchoconstriction; pretreat with 3 weeks of α-blockers and 3 days of β-blockers.

XX. Pediatric Tumors—Juvenile Pilocytic Astrocytoma, Medulloblastoma, Brainstem Glioma, and Ependymoma; in Children <1 year, Usually Teratoma and Glioblastoma (GBM)

XXI. Skull Tumors—Epidermoid (Scalloped Margins), Hemangioma (Sunburst Pattern), Eosinophilic Granuloma (Punched-Out Lesion with Clean Margins, Tender, Associated with Histiocytosis X), Osteoma (Sclerotic), and Meningioma (Hyperostotic)

A. Treatment—en bloc resection if symptomatic:

1. Consider radiating a hemangioma if patient unable to tolerate surgery.

B.   Tumors originating from various tissues—bone (osteoma and osteosarcoma), cartilage (chondroma and chondrosarcoma), fibrous (meningioma), marrow (multiple
myeloma and histiocytoma), vessel (hemangioma), and other (fibrous dysplasia,
Paget disease, metastatic tumors).

XXII. Metastases

A.   Most frequent lesions—lung, breast, kidney, colon, and melanoma.

B.   Tumors that frequently hemorrhage—choriocarcinoma, renal cell carcinoma, and
melanoma.

C.   Most common in children—neuroblastoma, rhabdomyosarcoma, and Wilms tumor.

D.   Drop mets—possible from medulloblastoma, ependymoma, pineal tumors.

E.   Evaluation—evaluate for primary tumor with CXR; CT of chest, abdomen, and
pelvis; mammogram; bone scan:

1.   Areas of diffuse ependymal enhancement are seen with leptomeningeal carci-
nomatosis or abscess.

F.   Treatment:

1.   Antiepileptic (e.g., Keppra) and steroids; possibly surgical resection and XRT.

2.   Solitary met—excision and whole brain radiation therapy (WBRT) or stereotactic radiosurgery (SRS) if inaccessible.

3.   3 or less mets—WBRT and SRS or surgery if accessible with one craniotomy.

4.   Greater than 3 mets—WBRT classically (evidence now demonstrating stereotactic radiosurgery (SRS) for up to 10 mets may have survival benefit while
limiting effects of WBRT.

5.   XRT—30 Gy over 2 weeks (sensitive tumors are small cell, germinoma, and
lymphoma).

6.   Postoperative XRT—questionable value.

G.   Survival—consider resection only if greater than 6 months.

XXIII. Neurofibromatosis Type I (NF-1)

A.   Inclusion criteria are at least two of the following:

1.   Six café au lait spots.

2.   Two neurofibromas.

3.   One plexiform neurofibroma.

4.   Axillary or inguinal freckling.

5.   An osseous lesion (sphenoid dysplasia or thinning of long bones).

6.   An optic glioma.

7.   Two Lisch nodules (iris hamartomas, only seen in NF-1).

8.   A relative with NF-1.

XXIV. Neurofibromatosis Type II (NF-2)

A. Associated tumors—bilateral vestibular schwannomas, meningiomas, astrocytomas, hamartomas, spinal ependymomas (spinal astrocytomas are more common in NF-1), and nerve root schwannomas.

B. Inclusion criteria—bilateral vestibular schwannomas or a relative with NF-2 and one vestibular schwannoma, or two of the following:

1. Neurofibroma, meningioma, glioma, schwannoma, or postcapsular cataract at a young age.

C. Treatment—attempt to remove the vestibular schwannomas when small and try to preserve hearing in at least one ear. Stereotactic radiosurgery may be of value.

XXV. Tuberous Sclerosis

A. Signs/symptoms—classical triad is adenoma sebaceum (rash-like facial angiofibromas), mental retardation, and seizures.

B. Associated lesions:

1. Cerebral hamartomas—tubers, frequently calcify, and usually don't enhance.
2. Subependymal giant cell astrocytoma—enhances and is located near the foramen of Monro.
3. Cardiac rhabdomyoma.
4. Renal angiomyolipoma.
5. Pancreatic adenoma.
6. Retinal hamartoma.
7. Cysts in the lung, liver, and spleen.

C. Treatment—resect the astrocytoma if symptomatic (usually by hydrocephalus).

XXVI. Sturge–Weber Syndrome

A. Signs/symptoms—ipsilateral V1 port-wine stain, cortical tram-track calcifications, and atrophy.

B. Treatment—anticonvulsants and a skin-colored tattoo on the nevus flammeus.

XXVII. Ring-Enhancing Lesion

A. Vascular, infectious, neoplastic, demyelinating (VIND).

XXVIII. Basal Ganglia Lesions

A. Infection, astrocytoma, lymphoma, metastatic tumor, demyelination.

XXIX. Transdural Nasal Mass

A. Juvenile angiofibroma, esthesioneuroblastoma (use chemotherapy before resection and XRT), mucormycosis, meningioma, and metastatic disease.

XXX. Radiation

A. Theory—X-rays and gamma rays deliver photons and particulate radiation to tumor cells to cause cell death and cessation of replication by freeing an electron to break bonds and produce free radicals to injure DNA.

1 Gy = 1 J of energy absorbed/kg
1 Gy = 100 rad
1 cGy = 1 rad

B. External beam radiation:

1. Fractionation divides the dose to increase the therapeutic ratio (effect on tumor cells/normal cells).

2. Results depend on dose, time, and field. The body repairs sublethal damage.

3. Three Rs are redistribution (cells are most susceptible in the mitotic phase), repopulation (cell types change), and reoxygenation (cells are more susceptible with increased oxygen).

4. Delay XRT until 10 days postsurgery to allow initiation of healing.

5. Germinomas and lymphoma melt away but recur.

C. Radiation necrosis:

1. Vascular endothelium and oligodendrogliomas are the most susceptible.

2. Usually occurs after 18 months.

3. Radiation therapy lowers IQ 25 points (especially doses > 40 Gy) and may injure the optic pathways (limited to 8 Gy) and the pituitary/hypothalamic system, cause demyelination after methotrexate, and produce new tumors (GBM, meningioma, or osteosarcoma).

4. Evaluation—MR-spectroscopy or positron emission tomography (PET) scan (increased glucose use in tumors decreases with necrosis).

5. Treatment:

   a. Only resect necrosis if there is mass effect.

   b. Prevent necrosis by keeping the radiation dose <60 Gy over 6 weeks; in the spinal cord avoid doses > 0.2 Gy/d.

D. Stereotactic radiosurgery.

1. General:

   a. Best for AVMs or tumors < 3 cm and inaccessible.

   b. 2-year latency with AVM therapy before the hemorrhage risk decreases.

   c. Use multiple ports with a steep gradient drop-off to decrease surrounding brain injury.

2. Linear accelerator (LINAC):

   a. Photon beam is made by electron acceleration (X-ray).

   b. More flexible and less expensive than gamma knife with nonspherical lesions.

   c. Results—similar to gamma knife.

   d. Modification of target—produced by changing arc paths and collimator size.

3. Gamma knife:

   a. Photon beam is made by natural radioactive decay (gamma ray).

   b. Narrower distribution of energy produces slightly better spatial accuracy than LINAC, but this is less than the error in target margins (LINAC has 1 mm error).

   c. Uses different-sized collimators and exposure times and > 1 isocenter.

   d. Target modification—performed by plugging collimators passing radiation through sensitive areas.

4. Fractionated stereotactic radiosurgery (radiotherapy):

   a. Reoxygenation helps kill more cells.

   b. Fractionation hits late responders and multiple cell cycles.

   c. Hypofractionation—1 fraction/d × 1 week; best for slow-growing benign tumors (meningioma, schwannoma, and AVM).

5. Planning:

   a. Use five arcs 100 degrees each to keep the drop-off optimal.

   b. Tissue 2.5 mm away will be injured.

   c. CT localizes better than MRI due to magnetic artifact, but accuracy can't be < 0.6 mm due to pixel size (MRI shift is 2 mm).

   d. Multiple isocenters help conform to an irregular shape.

6. Specific lesions:

   a. AVM—perform 30 days after embolization (avoid radiopaque dye). Use 15 Gy to the periphery of the lesion. Obliteration rate is 50% at 1 year and 86% at 2 years.

   b. Schwannoma—use 14 Gy at 80% isodense line; 40% shrink and 40% stop growing.

   c. Metastatic tumors—use 15 Gy at the center at 80% isodense curve.

7. Complications—headache, emesis, seizures (premedicate with Dexamethasone 10 mg and phenobarbital 90 mg), radiation necrosis 3%, symptomatic white matter changes 20%, vascular changes 5%, and CN dysfunction 1%.

Helpful Hints

1. DOG P—DNET, Oligo, Ganglioglioma, and PXA are cortically based tumors that present with seizures.

2. SATCHMO—Sarcoid, Astrocytoma/Aneurysm/Adenoma, Teratoma, Craniopharyngioma, Hamartoma, Met, Optic glioma are suprasellar lesions.

3. New onset headaches should be evaluated with CT, LP (don't miss infection or sentinel subarachnoid hemorrhage) and possibly angiogram (CT or MR angiography [CTA/MRA] are good fast choices).

4. History should suggest infection or tumor diagnosis.

5. Be aggressive with temporal tumors (prevent uncal herniation) and posterior fossa tumors (prevent central herniation; treat obstructive hydrocephalus with external ventricular drain immediately at beginning of surgery).

6. Rule out pulmonary embolism due to deep vein thrombosis in postop hypoxia.

Case 22

A 55-year-old man presents with sudden headache that is worse with Valsalva maneuvers. Past medical history is nonsignificant. Examination was normal except for ataxia (**Fig. 8.5**).

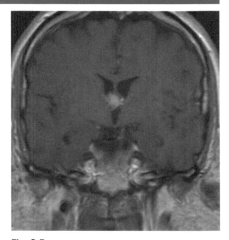

Fig. 8.5

Case 23

A 60-year-old woman presents with progressive right hemiparesis and diplopia over the past 6 weeks. Past medical history is significant for breast cancer. Examination was normal except right arm and leg motor strength was ⅘, and there was partial left abducens nerve palsy (**Fig. 8.6**).

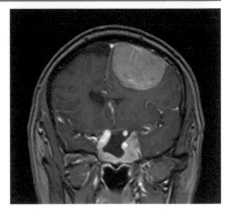

Fig. 8.6

Case 24

A 50-year-old man presents with visual difficulty and fatigue. Past medical history is significant for colon cancer, lung disease, and immunodeficiency. Examination revealed bitemporal hemianopsia (**Fig. 8.7**).

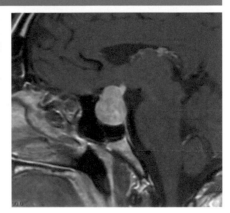

Fig. 8.7

9 Cerebrovascular Disease

I. Stroke

A. Transient ischemic attack (TIA)—deficit lasts <24 hours.

B. Reversible ischemic neurologic deficit (RIND)—deficit lasts <1 week.

C. Cerebrovascular accident (CVA)—stroke, deficit lasts >1 week.

D. Amaurosis fugax—transient monocular blindness usually due to a small fibrin embolus.

E. CVA risk after an ocular TIA—17% in 2 years.

F. CVA risk after a hemispheric TIA—43% in 2 years (usually within 3 months).

G. CVA etiologies:

   1. 60% from atherosclerosis—possibly from an embolic plaque or ischemia; usually 50% stenosis is necessary to be symptomatic.

   2. 20% lacunar—small-vessel lipohyalinosis.

   3. 15% from cardiac embolism.

   4. 15% of CVAs are hemorrhage; 85% are dry.

H. Cerebral autoregulation:

   1. Occurs with cerebral perfusion pressure (CPP) 50–150 mm Hg to keep cerebral blood flow (CBF) normal (around 55 mL/100 g of brain tissue/min).

   2. Ischemic penumbra—area where cells receive CBF of 18–23 mm Hg, enough to survive, but not enough to be functional (these cells may survive to restore function over time).

I. CVA symptoms:

   1. Carotid circulation—unilateral motor, sensory, visual, or speech deficit.

   2. Vertebral circulation—bilateral motor, sensory, or visual deficits, or syncope.

J. Evaluation:

   1. History—tobacco use, elevated cholesterol, hypertension (HTN), diabetes mellitus (DM), angina, and claudication.

   2. NIH Stroke Scale (NIHSS, standard bedside clinical tool).

   3. Laboratory evaluation—complete blood cell count (CBC), platelets, prothrombin time/partial thromboplastin time (PT/PTT), electrolytes, arterial blood gases (ABGs), rapid plasma reagin (RPR; syphilis), erythrocyte sedimentation rate (ESR), electrocardiogram (ECG), and 24-hour cardiac monitor.

   4. Radiologic evaluation.

      a. Computed tomography (CT): (1) Consider CT angiogram in initial workup if large vessel occlusion is possible etiology; (2) CT perfusion can determine areas at risk (ischemic penumbra), although utility still under active study; (3) ASPECTS score (10-point score highlighting CT findings of ischemia); (4) After 1 week shows gyral ribbon enhancement; (5) Many weeks later reveals atrophy.

      b. Carotid duplex—combines color flow Doppler and β-mode ultrasound: (1) Doppler effect—change in sound pitch as sound waves hit a moving target; the frequency decreases as it leaves and increases as it approaches.

      c. Carotid and cerebral magnetic resonance angiography (MRA) or angiogram—may demonstrate a string sign or occluded vessels as well as luxury perfusion (increased CBF adjacent to a CVA due to impaired auto-regulation from the acidosis). Don't operate if a tandem cerebral lesion is more stenotic than the carotid lesion.

K. Thrombolytic therapy:

  1. Recombinant tissue-plasminogen activator (t-PA) use does not change the deficit at 24 hours, but improves it at 3 months; 30% of patients are more likely to have little or no deficit.

  2. Must be administered within 4.5 hours of symptoms (see quick reference guide for acute stroke timeline for treatment and intravenous [IV] tPA contraindications).

  3. Use reserved for patients with NIHSS 6 or greater.

  4. Exclusion criteria—CT with edema or hemorrhage, systolic blood pressure (SBP) >185 mm Hg, seizures, anticoagulants, surgery within 14 days, CVA within 3 months, or glucose >400.

  5. Increased risk of intraparenchymal hemorrhage 6.4% from 0.6%, though the mortality stays at 20%.

  6. Dose—0.09 mg/kg IV over 1 minute and then 0.81 mg/kg over 60 minutes.

  7. Reverse t-PA for surgery—Amicar 5 g IV (acts in 15 minutes), cryoprecipitate, and fresh frozen plasma (FFP).

L. CVA treatment:

  1. IV fluid without dextrose.

  2. Aspirin (ASA)—325 mg orally daily (PO once a day). Consider adding statin therapy to reduce LDL-C to <70 mg/dL.

  3. Maintain SBP <180 mm Hg (but >130 mm Hg).

  4. The risk of another CVA is 1%/week with or without heparin (not recommended).

  5. Warfarin—use only for antiphospholipid antibody, atrial fibrillation, or verte-bral insufficiency.

  6. Hemicraniectomy—may be used for cerebellar or right middle cerebral artery CVAs with excessive mass effect.

  7. Avoid hyperthermia and hyperglycemia; they make the neurons more vulner-able to ischemia.

M. Best medical management:

  1. Start with ASA (325 mg one a day) or Ticlopidine to produce a 30% decrease in CVA rate after a TIA.

  2. Ticlopidine and Clopidogrel may lower the white blood cell (WBC) count.

  3. Control HTN, DM, cholesterol, and tobacco use.

  4. Anticoagulation—for atrial fibrillation or vertebrobasilar symptoms.

N. Surgical management:

1. Degree of stenosis—as per the North American Symptomatic Carotid Endarterectomy Trial (NASCET) (1 – a/b) × 100 is the percent stenosis (**Fig. 9.1** and **Fig. 9.2**).

2. Asymptomatic Carotid Atherosclerosis Study (ACAS):

    a. If there is >60% stenosis, surgery decreases the CVA rate only if the complication rate is <3%.

    b. The 5-year CVA rate decreased 66% in males and 17% in females (however, there was no decrease in major CVA rate or death).

    c. The 5-year CVA rate without surgery was 11% and with surgery was 5%.

3. NASCET:

    a. In the presence of a hemispheric or retinal TIA and stenosis >70%, surgery decreases the CVA rate 17% and the death rate 7% over 1.5 years.

    b. A 2-year CVA rate is 40% without ASA, 26% with ASA, and 9% with ASA and carotid endarterectomy (CEA).

    c. There is a 1%/month risk of CVA while waiting for surgery.

4. Recommendations:

    a. Asymptomatic carotid stenosis—only operate if >60% stenosis.

    b. Symptomatic carotid stenosis—operate if >50% stenosis.

5. CEA:

    a. Timing—following ischemic event, risk of stroke is 2% within 7 days and 4% within the first month. Revascularization should be performed as soon as safely possible.

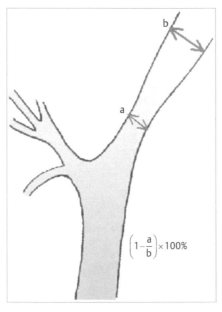

$$\left(1-\frac{a}{b}\right)\times 100\%$$

Fig. 9.1 Carotid stenosis diagram. (Source: Citow JS. Neurosurgery Oral Board Review. 1st ed. New York, NY: Thieme Medical Publishers; 2003: 88, Fig. 10.1.)

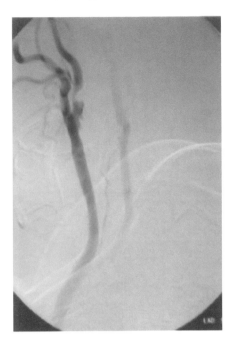

Fig. 9.2 Carotid artery stenosis. Angiogram demonstrates proximal internal carotid artery plaque. (Source: Citow JS. Neuropathology and Neuroradiology: A Review. New York, NY: Thieme Medical Publishers; 2001: 149, Fig. 194.)

b. Sundt morbidity and mortality scale—Risk factors are myocardial infarction (MI), HTN, chronic obstructive pulmonary disease (COPD), CVA within 7 days, carotid siphon stenosis, and contralateral stenosis.

c. Elective patients should receive aspirin (81 mg) 4 days preop and for 6 weeks postop. Emergent cases should receive loading dose of aspirin (325 mg) followed by 6 weeks postop: (1) Clopidogrel is used by some surgeons (75 mg daily 4 days preop and for 6 weeks postop for elective cases and with 300 mg loading dose for emergent cases).

d. Selective shunting—Based on electroencephalogram (EEG) changes (1–4% require a shunt): (1) EEG changes—Usually caused by a shower of cholesterol plaques, not blood clots; (2) Treatment—Heparin 5000 U, thiopental 3 mg/kg, raise the SBP to 170 mm Hg, shunt, and consider angiography with possible urokinase or embolectomy.

e. Patch implantation—If small vessel, long plaque, or repeat surgery (often patient/plaque characteristics and surgeon preference).

f. Exposure: (1) Make the skin incision over the medial border of the sternocleidomastoid (SCM); (2) Watch for the greater auricular nerve over the SCM (section causes numbness in the jaw and ear); (3) Expose the digastric muscle proximally and omohyoid muscle distally; (4) Divide the common facial vein; (5) Follow the descendent hypoglossi to cranial nerve (CN) XII; (6) Place loops around the common carotid artery (CCA), internal carotid artery (ICA), external carotid artery (ECA), and superior thyroid artery (**Fig. 9.3**).

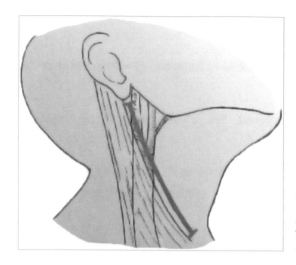

Fig. 9.3 Carotid endarterectomy incision. (Source: Citow JS. Neurosurgery Oral Board Review. 1st ed. New York, NY: Thieme Medical Publishers; 2003: 90, Fig. 10.3.)

g. Clamping: (1) Bolus with heparin 70 U/kg 5 minutes before clamping; (2) Clamp first the ICA, the CCA, the superior thyroid artery, and then the ECA (aneurysm clips on all but a vascular clamp on the CCA); (3) After the endarterectomy, suture the vessel closed with 5.0 Prolene; (4) Unclamp first the ECA and flush the CCA and ICA; (5) Open the CCA and finally the ICA.

h. Emergent CEA: (1) Only used if there is a sudden deficit with a lost bruit in the presence of known stenosis, during angiography, or after CEA; (2) Don't operate on a totally occluded carotid artery after 2 hours if there is a fixed deficit; (3) There is a 3%/year CVA risk from stump embolism with complete occlusion.

i. Complications: (1) Injuries to CN XII—near the facial vein; (2) Injuries to recurrent laryngeal nerve—near the trachea; keep the medial retractor at the platysma; (3) Injuries to superior laryngeal nerve—dysphasia; avoid by starting dissection lateral to the carotid artery; (4) Reactive cerebral hyperemia; (5) Recurrence—stenosis recurs in 20% of patients over 10 years.

j. Postop evaluation: (1) Look for pronator drift, dysphasia, pupillary reactivity, STA pulses (to find ECA or CCA occlusion), tongue deviation, hoarseness, and hematoma with dysphagia or tracheal deviation; (2) Beware of vessel leak, pseudoaneurysm, TIA/CVA, cerebral hemorrhage, or seizure; (3) CN injuries: (a) CN X—vocal cord paralysis or hoarseness; (b) CN XII—tongue deviation; (c) CN VII—lip depressor weakness from mandibular branch; (4) Possible HTN from loss of baroreceptor reflex; (5) Postop TIA—evaluate with CT and angiogram; (6) Fixed postop CVA: (a) Return to the operating room (OR) and reopen the vessel (clamp the CCA and ECA, open the ICA to see backflow, try to insert a Fogarty #4 catheter to remove the clot); (b) Use aggressive IV fluids to increase the SBP to 180 mm Hg, increase O_2, and use pressors if needed; (c) A neck hematoma may need to be removed to enable intubation (try once, don't paralyze the patient, open the neck in the OR); (d) Consider performing a CT if there is a nonlocalizing deficit; (7) Angioplasty: (a) CREST demonstrated non-inferiority between carotid stenting (CAS) and CEA. CAS has higher risk of periprocedural ischemic stroke and CEA has higher risk of MI; (b) CAS should be considered in cases of difficult surgical anatomy, revision, previous neck dissection, history of regional radiation, contralateral recurrent laryngeal nerve palsy, high anesthetic risk, and contralateral carotid occlusion.

O. CVA outcome—25% mortality, 25% disabled, 50% return home.

P. CVA from cardiac embolism:

1. Accounts for one-sixth of CVAs.

2. 2% of MIs develop a CVA within 2 weeks.

3. Without anticoagulation—Risk of CVA with atrial fibrillation is 4.5%/year and with a bioprosthetic heart valve is 3%/year.

4. With anticoagulation—Risk of CVA with a mechanical mitral valve is 3%/year and a mechanical aortic valve is 1.5%/year.

5. Evaluation:

   a. Rule out a paradoxical embolism from a patent foramen ovale in young patients who suffer a CVA.

   b. Rule out cerebrovascular disease and a source for an embolism (echocardiogram and ECG).

   c. There is frequent hemorrhagic transformation at 48 hours. (Up to 30% clinically silent hemorrhagic conversion by 10 days.)

6. Treatment:

   a. No proven benefit with early anticoagulation—12% CVA risk in 2 weeks versus risk of hemorrhagic transformation.

   b. Perform CT at 2 days—if no clot, use heparin and Warfarin together for 3 days until the international normalized ration (INR) is 2–3.

   c. Warfarin use with atrial fibrillation decreases the CVA risk 75% versus 40% with ASA.

Q. Young CVA patients—Search for deficiencies of protein C and S and antithrombin III, and the presence of factor V Leiden, antiphospholipid antibody, systemic lupus erythematosus (SLE), syphilis, tuberculosis, DM, HTN, tobacco use, and increased cholesterol.

R. Lacunar CVA—from small-vessel disease by lipohyalinosis of middle cerebral artery (MCA) branches:

1. Signs/symptoms:

   a. No cortical symptoms.

   b. Most common manifestation is pure sensory loss.

   c. Less common syndromes are pure motor hemiparesis or ataxic hemiparesis.

2. Treatment—Medical management (BP control, aspirin/statin therapy, lifestyle modification) CEA or angioplasty do not help.

S. Lateral medullary syndrome (Wallenberg syndrome):

1. Cause—vertebral or PICA occlusion.

2. Signs/symptoms—ipsilateral vertigo (CN VIII), facial numbness (CN V), dysphagia (CNs IX, X), Horner syndrome, cerebellar ataxia, loss of light touch in the

ipsilateral body (posterior columns), and contralateral loss of pain/temperature (spinothalamic tract).

T. Vertebrobasilar insufficiency:

1. Cause—usually subclavian steal or vessel stenosis; very poor natural history.

2. Signs/symptoms:

    a. 5 Ds—diplopia, dysarthria, defect visual, dizzy, drop attack.

    b. Bilateral motor, sensory, or visual symptoms.

3. Treatment—SAMMPRIS trial suggested first-line therapy should be medical management with antiplatelet agents. Endovascular intervention is only for those who fail medical therapy.

U. ICA dissection:

1. Signs/symptoms—pain, oculosympathetic Horner syndrome (sweat fibers travel with the ECA), CN XII deficit, TIA (due to artery to artery embolism or occlusion).

2. Evaluation:

    a. Angiogram with string sign or double lumen (dissection occurs 2 cm distal to the CCA bifurcation). Digital subtraction angiography (DSA) is gold standard, although MRA and CTA can be reliable alternative.

    b. Associated with cystic medial necrosis, fibromuscular dysplasia, Ehlers-Danlos syndrome, Marfan syndrome, and syphilis (**Fig. 9.4a, b**).

3. Treatment:

    a. CADISS trial compared antiplatelet therapy with anticoagulation, found no difference in rate of recurrent stroke. Consider 3 months of anticoagulation followed by single-agent antiplatelet therapy.

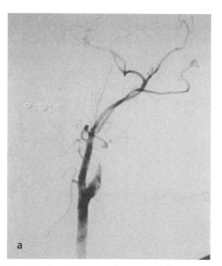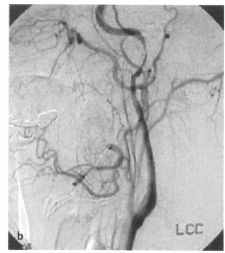

Fig. 9.4 Carotid artery dissection. **(a)** Angiograms demonstrate cervical internal carotid artery (ICA) and **(b)** petrous ICA tapered narrowings. (Source: Citow JS. Neuropathology and Neuroradiology: A Review. New York, NY: Thieme Medical Publishers; 2001: 155, Fig. 200.)

    b. If symptoms progress, consider direct surgical repair, ligation, stenting, or bypass (STA–MCA).

V. Vertebral dissection—usually occurs between C1 and 2 or at C6 (where the artery enters the foramen transversarium).

  1. Signs/symptoms:

    a. Neck pain, CVA (lateral medullary syndrome), or subarachnoid hemorrhage (SAH).

    b. Extradural lesions usually present with stroke from embolism or vessel occlusion, whereas intradural lesions present with SAH.

  2. Treatment—depends on neurologic status and location:

    a. If non flow-limiting stenosis, consider single-agent antiplatelet therapy. With flow-limiting stenosis, turbulent flow on angiogram or recurrent emboli, consider anticoagulation.

    b. For neurologically unstable patients with hypoperfusion, consider endovascular recanalization (**Fig. 9.5**).

    c. Trapping proximal to PICA can be considered if other treatments fail and patient tolerates balloon test occlusion.

W. Venous sinus thrombosis:

  1. Causes—related to infection, dehydration, pregnancy, oral contraceptive pill (OCPs), and deficiency of proteins C, S, antithrombin III, and factor V Leiden.

  2. Evaluation—CT and CT venogram (95% sensitivity) or magnetic resonance venography (MRV).

  3. Treatment:

    a. Address the primary imbalance in clotting factors, increase hydration, and consider anticoagulation in patients without contraindications.

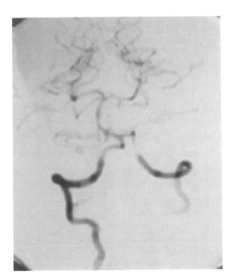

Fig. 9.5 Vertebral artery dissection. Angiogram demonstrates left distal vertebral artery narrowing. (Source: Citow JS. Neuropathology and Neuroradiology: A Review. New York, NY: Thieme Medical Publishers; 2001: 156, Fig. 201.)

b. ISCVT compared unfractionated heparin to low-molecular-weight heparin (LMWH) and found no difference in complete recovery/mortality, but patients who received LMWH had fewer hemorrhagic complications.

c. Antiplatelet agents have not shown clinical benefit.

d. Transition to oral anticoagulation for 3 to 12 months and repeat imaging.

e. In patients who are declining despite medical management, ICP interventions can be performed, up to and including decompressive hemicraniectomy if necessary.

f. Endovascular therapy with tPA or mechanical thrombectomy via venous approach has been reported and can be considered in refractory cases.

X. Moyamoya disease—bilateral distal ICA occlusion with rete mirabile (transdural ECA anastomoses causing a puff-of-smoke appearance).

1. Signs/symptoms—CVA in children; hemorrhage in adults.

2. Evaluation—magnetic resonance imaging (MRI) and angiogram (there are frequently aneurysms) (**Fig. 9.6**).

3. Treatment:

a. Medical therapy is of unknown benefit.

b. Surgical treatment—STA–MCA bypass, encephalomyosynangiosis (temporal muscle to brain), encephaloduroarteriosynangiosis (STA branches placed inside a dural opening), or an omental flap.

c. Encephaloduralsynangiosis: (1) Identify the STA and middle meningeal artery branches on the angiogram; (2) Palpate the STA and locate with a Doppler; incise around it with 15-blade knife; (3) Make two burr holes and connect with a craniotomy; (4) Open the dura where avascular and sew the STA adventitia to the pia with 10.0 Prolene; (5) Lay down the dura and bone; (6) Make a few more burr holes.

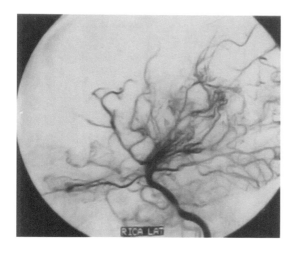

Fig. 9.6 Moyamoya disease. Angiogram demonstrates distal internal carotid artery occlusion with prominent leptomeningeal collaterals ("puff of smoke"). (Source: Citow JS. Neuropathology and Neuroradiology: A Review. New York, NY: Thieme Medical Publishers; 2001: 154, Fig. 199.)

II. Intraparenchymal Hemorrhage

A. Hypertensive hemorrhage—most common locations are putamen 60%, thalamus 20%, pons 10%, and cerebellum 5% (near the dentate nucleus).

   1. Signs/symptoms:

      a. Headache, weakness, and dysphasia.

      b. Pontine hemorrhages may produce pinpoint pupils and "locked—in syndrome."

      c. Cerebellar hemorrhages present with contralateral eye deviation, focal weakness but not hemiplegia, and a rapid loss of consciousness.

      d. Most patients have a history of HTN and usually present to the emergency room (ER) with an SBP over 180 mm Hg.

   2. Treatment:

      a. Lower the blood pressure 30% with Nipride (overaggressive lowering to a "normal range" may lead to hypoperfusion CVA).

      b. Anticonvulsants—usually not needed.

      c. Rehemorrhage—Relatively rare.

      d. Ventricular extension in up to 50% of cases—May require external ventricular drainage.

      e. Surgery—Not proven to improve functional outcome with putamen or thalamic clots, though mortality may be decreased.

      f. Surgical evacuation—for cerebellar clots >4 cm or with hydrocephalus (HCP).

      g. Functional outcome—Best with volumes 10–30 mL.

B. Amyloid angiopathy:

   1. Usually occurs in older patients.

   2. Most common cause of lobar hemorrhage in normotensive elderly patients.

   3. Clot typically extends from the centrum semiovale to the subarachnoid space.

   4. Cause of the hemorrhage is replacement of the contractile elements in the media of the arteries and arterioles of the leptomeningeal and superficial cortical vessels with noncontractile amyloid that is yellow-green with dichroism (birefringence) when stained with Congo red dye and viewed under polarized light.

C. Iatrogenic:

   1. Hemorrhage rate in CVA patients treated with t-PA is 6%; in those with MI treated with t-PA it is 2%.

   2. Risk of cerebral hemorrhage with Warfarin therapy for atrial fibrillation is 0.3%/year.

   3. Delay for 1week anticoagulation after intraparenchymal hemorrhage in patients with mechanical heart valves.

D. Evaluation—Consider evaluation of an intraparenchymal hemorrhage with an angiogram (to rule out vascular lesions) in patients <45 years and with no history of HTN.

E. Multiple intraparenchymal hemorrhages in young patients:

1. Causes—trauma, drug abuse (cocaine), vasculitis systemic lupus erythematosus, Wegener granulomatosis, polyarteritis nodosa, infection, or coagulopathy.

F. Multiple intraparenchymal hemorrhage in older patients:

1. Causes—amyloid angiopathy, embolic CVA, vasculitis, syphilis, or metastatic tumor.

III. Cerebral Aneurysms

A. Causes of spontaneous SAH:

1. Aneurysm 80% and vascular malformation 10%.

2. By far, the most common cause of SAH overall is trauma.

B. Conditions associated with aneurysms—HTN, atherosclerosis, fibromuscular dysplasia (FMD), polycystic kidney disease, Ehlers-Danlos syndrome, and Marfan syndrome.

C. Rupture rate—the rupture rate of unruptured aneurysms <10 mm is 0.05%/year and >10 mm is 1%/year. However, these numbers will vary significantly based on location, size, configuration, and patient factors, making it difficult to broadly state rupture risk across aneurysm types/sizes. 2015 AHA guidelines suggest 0.25%/year rupture risk for unruptured intracranial aneurysms.

1. Morbidity and mortality per rupture—5% in patients <30 years and 30% in patients >60 years.

2. The surgical mortality/morbidity for clipping is around 5%.

3. May consider screening first-degree relatives of patients with an aneurysm as there may be a familial predisposition.

D. Rerupture rate of ruptured aneurysms:

1. 4% in 24 hours, 20% in 2 weeks, 50% in 6 months, and then 3%/year.

2. Rerupture rate for a "dog ear" incompletely clipped aneurysm is 0.4%/year.

E. Outcome after SAH from ruptured aneurysm—40% mortality, 30% disabled, 30% normal, 10% die at home.

F. Hunt and Hess grade:

0—unruptured aneurysm.
1—asymptomatic or mild headache and slight nuchal rigidity.
1a—no acute meningeal/brain reaction, but with fixed neuro deficit.
2—cranial nerve palsy, moderate to severe headache, nuchal rigidity.
3—mild focal deficit, lethargy, or confusion.
4—stupor, moderate to severe hemiparesis, early decerebrate.
5—deep coma, decerebrate posturing, moribund appearance.
Add one grade for serious systemic disease (HTN, DM, etc.) or severe vasospasm on angiogram.

G. Evaluation:

1. History—sudden onset of worst headache in life.

2. CT, lumbar puncture (LP) (if CT negative).

3. Four-vessel angiogram:

   a. Gold standard, but CT angiogram and MRI/MRA are increasingly popular in the setting of aneurysmal SAH.

   b. Aneurysm location, neck/dome ratio as well as patient factors help in decision making regarding endovascular occlusion versus open surgical clip reconstruction.

H. Fisher grade (for vasospasm, per CT):

See quick reference guide for modified Fisher scale and associated risk of vasospasm.
1—no subarachnoid blood.
2—diffuse blood or vertical layers <1 mm thick.
3—localized clot and/or vertical layer ≥1 mm thick.
4—intracerebral or intraventricular clot with diffuse or no SAH Grades 1, 2, and 4 patients usually do not develop vasospasm. Grade 3 patients frequently develop vasospasm.

I. Treatments:

1. Nipride to keep SBP 120–130 mm Hg to prevent rehemorrhage prior to surgery.

2. Studies suggest that surgery should be performed the same day or the following morning.

3. Surgical clip reconstruction—lower rates of neck remnant at long term follow-up, but more invasive and higher perioperative risk.

4. Endovascular coiling:

   a. Continues to grow in popularity, with results nearing that of surgical clipping. Decision to clip or coil depends on multiple patient and aneurysm factors.

   b. Long-term results from multiple trials suggest that endovascular occlusion is better tolerated by patients but is associated with a significantly higher recurrence rate (14% over long-term follow-up).

   c. Advent of flow diverters and new endovascular techniques continue to improve outcomes of endovascular occlusion.

5. Muslin wrapping—not proven to be beneficial.

6. Trapping with or without bypass may be needed for unclippable aneurysms.

7. During surgery:

   a. Achieve brain relaxation with mannitol (1 g/kg bolus), Lasix, hyperventilation, and ventricular drainage (or lumbar drainage).

   b. Maintain normotension (but use mild HTN during temporary clipping) and mild hypothermia (to 32–34 °C with passive drift).

8. Temporary clipping time >5 minutes—consider Pentothal (4 mg/kg bolus and 2 mg/kg/h titrated to burst suppression if available), propofol (170 μg/kg/min), or etomidate, although best to avoid prolonged temporary clipping of parent vessel if possible.

9. Intraop angiography—useful when available to determine if clip placement is adequate.

J. Specific aneurysms.

1. Cavernous ICA aneurysm:

a. May not require surgical intervention because hemorrhage is not intra-dural and the tendency to rupture is low (ISUIA 5-year rupture rate is 0% for aneurysms from 1 to 13 mm, 3% for aneurysms from 13 to 24 mm, and 6.4% for >25 mm).

b. Signs/symptoms—may be caused by mass effect or carotid-cavernous fistula (CCF) formation after rupture.

c. Many are managed conservatively. If treatment is required, endovascular approach with flow diversion, coiling, or parent vessel sacrifice are performed. Due to morbidity, clipping has fallen out of favor.

2. Carotid cave segment ICA aneurysm:

a. Nearly 97% of carotid cave aneurysms are treated via endovascular coiling or flow diversion.

b. If open surgical clipping is indicated, proximal control via cervical carotid exposure should be considered. Anterior clinoidectomy will be required.

3. Ophthalmic artery aneurysm:

a. Endovascular coiling with or without flow diversion can be considered if aneurysm has favorable configuration.

b. If surgical clip reconstruction is required, consider proximal control of cervical carotid in the neck.

c. Aneurysm usually lies directly under the optic nerve and points up from the ICA. Visual symptoms are common.

d. May be safe to clip the parent vessel (ophthalmic artery) if necessary.

e. Anterior clinoid process may need to be drilled to the optic strut, the optic strut removed, and the falciform ligament cut.

f. If bilateral, both can be approached from one side.

g. May be suitable for flow-diverting stent placement via endovascular approach.

4. Posterior communicating (PCOM) artery aneurysm:

a. Signs/symptoms—presentation may be with a dilated pupil with spared ocular movements (**Fig. 9.7, Fig. 9.8,** and **Fig. 9.9**).

b. Exposure via pterional approach.

c. Aneurysm usually points laterally.

d. Sundt encircling clip should be available in case of tearing of the aneurysm from the ICA.

e. Avoid retracting the temporal lobe until near the end of the exposure because this may precipitate hemorrhage.

5. Anterior choroidal artery aneurysm—exposure via pterional approach.

6. ICA bifurcation aneurysm—exposure via pterional approach.

7. Middle cerebral artery aneurysm—exposure via pterional approach working from proximal to distal or by splitting the sylvian fissure and working distal to proximal.

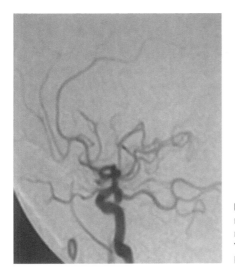

Fig. 9.7 Posterior communicating artery aneurysm; lateral angiogram. (Source: Citow JS. Neuropathology and Neuroradiology: A Review. New York, NY: Thieme Medical Publishers; 2001: 164, Fig. 209B.)

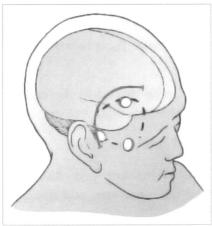

Fig. 9.8 Pterional craniotomy incision. (Source: Citow JS. Neurosurgery Oral Board Review. 1st ed. New York, NY: Thieme Medical Publishers; 2003: 102, Fig. 10.8.)

8. Anterior communicating artery aneurysm—exposure via pterional approach with resection of the gyrus rectus.

9. Distal anterior cerebral artery aneurysm—exposure via pterional approach if proximal at the orbitofrontal artery, but usually it requires an interhemispheric approach.

10. Posterior circulation aneurysms:

   a. Higher risk of rupture than anterior.

   b. For posterior cerebral artery (PCA) aneurysms, location compared to thalamic perforators can guide treatment decision-making. If proximal on PCA, perforators can make clip reconstruction difficult.

   c. Distal PCA aneurysms can be approached via subtemporal exposure with division of tentorium (**Fig. 9.10**).

   d. Other approaches include transsylvian and supracerebellar, infratentorial.

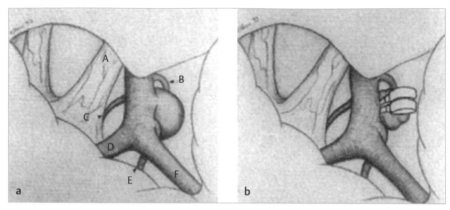

Fig. 9.9 (a, b) Posterior communicating (PCom) artery aneurysm exposure. A, optic nerve; B, PCom; C, superior hypophyseal artery; D, anterior cerebral artery; E, anterior choroidal artery; F, middle cerebral artery. (Source: Citow JS. Comprehensive Neurosurgical Board Review. New York, NY: Thieme Medical Publishers; 2000: 436, Fig. 5.1.)

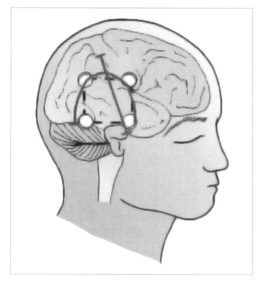

Fig. 9.10 Subtemporal craniotomy incision. (Source: Citow JS. Neurosurgery Oral Board Review. 1st ed. New York, NY: Thieme Medical Publishers; 2003: 104, Fig. 10.10.)

    e. PCA territory has rich collateral supply and is relatively resistant to infarction, therefore parent vessel occlusion is possible with large and/or difficult aneurysms.

    f. Endovascular occlusion via coils or flow diversion can be utilized.

11. Basilar artery apex aneurysm:

    a. Often coil first strategy—with rupture, may consider immediate but incomplete coil embolization to protect the aneurysm dome. After stabilization and recovery, the neck remnant can be treated with stent-assisted coiling or neck reconstruction devices.

    b. Surgical clip reconstruction has demonstrated high rates of occlusion, but also high morbidity.

    c. 6-year BRAT results suggested that for posterior circulation aneurysms, coiling showed sustained benefit over surgical clipping, but higher retreatment rates (not due to rehemorrhage).

    d. Surgical approaches included subtemporal (Drake), transsylvian (Yasargil) and pretemporal, transcavernous (Dolenc).

    e. Choice of surgical approach depends on configuration of aneurysm dome and association with thalamic perforators.

12. Midbasilar artery (AICA) aneurysms:

    a. Challenging aneurysms with high morbidity and mortality. Close association with basilar perforators make treatment difficult.

    b. Clip reconstruction often requires transpetrous, translabyrinthine or transcochlear approaches.

    c. If supratentorial approach is utilized, drilling of the posterior clinoid process will almost certainly be necessary.

    d. Endovascular approaches often utilized. Reports exist of flow diversion with or without concomitant coils leading to occlusion with continued patency of perforators, although morbidity and mortality remain high (10–15%).

13. Vertebrobasilar junction aneurysms:

    a. Exposure via a presigmoid approach with posterior petrosectomy.

    b. This approach exposes lesions >17 mm below the posterior clinoid process (middle and lower clivus).

14. Posterior inferior cerebellar artery (PICA) aneurysms:

    a. Unruptured PICA aneurysms can often be surgically clipped with excellent results. Ruptured PICA aneurysms have higher rates of surgical morbidity.

    b. Endovascular approaches including coiling, flow diversion, balloon-assisted remodeling can be utilized.

    c. Occasionally proximal occlusion with surgical bypass can be considered (PICA-PICA, OA-PICA bypass). PICA infarction causes significant neurological sequelae and treatment should focus on preservation of flow or bypass in order to avoid a PICA stroke.

15. Giant aneurysms (>2.5 cm):

    a. Often cause mass effect due to sheer size. Most require treatment due to aggressive natural history.

    b. Evaluation may include balloon occlusion tests for circle of Willis patency to assist in treatment decision-making (if trapping or hunterian ligation is considered).

    c. Endovascular occlusion limits the ability to address any mass effect that may be present. Coil occlusion can temporarily increase symptoms of mass effect and dexamethasone can be considered in select patients to decrease symptoms of mass effect.

16. Traumatic aneurysms:

    a. Cause—usually due to penetrating trauma involving the interhemispheric or sylvian fissure.

    b. Treatment—open trapping or balloon occlusion at the skull base.

17. Mycotic aneurysms:

    a. Cause—most often due to streptococcus associated with bacterial endocarditis.

    b. Treatment—6 weeks of antibiotics: (1) If aneurysm still present, surgical clipping/trapping is needed; (2) Follow patient with angiograms at 1, 3, 6, and 12 months; (3) Avoid anticoagulation.

K. Complications.

  1. Vasospasm:

    a. Occurs from days 4 to 14 (peak at day 7) as blood breakdown products irritate vessels near SAH.

    b. Risk is assessed by Fisher grade.

    c. Evaluation—Transcranial Doppler (>200 indicates spasm), cerebral blood flow studies, and angiography.

    d. Prevention—nimodipine 60 mg sublingual every 4 hours (q4h): (1) Some studies suggest using intraventricular t-PA 1 mg/d until the blood is dissolved.

    e. Treatment—Triple-H therapy: hypervolemia (central venous pressure [CVP] 12 and wedge 20), HTN, and hemo-dilution (if hematocrit [HCT] <30%, O_2 delivery impaired): (1) Maintain blood pressure at lowest level where the deficit disappears; (2) Refractory cases may be treated with intra-arterial papaverine or angioplasty.

  2. HCP:

    a. Many surgeons insert a ventricular catheter at the time of surgical clipping to minimize brain retraction and to monitor ICP after surgery to determine if a shunt will be needed.

    b. If catheter must be inserted before surgery for massive HCP, it should be set to drain at 15 cm of water to prevent detamponading of the aneurysm.

    c. Patients with aneurysmal SAH may ultimately require a shunt due to communicating HCP.

  3. Hyponatremia—usually due to cerebral salt wasting (CSW) by atrial natriuretic factor (patients are hypovolemic) versus syndrome of inappropriate antidiuretic hormone (SIADH; normo- or hypervolemic).

    a. Treatment for CSW—fluid replacement with normal saline b. Treatment for SIADH—fluid restriction.

  4. Postop focal deficit—evaluate with angiography (to check for parent vessel occlusion) and CT (to search for clot) and then possibly surgery for clip adjustment.

L. Benign perimesencephalic hemorrhage—SAH in prepontine or perimesencephalic cisterns possibly due to rupture of a small vein.

  1. Evaluation—CT, angiogram, MRA:

    a. Consider repeat angiogram in 10 days if blood not at the perimesencephalic cistern or anterior brainstem.

    b. Also consider cervical spine MRI to rule out arteriovenous malformation (AVM).

  2. Seldom recurs (**Fig. 9.11**).

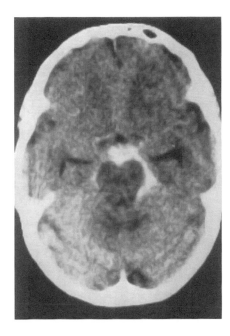

Fig. 9.11 Benign perimesencephalic hemorrhage. Computed tomography demonstrates typical subarachnoid hemorrhage extending into the left ambient cistern (angiogram was normal). (Source: Citow JS. Neuropathology and Neuroradiology: A Review. New York, NY: Thieme Medical Publishers; 2001: 171, Fig. 225.)

IV. Vascular Malformations

A. AVM hemorrhage:
1. Mortality—1%/year and 10%/bleed.
2. Morbidity—2.5%/year and 40%/bleed.
3. Initial hemorrhage rate—3%/year.
4. Rehemorrhage rate—as high as 7–10%/year, highest in initial 2 years then declines over subsequent 5 years.
5. ARUBA trial suggested that medical management (essentially just natural history) has better outcome than surgery; however, patients were only followed for 3 years and included all grades of AVM.
6. Natural history after 30 years of follow-up compared to general population suggest that treatment improves long-term survival (0.49: untreated vs. 0.87: obliterated).

B. Spetzler—Martin grading scale:
1. Size—<3 cm (1), 3–6 cm (2), >6 cm (3).
2. Eloquent location—noneloquent (0), eloquent (1).
3. Venous drainage—superficial (0), deep (1).
4. Total—1 and 2 (95% good outcome), 3 (84%), 4 (73%), 5 (69%).

C. Treatment.
1. Surgery:
   a. Identify and ligate feeding arteries with care to avoid sacrificing vessels just passing through.

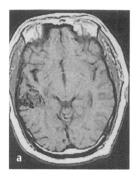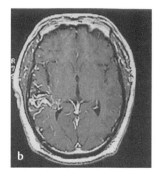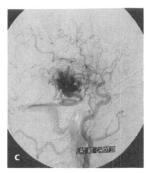

Fig. 9.12 Arteriovenous malformation (AVM). **(a)** Axial T1-weighted magnetic resonance images of noninfused and **(b)** infused AVM demonstrating serpentine vessels. **(c)** Angiogram demonstrating early-draining veins and AVM nidus. (Source: Citow JS. Neuropathology and Neuroradiology: A Review. New York, NY: Thieme Medical Publishers; 2001: 172, Fig. 228.)

    b. Avoid entering the malformation during dissection and ligate the draining veins as the last step.

    c. Perform surgery 1 week after embolization.

    d. To decrease the likelihood of normal perfusion pressure breakthrough, which can cause postop edema and hemorrhage, try 3 days of preop treatment with propranolol 20 mg orally daily (PO 4 times a day).

    e. Surgical risks: (1) Consider Spetzler–Martin grading scale; (2) Aneurysms (feeding, draining, or intranidal); (3) High- or low-flow AVMs; (4) Recent hemorrhage—may make the dissection plane more obvious; (5) 10% of AVMs have aneurysms; (6) Higher risk of hemorrhage with intranidal aneurysms and venous stenosis (**Fig. 9.12a–c**).

2. Radiation:

    a. Stereotactic radiosurgery—Proven useful for lesions <3 cm.

    b. Complete obliteration rate—80% (only 50% for larger lesions).

    c. 18-month delay before vessels become occluded and hemorrhage risk decreases.

    d. Risk of increased neurologic deficit from therapy is 3%.

    e. Incomplete obliteration—Radiosurgery can be repeated.

    f. Consider for deep lesions or around eloquent cortex.

    g. Radiosurgery best performed 30 days after embolization.

3. Endovascular embolization:

    a. Mostly useful as an adjuvant to other therapies, but some suggest that select Grade I and II AVMs can be obliterated via endovascular approaches alone.

    b. Risk of complications (i.e., CVA)—5%.

    c. Most useful for dural arteriovenous fistula (AVF), CCF, or vein of Galen malformation.

D. Angiographically occult AVM (cryptic)—due to either a small feeding vessel (beyond the resolution of angiography) or a vessel compressed by a hemorrhage.

E. Cavernous malformation:

1. Not visualized on angiogram.

2. Frequently associated with seizures.

3. 50% are multiple.

4. Hemorrhage—Population-based studies suggest 0.25–2.3% per patient year. Initial period of increased risk after hemorrhage (2% rehemorrhage per month initially) decreases until baseline again achieved approximately 2 years after initial bleed.

5. Treatment:

a. Surgery if symptomatic.

b. Radiation—cavernous malformations lack endothelium responsive to radiation. Response rates are controversial.

c. Brainstem cavernous malformations have higher risk of hemorrhage (4.6–6.5% annual). Surgical resection is on a case-by-case basis. Likely better results when cavernous malformation reaches pial surface of the brainstem.

d. Approaches transgressing the floor of the fourth ventricle often lead to significant postoperative deficits.

e. Potential surgical corridor between CN V and VII/VIII complex.

F. Dural AVM—actually an AVF because there is no nidus:

1. May arise from carotid or vertebral circulation (especially occipital artery) and drain into dural sinuses (usually the transverse–sigmoid junction).

2. Believed to be acquired by collateral revascularization after sinus thrombosis.

3. Signs/symptoms—pulsatile tinnitus, bruits, headaches.

4. Hemorrhage—risk is 4%/year.

5. Most behave benignly, but hemorrhage risk increases with cortical drainage or lesions in tentorial apex (as high as 80%) or anterior fossa (70%).

6. Treatment:

a. Initially—endovascular embolization of the fistulous connection via transarterial or transvenous (or combined) approaches.

b. Blockage of arterial feeders has relatively low success rate because there is frequently vessel recruitment: (1) If this fails, consider surgery to skeletonize the sinus (**Fig. 9.13a, b**).

G. CCF:

1. May either be post-traumatic or spontaneous.

2. Connection may be from ICA to cavernous sinus (high flow) or meningeal branches of ICA or ECA to cavernous sinus (low flow).

3. Signs/symptoms—Chemosis, proptosis, bruit, eye pain, visual loss, ophthalmoplegia.

4. 50% of low-flow lesions spontaneously thrombose.

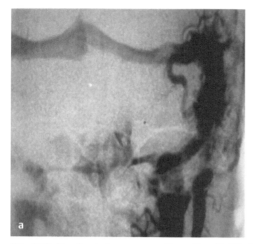
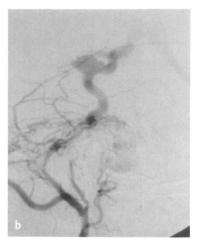

Fig. 9.13 Dural arteriovenous malformation (AVM). **(a)** Anteroposterior and **(b)** lateral external carotid artery (ECA) angiograms demonstrate supply from the ECA with early filing into the sigmoid sinus. (Source: Citow JS. Neuropathology and Neuroradiology: A Review. New York, NY: Thieme Medical Publishers; 2001: 175, Fig. 232.)

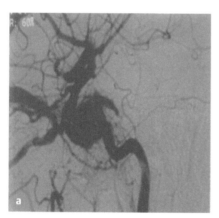
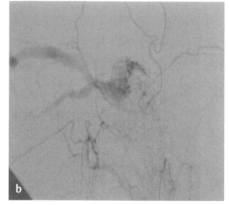

Fig. 9.14 Carotid-cavernous fistula. **(a)** Lateral angiograms of the common carotid artery demonstrating early filling of the cavernous sinus with dilated superior and inferior ophthalmic veins and **(b)** of the external carotid artery (ECA) demonstrating filling from the ECA. (Source: Citow JS. Comprehensive Neurosurgical Board Review. New York, NY: Thieme Medical Publishers; 2000: 441, Fig. 5.2.)

5. Low-flow lesions may be observed if vision is normal and intraocular pressure <25 (though frequent visual exams are needed).

6. Treatment:

    a. Initially—balloon occlusion: (1) Through ICA to fistula; (2) Two balloons to trap the ICA; (3) Or cavernous sinus occlusion via superior ophthalmic vein.

    b. Before trapping the ICA, test tolerance with a balloon occlusion under controlled hypotension to SBP 80 mm Hg and evaluate for symptoms or evaluate with SPECT scan to determine ischemia.

    c. If patient cannot tolerate trapping or other endovascular occlusion techniques, consider ECA–ICA bypass (**Fig. 9.14a, b**).

V. Neonatal Hemorrhage

A. Germinal matrix hemorrhage:

1. Located in subependymal region and may extend into ventricle.

2. Due to impaired autoregulation before 34 weeks and found in 40% of children born before 35 weeks.

3. Frequency increases with asphyxia due to HTN and hypercapnia.

4. Prevention may be accomplished with indomethacin to close patent ductus arteriosus and increase pO_2.

5. 75% of grade II hemorrhages have normal IQ.

6. Full-term children usually develop intraventricular hemorrhages.

B. Evaluation—ultrasound, occipital-frontal circumference (OFC; 35% develop hydrocephalus), CSF; protein <100 may resolve spontaneously.

C. Treatment:

1. Acetazolamide.

2. Daily removal of CSF with ventricular taps (<800 g).

3. Serial LPs (>800 g).

4. Ventricular access device (>1100 g).

5. Amount of CSF to remove is 10 mL/kg/tap or until the manometer lowers to 3 cm water (tap before it exceeds 10 cm water).

6. Consider VP shunt if >2500 g (earlier may cause necrotizing enterocolitis).

Helpful Hints

1. Focus on the basics for the most common aneurysms-anterior communicating artery (ACom), PCom, MCA, basilar.

2. Safe aneurysm surgery requires proximal control (even if you have to access the ICA in the neck).

Case 25

A 25-year-old medical student presents with new onset of frontal headache and was found to have sinusitis on head computed tomography (CT). Past medical history is significant for seasonal allergies. Examination was unremarkable (**Fig. 9.15**).

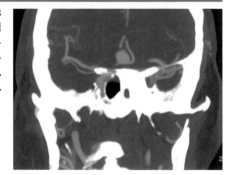

Fig. 9.15

Case 26

A 60-year-old farmer undergoes workup for persistent dizziness. Past medical history includes hypertension (HTN), diabetes mellitus (DM), post coronary artery bypass surgery (CABG) with stenting, and peripheral vascular disease. Examination found the patient neurologically intact (**Fig. 9.16**).

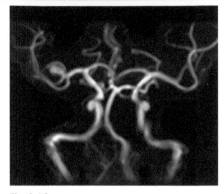

Fig. 9.16

Case 27

A 20-year-old man presents with progressively worsening headaches. Past medical history is negative. Examination found the patient neurologically intact (**Fig. 9.17a, b**).

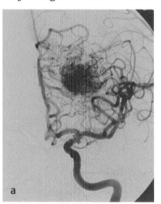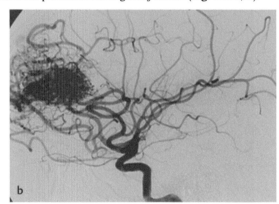

Fig. 9.17

10 Other Cranial Disorders

I. Hydrocephalus (HCP)

A. Evaluation:
1. Occipitofrontal circumference.
2. Computed tomography/magnetic resonance imaging (CT/MRI).
3. Pump shunt.
4. Shunt series—anteroposterior and lateral skull X-ray; chest and abdominal X-ray.
5. Shunt-o-gram:
   a. Radionucleotide.
   b. 1 mL technetium injection while occluding distal tube.
   c. Flush with 3 mL cerebrospinal fluid (CSF).
   d. Immediate abdominal image with gamma camera to rule out distal injection.
   e. Image cranium to see proximal patency.
   f. Image abdomen in 10 minutes.

B. Treatment:
1. Shunts—ventriculoperitoneal, pleural, or atrial:
   a. Frontal ventricular access: (1) 1 cm anterior to coronal suture and 3 cm lateral to midline; (2) Aim catheter toward external acoustic meatus and medial canthus (perpendicular to skull usually works) and insert 5–6 cm.
   b. Occipital ventricular access: (1) 7 cm above external occipital protuberance and 3 cm lateral to midline; (2) Aim catheter toward 3 cm above nasion and insert 10 cm.
   c. Ventriculoatrial placement: (1) Place occipital burr hole, sagittal incision over medial sternocleidomastoid; (2) Tunnel between the two incisions, cut down 3 cm proximal to the neck incision; (3) Pass atrial catheter, place ventricular catheter, perform internal jugular stick; (4) Connect tubing after flushing.
2. Third ventriculostomy—to treat aqueductal stenosis:
   a. Foramen of Monro—must be 4.5 mm to fit endoscope.
   b. Access—may be same location as for frontal ventricular catheter, but must check mid-sagittal view for trajectory.
   c. Penetrate floor of third ventricle anterior to mamillary bodies and posterior to infundibular and suprachiasmatic recesses.
   d. Consider Bugby—Bovie catheter, #3 Fogarty balloon catheter, grasper, and irrigation (**Fig. 10.1a–c**).
3. Lumboperitoneal shunt—best used for pseudotumor cerebri; shown to increase risk of Chiari malformation in children (70%).
4. Emergent access to ventricles in the office setting—push down optic globe and insert spinal needle through roof of orbit in midpupillary line.

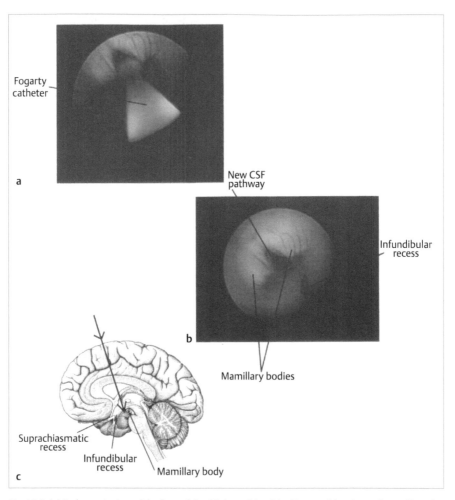

Fig. 10.1 **(a)** Endoscopic view of the floor of the third ventricle with a Fogarty #4 catheter directed into the floor of the ventricle. **(b)** View after third ventriculocisternostomy. **(c)** Ventriculostomy anatomy diagram. (Source: Citow JS. Neurosurgery Oral Board Review. 1st ed. New York, NY: Thieme Medical Publishers; 2003: 35, Fig. 5.1A–C.)

C. Complications:

1. Malfunction rate—17% in first year; 50% in 5 years, usually by infection or obstruction.

2. Craniosynostosis.

3. Subdural collections—treat by increasing the valve pressure, adding an antisiphon device, or shunting the subdural space to the peritoneum.

4. Visual loss—after shunt placement or with hydrocephalus it may be from posterior cerebral artery (PCA) occlusion from downward herniation, papilledema, or an enlarged third ventricle compressing the optic chiasm.

5. Slit ventricle syndrome—may be due to overdrainage, intermittent underdrainage, or constant underdrainage.

6. Positional headaches relieved by lying down—suggest overdrainage; treat with high valve pressure or antisiphon device.

7. Nonpositional headaches—suggest shunt obstruction.

8. Noncomplicant ventricles-ependyma scars and adheres to itself thus allowing increased pressure without a change in ventricular size.

9. Shunt unable to be tapped—replace using the same trajectory and consider using an endoscope or image-guided assistance.

10. Catheter adheres to choroid or ependyma—remove by inserting a stylet and coagulating with a Bovie.

D. Normal-pressure HCP:
   1. Signs/symptoms—apraxic, wide-based gait, urinary incontinence, dementia (impaired memory, usually not severe).
   2. Evaluation—CT/MRI and lumbar puncture (LP) (lumbar drain × 3 days at 10 cc/h and have physical therapy access for gait improvement).
   3. Treatment—best results for shunting obtained in patients presenting with ataxia:
      a. Urinary control improves first.
      b. 35% of patients develop subdural hematoma, so set value high and slowly titrate setting down.

II. Meningitis

A. Neonates (< 1 m)—group B *Streptococcus* and *Escherichia coli*.

B. Newborns (1–3 m)—strep pneumonia.

C. Children (3–7 years)—*Haemophilus influenza*.

D. Older children and adults (>7 years)—*Neisseria meningitidis, Listeria*.

E. Elderly—strep pneumonia.

F. Postop or wound infection—usually staph.

G. Chronic meningitis—usually tuberculosis, fungus, cysticercosis, tumor, or sarcoid.

III. Skull Osteomyelitis

A. Treatment—3 months of antibiotics; replace bone in 6 months.

IV. Brain Abscess

A. Causes—usually strep, fungus (immunocompromised), and gram-negative rods (infants).

B. Evaluation—complete blood count (CBC), erythrocyte sedimentation rate (ESR), C-reactive protein (CRP), MRI, Gram stain, culture (also for fungus and acid fast bacillus [AFB]).

C. Treatment:
   1. Antibiotics—6 weeks intravenous (IV) and 6 weeks orally (PO).

2. Surgery (to aspirate or excise)—in cases with abscess >3 cm, unknown organism, location near the ventricle (80% mortality with rupture into ventricle), increased intracranial pressure (ICP), or failed antibiotic therapy.

   a. Use anticonvulsants.

   b. Antibiotics may be stopped 1 week after capsule is excised.

   c. Follow-up CTs at 2, 4, and 6 weeks during antibiotic therapy.

V. Subdural Empyema

A. Causes—usually strep and related to recent surgery or adjacent infection.

B. Signs/symptoms—caused by venous thrombosis and infarction.

C. Treatment—urgent craniectomy or burr-hole drainage.

VI. Herpes Simplex Virus

A. Signs/symptoms—hemorrhagic inflammation of medial temporal lobes followed by rapid decline into coma.

B. Evaluation:

   1. MRI—edema.

   2. LP—increased lymphocytes and protein.

   3. Biopsy—if unsure of diagnosis; start IV acyclovir before biopsy.

   4. Polymerase chain reaction—usually returns too late to help.

C. Treatment—acyclovir.

VII. Acquired Immunodeficiency Syndrome (AIDS)—Focal Lesions Are due to Toxoplasma, Progressive Multifocal Leukoencephalopathy (PML), Lymphoma, and Cryptococcus. There May Also Be AIDS Encephalitis and Dementia

A. Toxoplasmosis:

   1. Evaluation—detected by a change in baseline titers.

   2. Treatment—pyrimethamine and sulfadiazine.

B. Progressive multifocal leukoencephalopathy (PML):

   1. Cause— John Cunningham virus (JCV).

   2. Signs/symptoms—presents with mental changes.

   3. Evaluation:

      a. MRI with nonenhancing increased T2 signal.

      b. Loss of myelin in the white matter.

      c. LP may be sent for polymerase chain reaction (PCR) for JCV.

   4. Treatment—none.

C. Lymphoma:
1. Evaluation—enhances on MRI and is usually near the third ventricle; LP for PCR for Epstein–Barr virus.
2. Treatment—radiation and steroids; survival is 3 months.

D. Brain masses:
1. Treatment—antitoxoplasma medications for 2 weeks and biopsy if there is no decrease in size.

VIII. Creutzfeldt–Jakob Disease

A. Cause—prion or slow virus.

B. Signs/symptoms—dementia, ataxia, visual loss, and myoclonus.

C. Evaluation:
1. MRI—hyperintense on T2 in basal ganglia.
2. LP—rule out syphilis, may see increased protein.
3. Electroencephalography (EEG)—periodic spikes.
4. Biopsy—spongiform encephalitis with decreased cells and no inflammation, stain for protease-resistant protein. Sterilize biopsy equipment with steam and sodium hydroxide.

D. Treatment—none; death usually within 1 year.

IX. Lyme Disease

A. Cause—Borrelia burgdorferi.

B. Signs/symptoms—many symptoms, including bilateral VIIth nerve dysfunction. Neurologic symptoms are usually preceded by erythema chronicum migrans rash.

C. Evaluation—serum antibody titer.

D. Treatment—antibiotics.

X. Cysticercosis

A. Evaluation—serum or CSF enzyme-linked immunosorbent assay (ELISA) study and CT/MRI.

B. Treatment:
1. Praziquantel or albendazole for 30 days.
2. Ocular or spinal cysts—avoid antibiotics.
3. Large or intraventricular lesions—consider surgical resection.
4. Ventricular shunting—often required (**Fig. 10.2a, b**).

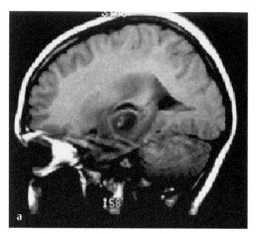
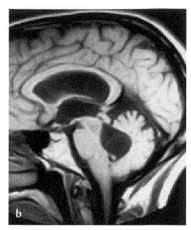

Fig. 10.2 Cysticercosis. **(a)** Noninfused sagittal T1-weighted magnetic resonance images demonstrate cystic lesions with a scolex in the left temporal lobe and **(b)** in the fourth ventricle. (Source: Citow JS. Neuropathology and Neuroradiology: A Review. New York, NY: Thieme Medical Publishers; 2001: 30, Fig. 32.)

Helpful Hints

1. In HCP, some ventricles are noncompliant (especially in slit ventricle syndrome and long-term shunting).
2. Pick one shunt valve system and understand it well.
3. If history is consistent for intracranial infection, rule it out emergently with LP. Even if scans look unremarkable, have low suspicion for subdural empyema and be ready to culture and washout quickly.

Case 28

A 75-year-old man presents with new-onset gait difficulty and urinary incontinence. Past medical history is significant for lung cancer post chemotherapy and radiation therapy, high blood pressure, type 2 diabetes, and degenerative spine disease. Examination revealed difficulty with higher cognitive function and ataxia (**Fig. 10.3**).

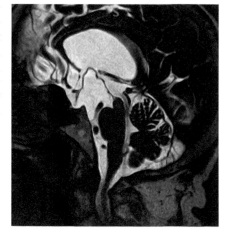

Fig. 10.3

Case 29

A 45-year-old woman presents with progressive right headache, hearing loss, and tinnitus for 1 year. Past medical history is significant for numerous childhood episodes of right otitis externa. An audiogram showed 20% high-frequency sensorineural healing loss (SNHL) and 50% speech discrimination (**Fig. 10.4**).

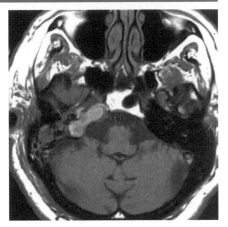

Fig. 10.4

Case 30

A 38-year-old woman presents with progressive right-sided headache and enlarging mass. Past medical history is significant for bilateral mastectomy for breast cancer, chronic back pain, and minor head trauma. Examination was unremarkable except for a soft, tender to palpation, nodule on the right parietal boss (**Fig. 10.5**).

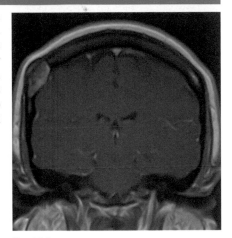

Fig. 10.5

Part 3

Miscellaneous Topics

11 Congenital and Pediatric Lesions

I. Arachnoid Cyst—Frequently Associated with Subdural Hematomas

A. Treatment—only if symptomatic:
   1. Craniotomy and fenestration into medial cerebrospinal fluid (CSF) cisterns (consider a shunt if this fails).
   2. Consider endoscopic third ventriculostomy and fenestration for a suprasellar cyst.

II. Neurenteric Cyst—Lined by Gastrointestinal or Respiratory Endothelium and Usually Occurs in the Cervical or Thoracic Spine

A. Treatment—Resection is required.

III. Encephalocele—Most Children Do Not Develop Normally

A. Cranial vault (occipital)—most common variety in the Western hemisphere.
   1. Treatment—excision and closing of dura (**Fig. 11.1a, b**).
B. Sincipital—nasofrontal, nasoethmoidal, and naso-orbital.
C. Basal—transethmoidal, transsphenoidal, sphenoethmoidal, and spheno-orbital. There is no visible mass.
   1. Treatment—combination nasal and subfrontal closure.

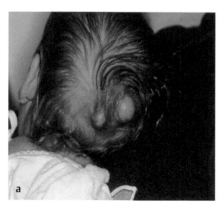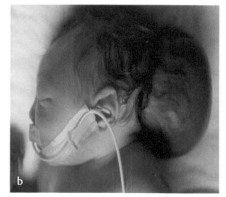

Fig. 11.1 Encephaloceles. (a) Two small occipital encephaloceles. (b) Large occipital encephalocele. (Source: Citow JS. Neuropathology and Neuroradiology: A Review. New York, NY: Thieme Medical Publishers; 2001: 7, Fig. 4.)

IV. Chiari Malformation

A. Type 1—cerebellar tonsil herniation 5 mm below foramen magnum (varies with age); presentation is usually around 40 years.

   1. Signs/symptoms—headaches, paresthesias, or syringomyelia.

   2. Treatment—suboccipital craniectomy and C1 laminectomy with duraplasty (**Fig. 11.2**).

B. Type 2—always present at birth if the patient has a myelomeningocele (MM).

   1. Signs/symptoms—due to brainstem and cranial nerve (CN) dysfunction (dysphagia, stridor, apnea, and nystagmus).

   2. Evaluation—magnetic resonance imaging (MRI) shows vermis herniation with tectal beaking, elongated medulla, hydrocephalus (HCP), and bony abnormalities.

   3. Treatment—initially with a ventriculoperitoneal (VP) shunt; 20% will eventually require a suboccipital decompression (**Fig. 11.3**).

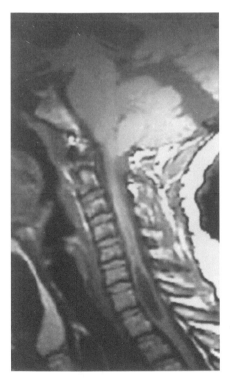

Fig. 11.2 Chiari 1 malformation. Sagittal T1-weighted magnetic resonance image demonstrates peg-like tonsils extending below foramen magnum with an associated syrinx. (Source: Citow JS. Neuropathology and Neuroradiology: A Review. New York, NY: Thieme Medical Publishers; 2001: 13,Fig. 11.)

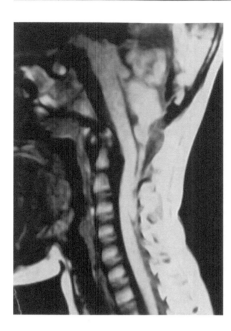

Fig. 11.3 Chiari 2 (Arnold-Chiari) malformation. Sagittal T1-weighted magnetic resonance image with tectal beaking, low-lying torcula, and vermian descent. (Source: Citow JS. Neuropathology and Neuroradiology: A Review. New York, NY: Thieme Medical Publishers; 2001: 13, Fig. 12.)

V. Dandy–Walker Malformation

A. Cause—atresia of the foramen of Magendie and Luschka with agenesis of the vermis and a posterior fossa cyst communicating with a large fourth ventricle.

B. Signs/symptoms—associated HCP (90%) as well as cardiac and multiple other abnormalities; 50% of patients have normal IQs.

C. Treatment—shunting the cysst (**Fig. 11.4a–c**).

VI. Aqueductal Stenosis

A. Treatment—VP shunt or third ventriculostomy.

VII. Myelomeningocele

A. Facts—80% have HCP, most have Chiari 2 malformation, 80% have normal IQ, and 10% have normal urinary continence (**Fig. 11.5a, b**).

B. Prevention:
   1. Folic acid supplements during the first trimester.
   2. Avoid valproic acid, saunas, and hot tubs in the first trimester.

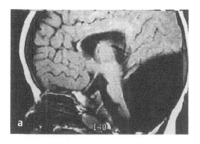

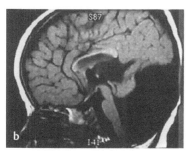

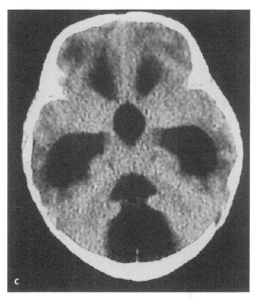

Fig. 11.4 Dandy–Walker malformation. **(a, b)** Sagittal T1-weighted magnetic resonance images and **(c)** axial computed tomography scan demonstrate vermian agenesis and connection of fourth ventricle to posterior fossa cyst. (Source: Citow JS. Neuropathology and Neuroradiology: A Review. New York, NY: Thieme Medical Publishers; 2001: 15, Fig. 15.)

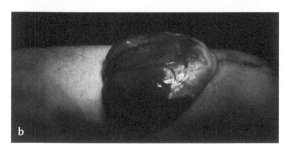

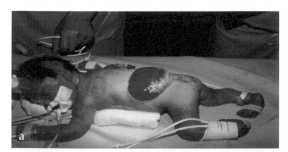

Fig. 11.5 Myelomeningocele. **(a)** Neuralplacode noted on center of dorsal aspect. **(b)** Close-up image. (Source: Citow JS. Neuropathology and Neuroradiology: A Review. New York, NY: Thieme Medical Publishers; 2001: 7, Fig. 3.)

C. Evaluation:

1. 3% risk after a prior abnormal birth.

2. Maternal serum α-fetal protein (AFP), ultrasound, and amniocentesis for AFP.

3. Evaluate the child for spontaneous leg movement, scoliosis, hip and knee abnormalities (X-rays).

4. Genitourinary evaluation—15% have abnormalities such as one kidney or a horseshoe kidney; perform a straight catheterization.

5. Cardiac echo—15% have abnormalities such as atrial or ventricular septal defects.

6. Head ultrasound—most have HCP.

D. Treatment—85% survival:

1. Cover the lesion with Telfa and sponges soaked with normal saline (consider connecting intravenous [IV] tubing running at 5 mL/h to the gauze).

2. Maintain prone Trendelenburg position.

3. If ruptured, use nafcillin and gentamicin until 6 hours after closure.

4. If unruptured don't use antibiotics.

5. Closure within 24 hours.

6. If no HCP by ultrasound and occipital-frontal circumference (OFC) measurements, repair the MM and shunt in 3 days if needed.

7. If there is HCP, operate in the prone position with the head turned.

   a. Shunt the ventricles to the peritoneum via the flank.

   b. Begin MM repair by isolating the placode and removing the tissue between the placode and skin.

   c. Suture the cord into a cylinder.

   d. Close the dura, fascia, and skin.

   e. Complications include shunt malfunction, syrinx, and tethered cord.

   f. There is no proof that birth by C-section alters outcome.

VIII. Lipomyelomeningocele—Skin-Covered Lesion

A. Signs/symptoms—most have cutaneous stigmata of spina bifida such as a hair patch, dimple, or red mark.

B. Evaluation—MRI.

C. Treatment:

1. Untether the cord and debulk the fat.

2. Use intraop somatosensory evoked potential (SSEP) and nerve root stimulation.

3. Surgical outcome—Unchanged (75%), improved (20%), worse (5%).

IX. Dermal Sinus Tract

A. Signs/symptoms:

1. Cutaneous indication is a dimple with hair.

2. Often meningitis.

B. Evaluation—MRI and X-ray (to find spina bifida).

C. Treatment—repair with resection of tract and dural closure.

X. Tethered Cord—Low-Lying Conus Below L2 with Thickened Filum or Mass; Frequently Associated with Myelomeningocele (MM); Cutaneous Manifestations in 50%

A. Signs/symptoms—gait dysfunction (90%), sensory loss (70%), bladder dysfunction (40%), scoliosis, pain.

B. Evaluation—cystometrogram, X-ray (spina bifida is seen in 98%), MRI.

C. Treatment—stimulate the filum before sectioning.

1. Filum terminale is whiter than the nerve roots and has ligamentous fibers with a squiggly vessel on the surface.

2. Intraop anal sphincter electromyogram (EMG).

XI. Diastematomyelia—Spinal Cord Split Malformation (SCM)

A. SCM type I—Two hemicords in separate dural sleeves and separated by osseous septum that has to be removed to untether the cord.

B. SCM type II—Single dural sac with a fibrous band splitting the tethered cord.

XII. Klippel–Feil Syndrome—Congenital Fusion of At Least Two Cervical Vertebrae; Associated with Multiple Systemic Anomalies (One Kidney, Cardiac Irregularities, etc.)

A. Evaluation—electrocardiogram (ECG), chest X-ray (CXR), and renal ultrasound.

B. Treatment:

1. Fuse from an anterior and posterior approach if unstable after trauma.

XIII. Craniosynostosis

A. Fontanelles—anterior closes at 18 months; posterior closes at 3 months.

B. Skull diploë—forms at 4 years in unilaminar bone.

C. Evaluation:

1. Palpate the prominent suture.

2. X-ray may fail to demonstrate a normal lucent suture.

3. 3-D computed tomography (CT) reconstruction demonstrates the abnormal shape.

D. Sagittal synostosis—most common variety; more often seen in males.

1. Signs/symptoms—dolichocephalic or scaphocephalic shape with decreased biparietal distance.

2. Treatment:

   a. Prone position with a strip craniectomy from coronal suture to lambdoid suture 3 cm wide at 3 to 6 months.

   b. Skull remodeling—required after 1 year to make the skull shorter and wider.

   c. Be careful about blood loss and hypothermia.

E. Coronal synostosis—more common in females:

   1. Unilateral—plagiocephaly.

      a. Normal side bulges; abnormal side has a harlequin eye due to elevated supraorbital margin (**Fig. 11.6**).

   2. Bilateral—brachycephaly with proptosis and maxillary hypoplasia.

   3. Crouzon syndrome—bilateral synostosis with midface hypoplasia of sphenoid, orbital, and facial bones.

   4. Apert disease—as with Crouzon syndrome syndactyly, HCP, low IQ.

   5. Treatment—Strip craniectomy or frontal craniotomy with lateral canthal advancement at 3 to 6 months with absorbable plates.

F. Metopic synostosis—trigonocephaly.

G. Lambdoid synostosis—more common in males and on the right side:

   1. Evaluation—Rule out positional plagiocephaly due to the child lying on one side too much.

   2. Treatment—Molding helmet (if positional) or strip craniectomy at 6 to 18 months.

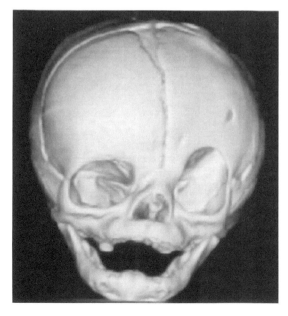

Fig. 11.6 Unilateral coronal synostosis (plagiocephaly). Computed tomography reconstruction with harlequin eye on the left. (Source: Citow JS. Neuropathology and Neuroradiology: A Review. New York, NY: Thieme Medical Publishers; 2001: 17, Fig. 17.)

XIV. Shunt Infection—50% Occur by 2 Weeks

A. Causes—most common organisms are *Staphylococcus epidermidis* and *S. aureus* and gram-negative rods.

B. Signs/symptoms—fever, leukocytosis, and headache.

C. Treatment—externalization of shunt, vancomycin (until cultures back), and shunt replacement after 10 days of antibiotics when CSF is sterile.

XV. Child Abuse (Nonaccidental Trauma)

A. Search for retinal hemorrhages, long bone fractures, subdural hematomas (especially interhemispheric), and nonparietal skull fractures.

Helpful Hints

1. No matter what the problem is, if there is a shunt, rule out shunt failure first.

2. Posterior fossa cysts—arachnoid cyst, Dandy–Walker, mega cistern magna, pilocystic astrocytoma.

3. No matter what the spinal problem is, look at conus level for tethering.

4. Noncompliant ventricles are common in pediatric HCP, especially after multiple procedures.

5. Look at entire neuraxis in congenital disorders.

Case 31

This baby girl was born with macrocephaly. Past medical history is significant for prematurity and lack of maternal prenatal care. Examination revealed a quiet girl who coos appropriately, opens eyes spontaneously, moves all extremities well (MAEW), with a soft anterior fontanelle, large, soft, skin-covered occipital protrusion (**Fig. 11.7**).

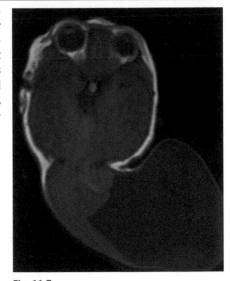

Fig. 11.7

Case 32

A 10-year-old boy presents with progressive headaches, especially during a Valsalva. Past medical history is significant for multiple episodes of pneumonia during childhood. Examination revealed left upper extremity hypertrophy, downbeat nystagmus, uvula deviation, and diminished gag reflex (**Fig. 11.8**).

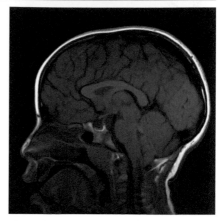

Fig. 11.8

Case 33

A 1-year-old boy presents with an abnormally shaped head. Past medical history is significant for full-term birth and normal development milestones. Examination revealed flattened left frontotemporal region (**Fig. 11.9**).

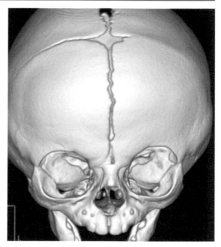

Fig. 11.9

12 Functional and Pain Neurosurgery

I. Parkinsonism

A. Treatment:
1. Thalamotomy—ventral intermediate (VIM) thalamic nucleus to treat tremor.
2. Pallidotomy—globus pallidus interna (GPi) lesion to treat rigidity or bradykinesia. Also useful for levodopa-induced dyskinesias and on–off problems.
3. Stimulation—of thalamus, globus pallidus, or subthalamic nucleus.
4. Surgery—avoid if the patient has dementia, a coagulation disorder, contralateral hemianopsia, or secondary parkinsonism.
5. Remember to create a lesion contralateral to the symptomatic side.
   a. 80% of patients are improved.
   b. Microelectrode recording helps determine the location of the radiofrequency (RF) lesion.
6. Complications—visual field cut, hemiparesis, blood clot, and dysarthria (especially if bilateral).

II. Spasticity

A. Treatment.
1. Medical:
   a. Prolonged stretching to decrease contractures.
   b. Diazepam.
   c. Baclofen.
   d. Dantrolene.
2. Surgical:
   a. Intrathecal (IT) baclofen.
   b. Neurectomy or blocks.
   c. RF rhizotomy or open selective dorsal rhizotomies—electromyogram (EMG) intraop.
   d. Midline thoracic myelotomy with T11–L1 laminectomy—cut the T12–S1 cord to spare the S2–4 bladder reflex 4 mm deep.

III. Torticollis

A. Cause—dystonia by spasm of the sternocleidomastoid muscle.
B. Evaluation—rule out C1–2 rotatory subluxation, 11th nerve compression, infection, or tumor.
C. Treatment—physical therapy, transcutaneous electrical nerve stimulation (TENS) unit, spinal cord stimulator, Botox injection, section spinal accessory nerve (XI), or microvascular decompression of XI from the vertebral artery.

IV. Hemifacial Spasm

A.   Cause—compression of VII by the anterior inferior cerebellar artery (AICA) at the root entry zone (REZ).

1.   Compression of VIII causes tinnitus.

2.   Brainstem glioma or multiple sclerosis can cause facial myokymia (continuous facial spasm).

3.   Blepharospasm is bilateral eyelid spasms.

B.   Treatment—Botox injections or a microvascular decompression.

V. Hyperhidrosis—Increased Sweating (Especially in the Palms)

A.   Evaluation—rule out hyperthyroidism, diabetes, pheochromocytoma, Parkinson disease, and menopause.

B.   Treatment—Antiperspirants, anticholinesterases, or sympathectomy.

VI. Sympathectomy—Used to Treat Hyperhidrosis, Raynaud Syndrome, Angina, or Reflex Sympathetic Dystrophy (RSD)

A.   For upper extremity symptoms—remove the sympathetic ganglia at T2 (to avoid Horner syndrome) via an open midline T3 costotransversectomy or thoracoscopic approach.

VII. Chronic Pain

A.   Conservative management options—physical therapy, oral medications (nonsteroidal anti-inflammatory drugs [NSAIDs], steroids, Amitriptyline, Gabapentin, narcotics), and epidural steroid injections.

B.   Deep brain stimulation (DBS)—placed in the periaqueductal or periventricular gray.

C.   Spinal cord stimulator—for RSD, failed back syndrome, arachnoiditis, and refractory angina.

1.   Place the electrodes percutaneously or open and connect to an internal pulse generator.

D.   Intrathecal pumps:

1.   May use subcutaneous (SQ) reservoir or pump (if >3-month survival).

2.   Test with 2 mg cerebrospinal fluid (CSF) injection.

a.   Watch for decreased breathing <10/min and have Naloxone 0.4 mg ready (1 A [ampule]): (1) IT dose—1/10 the epidural dose, 1/100 the intravenous (IV) dose, and 1/300 the oral dose; (2) Bolus 0.4 mg postoperative.

3.   Most (90%) patients have significantly improved pain control.

E. Cordotomy—useful for cancer pain involving one limb or one side of the body.

  1. Performed on the side contralateral to the pain because the crossed lateral spinothalamic tract is severed.

  2. C1–2 percutaneous method usually used with fluoroscopic guidance.

  3. Needle should be anterior to the dentate ligament.

  4. Open procedure may be done in the thoracic spine.

  5. Complications—ipsilateral weakness, urinary incontinence, and Ondine curse (failure of involuntary respiration with bilateral cervical procedures).

F. Midline myelotomy—for bilateral pain below the thoracic region:

  1. After laminectomy, the midline sulcus is penetrated with a Penfield #4 down to the central canal extending from T10 to two levels above the conus (to avoid bladder dysfunction).

G. Hypophysectomy—for severe bone pain related to breast or prostate cancer:

  1. May be performed with radiosurgery, open resection, or insertion of alcohol.

H. Cingulotomy—for diffuse pain; a last resort.

I. Dorsal root entry zone (DREZ) lesion—for deafferentation pain due to nerve root avulsion.

VIII. Reflex Sympathetic Dystrophy (Complex Regional Pain Syndrome, Causalgia)

A. Cause—unknown.

B. Signs/symptoms:

  1. Burning pain—usually in the median, ulnar, and sciatic nerves.

  2. Vasomotor changes—pink or cold and with increased or decreased sweating.

  3. Trophic changes—dry and thin skin, stiff joints, possibly due to immobility.

C. Evaluation—clinical and with sympathetic blocks; nerve conduction velocity (NCV) may be useful to rule out nerve compression.

D. Treatment:

  1. Physical therapy—most useful option, with muscle stretching.

  2. Amitriptyline, Gabapentin, phentolamine IV.

  3. Stellate ganglion block—better at T2 to avoid Horner syndrome.

  4. Lumbar sympathetic blocks.

  5. Surgical sympathectomy.

  6. Spinal cord stimulator.

Helpful Hints

1. Body pain treatments—cordotomy if <3-month survival, unilateral pain; IT morphine pump or spinal cord stimulation (SCS) if >3-month survival, bilateral pain; SCS for radiculopathy, postherpetic pain, complex regional pain syndrome (CRPS); DREZ for brachial plexus avulsion pain.

2. Face pain treatments—microvascular decompression (MVD) or percutaneous treatments for tic (thermocoagulation, balloon compression, glycerol).

3. Basic DBS targets:
   a. VIM—lateral (X):11.5 mm + half third ventricle width (14.5–15.5 mm off midline) front back; (Y): 4–6 mm in front of posterior commissure (PC; in front of the sensory nucleus), officially 2/12–3/12 of anterior commissure–posterior commissure (AC–PC) distance in front of PC depth; (Z): on the AC-PC line (which is the bottom of thalamus) usually for tremor, either essential, cerebellar or Parkinson disease (PD; when tremor is dominant).
   b. Subthalamic nucleus (STN)—lateral (X) 10.5–11.5 off midline; (Y) 3 mm behind midpoint of AC–PC; (Z) 4 mm deep to AC–PC for akinetic-rigid and mild tremor PD patients (dyskinesias, etc.).
   c. GPi—lateral (X) 19–21 off midline (just above optic tract as courses lateral to midbrain); (Y) 2–3 mm anterior to midpoint AC-PC; (Z) 4–6 mm deep to AC-PC (best target is 2 mm above optic tract at 20 mm off midline), equally good for PD (from recent randomized trial) as STN, commonly used for dystonia.

4. Hemifacial spasm (HFS)—rule out seizure.

Case 34

A 38-year-old woman presents with episodes of lancinating pain in her left cheek and jaw when brushing her teeth. Past medical history is significant for two episodes of visual alterations 1 year earlier, a family history of migraines, and post-traumatic stress disorder. Examination was unremarkable (**Fig. 12.1**).

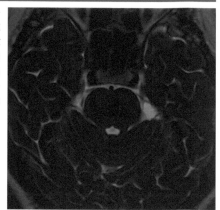

Fig. 12.1

Case 35

A 65-year-old man presents with troubling jerky, dance-like movements in the left arm that have worsened over the past 3 years. Past medical history is significant for a 10-year history of Parkinson disease treated with Levodopa, transient ischemic attacks (TIAs), coronary artery disease (CAD), and carotid stenosis. Examination revealed normal mental status, diffuse bradykinesia, rigidity, pill-rolling tremors, and shuffling gait (**Fig. 12.2**).

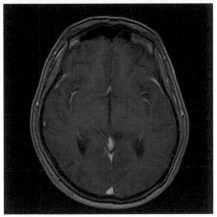

Fig. 12.2

Case 36

A wheelchair-bound, 30-year-old woman presents with worsening difficulty using her hands and sitting in the wheelchair due to pain and scissoring of legs. Past medical history is significant for spinal cord injury (SCI) 15 years earlier and multiple antispasmodic medications. Examination revealed marked rigidity throughout body (Ashworth score ⅘), 3+ deep tension reflexes (DTRs) throughout, Hoffman syndrome, and clonus.

13 Peripheral Nerves

I. Anatomy

A. Upper extremity.

B. Brachial plexus (**Fig. 13.1**).

C. Dorsal scapular nerve—rhomboids and levator scapulae.

D. Long thoracic nerve—serratus anterior.

E. Suprascapular nerve—supra- and infraspinatus.

F. Thoracodorsal nerve—latissimus dorsi.

G. Phrenic nerve (C3–5)—diaphragm.

H. Axillary nerve—deltoid and teres minor.

I. Musculocutaneous nerve—coracobrachialis, biceps, and brachialis.

J. Radial nerve—triceps, brachioradialis, and extensor carpi radialis longus and brevis:

   1. Posterior interosseous nerve—supplies the supinator, extensor carpi ulnaris, extensor digitorum, extensor digiti minimi, extensor pollicis longus and brevis, extensor indicis, and abductor pollicis longus (not median nerve).

K. Median nerve—pronator teres, flexor carpi radialis, palmaris longus, flexor digitorum superficialis (flexes proximal interphalangeal joints of all fingers):

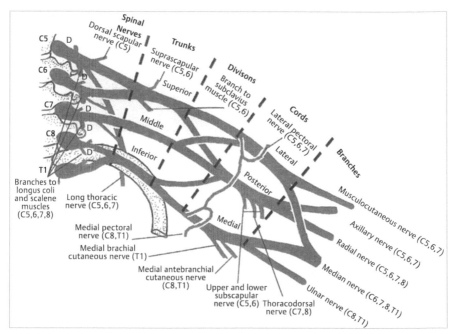

Fig. 13.1 Brachial plexus anatomy. (Source: Ciow JS. Comprehensive Neurosurgical Board Review. New York, NY: Thieme Medical Publishers; 2000: 80, Fig. 1.44.)

1. Anterior interosseous nerve—supplies the flexor digitorum profundus (flexes distal interphalangeal joints to index and/or middle fingers), flexor pollicis longus, and pronator quadratus.

2. Recurrent (thenar) branch—LOAF muscles—lumbricals 1 and 2, opponens pollicis, abductor pollicis brevis, flexor pollicis brevis (half).

L. Ulnar nerve—flexor carpi ulnaris, flexor digitorum profundus 3 and 4:

1. Divides into two branches in Guyon's canal at wrist.

2. Deep branch—abductor digiti minimi, opponens digiti minimi, flexor digiti minimi, lumbricals 3 and 4, dorsal and palmar interosseous, flexor pollicis brevis (also by the median nerve), and adductor pollicis.

3. Superficial branch—sensation to ulnar 1½ digits.

M. Note—dorsal cutaneous branch arises 6 cm above wrist and supplies dorsoulnar aspect of hand.

N. Lower extremity:

1. Superior gluteal nerve (L4–S1)—gluteus medius and minimus and tensor fasciae latae.

2. Inferior gluteal nerve (L5–S2)—gluteus maximus.

3. Femoral nerve (L2–4)—iliacus, psoas, quadriceps femoris (rectus femoris and vastus lateralis, intermedius, and medialis), and sartorius. There is also sensory innervation to the knee (anterior femoral cutaneous nerve) and medial leg to foot (saphenous nerve).

4. Obturator nerve (L2–4)—adductor brevis, adductor longus, adductor magnus (also by sciatic nerve), gracilis, and obturator externus.

5. Sciatic nerve (L4–S3)—exits through the greater sciatic foramen to innervate the semimembranosus, semitendinosus, biceps femoris (long head, tibial division of sciatic nerve; short head, peroneal division of sciatic nerve), and adductor magnus (also by the obturator nerve).

6. Tibial nerve—gastrocnemius, soleus, tibialis posterior, flexor hallucis longus, and flexor digitorum longus:

   a. Medial plantar nerve—abductor hallucis, flexor digitorum brevis, and flexor hallucis brevis.

   b. Lateral plantar nerve—abductor digiti minimi, flexor digiti minimi, adductor hallucis, and interosseus muscles.

7. Common peroneal nerve:

   a. Superficial peroneal nerve—peroneus longus and brevis.

   b. Deep peroneal nerve—tibialis anterior, extensor digitorum longus, extensor hallucis longus, peroneus tertius, and extensor digitorum brevis.

8. Sensory branches—posterior femoral cutaneous nerve (posterior thigh from lumbosacral plexus), tibial nerve (most of lower leg and sole of foot), and sural nerve (a small patch of dorsolateral foot); peroneal nerve (dorsal foot [superficial peroneal nerve] and first web space [deep peroneal]).

9. Lateral femoral cutaneous nerve (L2, L3)—sensation to lateral thigh.

10. Pudendal nerve (S2–S4)—sensation to perineum and external genitalia and motor to the external anal and urethral sphincters.

11. Pelvic nerves (S2–4)–parasympathetic input for bowel, bladder, and sexual function.

12. Miscellaneous sensory nerves–subcostal (T12), iliohypogastric (L1), ilioinguinal (L1), and genitofemoral (L1, 2).

II. Entrapment Syndromes—Upper Extremity

A. Carpal tunnel syndrome–median nerve entrapment at the wrist by the transverse carpal ligament.

1. Anatomy:

   a. Median nerve–passes between the two heads of the pronator teres in the upper forearm.

   b. Anterior interosseus nerve branch–supplies motor innervation for thumb and finger flexion and some pronation (pronator quadratus, not pronator teres which is supplied by main median nerve more proximally).

   c. Median nerve–passes under transverse carpal ligament (TCL) medial to flexor carpi radialis tendon, lateral to palmaris longus tendon, and above tendons of flexor digitorum superficialis and profundus.

   d. Recurrent motor branch–normally arises under TCL (though rarely it runs through it) to supply LOAF muscles.

   e. Digital nerves–arise in palm and supply sensation to radial 3½ digits.

   f. Palmar cutaneous branch–arises from radial side of nerve, 5 cm proximal to TCL and passes above it.

   g. TCL–extends from palm to 3 cm beyond distal wrist crease; 9 tendons and median nerve pass in carpal tunnel.

2. Cause–most cases related to repetitive hand motion:

   a. Acute severe carpal tunnel syndrome may be caused by thrombosis of a persistent median artery or a local hematoma.

   b. Associated conditions–acromegaly, amyloid, multiple myeloma, hypothyroidism, diabetes, mucopolysaccharidosis, rheumatoid arthritis, and pregnancy.

3. Symptoms/signs:

   a. Dysesthesias (usually nocturnal) involving the palmar side of the thumb, index and middle fingers, and half of the ring finger.

   b. Sensory loss (radial 3½ digits).

   c. Weakness of the LOAF muscles.

   d. Thenar atrophy.

   e. Characteristic splitting of sensation of the fourth finger does not occur with nerve root or plexus lesions.

4. Classic symptoms–nocturnal (improved with shaking hands); worse with positions that involve wrist dorsiflexion or palmarflexion, such as driving a car.

5. Evaluation:

    a. History.

    b. Motor evaluation—especially opposition of thumb to little finger and thumb elevation/abduction.

    c. Tinel sign—tapping over TCL.

    d. Phalen's maneuver—symptoms reproduced by wrist flexion or reversed Phalen's maneuver; symptoms reproduced by wrist dorsiflexion.

    e. Nerve conduction velocity (NCV)—prolonged distal latency >3.7; electromyogram (EMG) may show fibrillations in abductor pollicis brevis with severe compression.

    f. Thyroid panel, growth hormone, complete blood cell count (CBC; for myeloma), glucose, and renal panel.

    g. Laboratory evaluation—usually reserved for young patients with no history of repetitive hand movements.

    h. Ultrasound (US) (or magnetic resonance imaging [MRI]) may show enlargement of median nerve at carpal tunnel.

6. Treatment:

    a. Most cases resolve with conservative management such as rest, nonsteroidal anti-inflammatory drugs (NSAIDs), neutral position splinting, and steroid injections (in line with the ring finger medial to the palmaris longus tendon to avoid injuring the nerve).

    b. Surgery—involves division of the TCL.

    c. Incision—from distal wrist crease to base of thumb in line with web space between third and fourth digits (**Fig. 13.2**).

    d. Care is taken to avoid sectioning the palmar cutaneous branch on the radial side of the nerve.

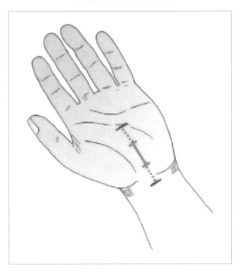

Fig. 13.2 Carpal tunnel incision. (Source: Citow JS. Neurosurgery Oral Board Review. 1st ed. New York, NY: Thieme Medical Publishers; 2003: 163, Fig. 14.2.)

      e. To section entire TCL—scissors should be used to undercut 3 cm proximal to wrist crease (under direct vision) and distally into hand until there is loss of resistance and fat is seen.

      f. Endoscopic division of TCL—also an option.

  7. Complications:

      a. Incorrect diagnosis (carpal tunnel syndrome is frequently seen on EMG; it is not always symptomatic or the cause of the symptoms may be due to other diagnoses).

      b. Incomplete division of TCL.

      c. Section of palmar cutaneous branch or motor branch.

      d. Damage to median nerve.

      e. Delayed neuroma or hypertrophic scar formation.

      f. Complex regional pain syndrome (CRPS)—rare, usually self-limited in 2 weeks, and treated with phentolamine intravenously (IV) or a sympathetic block.

      g. Deep infection.

      h. Injury to superficial palmar arch.

B. Pronator teres syndrome—entrapment of median nerve in forearm between the two heads of the pronator teres:

  1. Causes—repetitive pronation or direct trauma.

  2. Symptoms/signs—aching and fatiguing with grip weakness and median distribution paresthesias:

      a. No characteristic nocturnal exacerbations.

      b. Numbness in the palm; not seen with carpal tunnel syndrome because the palmar cutaneous branch travels over the TCL.

  3. Treatment—conservative, with surgery reserved for rare progressive cases.

C. Anterior interosseous nerve (AIN) syndrome—dysfunction of the anterior interosseous nerve, a branch of the median nerve innervating the flexor digitorum profundus 1 and 2, flexor pollicis longus, and pronator quadratus.

  1. "Pinch sign" may be seen with poor flexion of the thumb and index finger distal phalanges. The pinch is "square" rather than an "O".

  2. No sensory loss.

  3. When spontaneous, often inflammatory; most cases resolve by 12 weeks with conservative management.

  4. Evaluation should include imaging (elbow MRI) to rule out mass lesion.

D. Ligament of Struthers/supracondylar process compression:

  1. The median nerve may also rarely be compressed just above the elbow by the Struthers' ligament connecting the medial epicondyle and the supracondylar process (an anatomic variant located 5–7 cm proximal to the medial epicondyle).

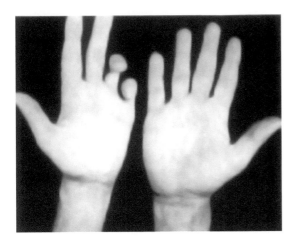

Fig. 13.3 A left claw hand. (Source: Citow JS. Neurosurgery Oral Board Review. 1st ed. New York, NY: Thieme Medical Publishers; 2003: 165, Fig. 14.3.)

E. Ulnar nerve entrapment—usually occurs at the elbow (cubital tunnel syndrome):

1. Symptoms/signs—hand (pinch) weakness, hypothenar and interosseus wasting, claw deformity (by weakness of lumbricals 3 and 4), and sensory loss and paresthesias of the medial hand, pinky, and medial half of the ring finger (**Fig. 13.3**).

2. Evaluation—Tinel sign at the elbow, examination of finger abduction and digits 4 and 5 flexion, sensory examination (two-point discrimination is the most sensitive), and EMG/NCV; US and MRI may be helpful on occasion and demonstrate an enlarged ulnar nerve in the cubital tunnel or T2 signal change.

3. Treatment:

a. In situ decompression or neurolysis and transposition—subcutaneous (SC), intramuscular (IM), or submuscular.

b. Medial epicondylectomy—seldom performed at this time.

c. Results appear similar with decompression or with transposition techniques in several prospective, randomized studies—excellent 60%, fair 25%, poor 15% (no improvement or continued worsening): (1) Technique for submuscular transposition—lazy incision ventral to medial epicondyle or posterior to it. Neurolysis of nerve across elbow; (2) Opening cubital tunnel between the two heads of the flexor carpi ulnaris distally; (3) Pening the arcade of Struthers proximally (a flat band of aponeurotic tissue anterior to the medial head of the triceps); (4) Flexor-pronator origin is then divided and the nerve tucked underneath along the bone; (5) Flexor-pronator origin is then repaired in a relaxed fashion to avoid compression of the nerve; (6) Care should be taken to avoid sectioning branches to the flexor carpi ulnaris (**Fig. 13.4**). Articular branches to the elbow may need to be divided.

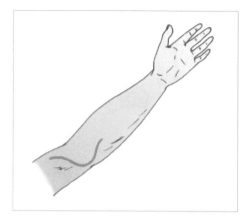

Fig. 13.4 Ulnar nerve incision. (Source: Citow JS. Neurosurgery Oral Board Review. 1st ed. New York, NY: Thieme Medical Publishers; 2003: 166, Fig. 14.4.)

F. Entrapment at the Wrist—in Guyon canal above the transverse carpal ligament:

1. Rare and may be due to compression by a ganglion cyst.

2. Known in carpenters due to wrist trauma.

3. Compression may produce motor, sensory or combined symptoms; isolated motor paralysis of the deep branch can occur and may mimic amyotrophic lateral sclerosis (ALS).

4. Clawing of the hand may be more profound than when compression of the ulnar nerve is at the elbow.

5. No sensory loss in the dorsal hand and fingers because this branch arises proximally and does not pass through the canal.

6. Differentiate from C8 radiculopathy:

    a. Radiculopathy is associated with neck pain, referred medial scapular pain, and more proximal arm pain.

    b. All of the intrinsic hand muscles should be weak, including the median nerve-innervated muscles.

    c. Some extrinsic muscles should also be weak, including radial nerve-innervated muscles (finger extensors) and other median innervated muscles (finger flexors).

    d. No sensory loss splitting the ring finger.

    e. Spurling's test would be positive (vs. positive elbow flexion test or Tinel sign at the elbow for cubital tunnel syndrome).

G. Radial nerve entrapment—usually in the mid-upper arm:

1. Cause—positioning (e.g., Saturday night palsy) or a humerus fracture (particularly with fracture near spiral groove).

2. Symptoms/signs—wrist drop and fingerdrop without triceps weakness.

3. Rule out lead poisoning.

4. Entrapment in the proximal forearm at the arcade of Frohse (superficial head of supinator) may cause a posterior interosseous syndrome with finger extension weakness, but no wristdrop or sensory loss. Wrist is in radial deviation. Evaluation—NCV; imaging; often inflammatory (similar to AIN syndrome). Exploration recommended by many if no improvement by 3–6 months.

5. Radial tunnel syndrome is due to compression in the supinator tunnel at and below the elbow region and causes elbow pain with little muscle weakness. It may respond to decompression.

   a. Evaluation—NCV; US/MRI; nerve block; exploration considered if there is no improvement in 3–6 months.

H. Suprascapular nerve entrapment—occurs in the suprascapular notch under the transverse scapular ligament; due to "sling effect." Well known in overhead athletes. Also, may be inflammatory:

   1. Symptoms/signs—deep shoulder pain and supraspinatus and infraspinatus muscle atrophy.

   2. Evaluation—EMG/NCS may help distinguish from C5 radiculopathy; Shoulder MRI can demonstrate a ganglion cyst or reveal rotator cuff disease which needs to be differentiated from suprascapular neuropathy.

   3. Treatment—surgical decompression of suprascapular ligament is effective if conservative management fails.

III. Entrapment Syndromes—Lower Extremity

A. Meralgia paresthetica (lateral femoral cutaneous nerve syndrome):

   1. Cause—nerve entrapment under lateral portion of inguinal ligament near anterosuperior iliac spine (ASIS).

   2. Usually seen with obesity, diabetes, pregnancy, and after surgery.

   3. Symptoms/signs—burning dysesthesias over the anterolateral upper thigh; Tinel sign near ASIS.

   4. Evaluation—US or MRI and electrophysiology; EMG is normal; NCS may be asymmetric from other side but is technically difficult, especially in obese patients. Differential may include L3 radiculopathy.

   5. Treatment—weight loss, NSAIDs, steroid injections, or surgery (nerve decompression by section of the inguinal ligament); some prefer neurectomy.

B. Sciatic neuropathy:

   1. Extraspinal causes of sciatica may be due to compression or trauma.

   2. Piriformis syndrome—due to compression as the sciatic nerve penetrates the piriformis muscle; remains controversial and difficult to diagnose definitively. Evaluate with EMG/NCS and high resolution MRI to show focal nerve hyperintensity and to rule out mass lesion. Rule out spinal origin. Treatment is nonoperative with physical therapy, steroid and/or Botox injuries; surgical decompression may be performed for refractory cases.

C. Peroneal nerve entrapment—usually due to compression of the common peroneal nerve at the fibular neck:

   1. Cause—may occur following squatting (e.g., strawberry picking).

   2. Symptoms/signs include pain radiating from knee to dorsal foot associated with weakness of foot dorsiflexion and toe extension and less often foot eversion. Sensory loss is less common and involves the lateral aspect of the lower half of the leg. Tinel at the fibular neck.

3. Evaluation—knee MRI or US peroneal nerve (to show nerve abnormality and rule out mass (an intraneural cyst may be present in 20% of patients with peroneal nerve palsy; these cysts arise from the superior tibiofibular joint and dissect intraneurally along the articular branch into the common peroneal nerve. Surgery needs to address the articular branch connection); EMG/NCV.

4. Differential diagnosis of footdrop has a broad differential. Most common lower motor neuron differential would be an L5 radiculopathy; back pain would radiate to foot; weakness would include inversion from posterior tibialis muscle (normal with peroneal nerve but abnormal with L5 radiculopathy); lumbar MRI and EMG would help distinguish. Footdrop may be seen in upper motor neuron disease as well (from stroke or rarely from a parasagittal brain tumor) or from spinal cord compression.

5. Treatment of peroneal nerve entrapment is with decompression of the common peroneal nerve posterior to the fibular head, near the fibular neck under the fascia of the peroneus longus and above the soleus (**Fig. 13.5**).

D. Tarsal tunnel syndrome:

1. Cause—tibial nerve entrapment beneath the arcuate ligament by the medial malleolus (tarsal tunnel) or more distally involving the medial and lateral plantar nerves within the plantar tunnels.

2. Symptoms/signs—pain and paresthesias of the toes and sole of the foot and weakness of intrinsic foot muscles.

3. Evaluate with EMG/NCS and MRI/US.

4. Treatment—surgical decompression indicated if conservative management (i.e., ankle support) fails.

IV. Miscellaneous

A. Greater occipital neuralgia—from a C2 sensory branch:

1. Superior nuchal trigger point—2.5 cm lateral and below the external occipital protuberance near the occipital artery.

2. C1 or C2 fracture or subluxation—may crush the dorsal root ganglia.

3. Treatment—usually with a nerve block using local anesthesia and steroids (10 mL 1% Bupivacaine and 40 mg Depo-Medrol).

4. Surgery—can be performed to avulse the nerve beyond the transverse process of C2 and the inferior oblique muscle (rarely needed).

V. Peripheral Neuropathy

A. Causes—DANG THE RAPIST—diabetes and drugs, amyloid, neoplasm and nutritional (B_{12}), Guillain–Barré syndrome, trauma, heredity, endocrine, electrolytes, and entrapment, renal and radiation, alcohol and AIDS, porphyria and paraneoplastic syndrome, infectious, immunologic, and ischemic, sarcoid, and toxins (i.e., lead).

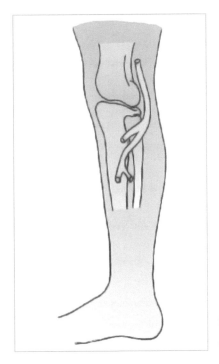

Fig. 13.5 Peroneal nerve exposure. (Source: Citow JS. Neurosurgery Oral Board Review. 1st ed. New York, NY: Thieme Medical Publishers; 2003: 168, Fig. 14.5.)

B.   Evaluation—glucose, Hgb1AC, thyroid stimulating hormone test (TSH), erythrocyte sedimentation rate (ESR), B_{12}, NCV, EMG, and muscle and nerve biopsies.

VI. Diabetic Neuropathy—May Be Sensory, Motor, or Autonomic

A.   Most commonly involves the distal sensory nerves (stocking-glove sensory loss) or femoral nerve.

B.   Femoral neuropathy (which also may be caused by a psoas hematoma) is distinguished from an L4 radiculopathy by the presence of hip flexion weakness.

VII. Charcot–Marie–Tooth Disease—Inherited Peroneal Hypertrophic Neuropathy Causing Peroneal-Innervated Muscle Atrophy

A.   Onset—in adolescence.

B.   Distal muscle atrophy occurs first in the feet and then the hands (claw hand).

C.   There is also sensory ataxia and weakness without autonomic dysfunction.

VIII. Brachial Plexitis

A. Idiopathic (Parsonage-Turner syndrome).

B. Cause—autoimmune attack on the brachial plexus, 2 weeks typically after an infection, immunization, surgery. Pain usually resolves within weeks. Weakness affecting certain muscles (shoulder girdle [rhomboid, spinatii]; deltoid; serratus anterior) or AIN or PIN-innervated muscles; may occur affecting several or occasionally in isolated nerve territories.

C. Evaluate with NCS/EMG and shoulder, brachial plexus or C spine MRI.

D. Treat pharmacologically and with PT. 80% of patients improve over 2 years. No defined role of steroids.

IX. Radiation Plexitis

A. May also be seen after radiation treatment.

B. Symptoms/signs—usually painless, numbness, paresthesias, and polyradicular weakness.

C. Evaluation—EMG (demonstrates demyelination after 3 weeks) may show myokymia. Brachial plexus MRI and chest X-ray (CXR) (to rule out a structural lesion such as a Pancoast or plexus tumor, usually involves the lower plexus).

D. Treatment—None. Usually slowly progressive over time.

X. Traumatic Neuropathy

A. Brachial plexus traumatic injury.

B. Stretch injury.

1. Preganglionic:
   a. Proximal to dorsal root ganglia.
   b. Avulsion—Not "fixable"; but reconstructable with nerve transfers.
   c. Associated with Horner syndrome, serratus anterior paralysis with scapular winging, and rhomboid weakness from dorsal scapular injury.

2. Postganglionic:
   a. May be amenable to neurolysis (in continuity) or nerve grafting (when advanced nerve injury or rupture). Evaluation—EMG/NCV after 3 weeks; high-resolution MRI or CT-myelogram.
   b. Erb-Duchenne palsy—C5–C6. No shoulder abduction/external rotation or elbow flexion; normal triceps, wrist and hand function.
   c. Adult—Usually posttraumatic.
   d. Birth injury and "waiter tip" posture.

3. Klumpke palsy—C8-T1 injury from a fall or Pancoast tumor causing a weak hand with claw deformity. T1 lesion may cause Horner syndrome.

C. Pan plexus (complete) C5-T1 palsy associated with high-speed trauma; often with preganglionic injury.

1. Treatment:
   a. Explore plexus.
   b. Record with nerve action potentials (NAPs); some may use somatosensory evoked potentials (SSEPs) or motor evoked potentials (MEPs).
   c. Priorities shoulder, elbow. Hand function generally not obtainable with nerve grafting or nerve transfer techniques.
   d. For flail arm, consider distal spinal accessory nerve transfer to supras-capular nerve (or shoulder fusion) and 3 intercostal nerve transfer to musculocutaneous nerve.

XI. Types of Nerve Injuries

A. Neurapraxia—Functional loss without structural damage that lasts 6–8 weeks. Motor function usually affected more than sensation.

B. Axonotmesis—Interruption of axons and myelin with intact perineurium and epi-neurium. Spontaneous regeneration may occur at 1–2 mm/d.

C. Neurotmesis—Complete transection of the nerve and nerve sheath. Axonal regen-eration may lead to neuroma formation.

D. Open injuries:
   1. Perform immediately within several days (to prevent retraction) for a clean laceration with a very sharp object (i.e., razor, scalpel, knife).
   2. Nerve repair—trim back ends to normal appearing fascicular structure; several sutures without tension using standard microsurgical technique; nerve graft if necessary.
   3. For blunt transection may wait 3weeks to explore, to allow the scar to heal and the inflammation to resolve.
   4. Evaluation—May include physical examination to determine the injured nerve, and US (to visualize continuity). Early electrophysiology may not be indicated.

E. Closed injuries:
   1. Typically nerves in continuity, rarely ruptured/transected. This includes gun-shot wounds. Most commonly observe for clinical/electrical recovery for 3–6 months. EMG and US (determines continuity).

F. Treatment:
   1. In surgery, perform NAPs over the neuroma to determine nerve recovery, and if positive, do only a neurolysis.
   2. Distal stump stimulation may be negative due to Wallerian degeneration, thus should not inhibit repair.
   3. If NAP is negative, resect the neuroma until clean fascicles are seen and repair. If short gap exists, this may be amenable to direct repair. Mobilize nerve ends. Transpose nerve if possible.
   4. If gap exists despite mobilization or if undue tension, then use nerve grafts (sural nerve, radial cutaneous nerve, etc.). Cable grafts (several nerves) may be interposed to match the cross-sectional diameter.

5. 8–0, 9–0 suture, microsurgical repair; may be reinforced with fibrin glue.

6. Earlier surgery preferred and if performed after 18 months, the muscle end plates may no longer be functional and the muscle may be fibrotic.

7. When cable grafting, shorter distances are more successful, and be sure to avoid tension.

8. Bioabsorbable tubes are now being introduced and used by some in place of nerve grafts; most commonly for small nerves (digital nerves). They are not commonly used for major nerves.

9. Immobilize the limb for several weeks (e.g., apply a splint if the repair crosses over a joint with joint gently flexed).

G. Knee dislocation—peroneal nerve stretch injury:

1. This is more severe than typical compression syndrome. Results tend to be poorer than with surgery for typical compression syndrome.

2. Refractory footdrop may be treated with a posterior tibialis tendon transfer (assuming tibial innervated muscle is functioning and heel cord is passively supple).

H. Hip dislocation—sciatic nerve injury.

1. Usually affects peroneal division more than tibial division. Difficult for peroneal nerve to recover.

2. Tibial nerve dysfunction recovers better than peroneal nerve.

I. Shoulder dislocation—axillary nerve:

1. Sometimes infraclavicular injury affecting other terminal branches or cords. EMG/NCS.

2. Assess rotator cuff with shoulder MRI for combined injury.

3. Results of repair will usually not be evident for 6 months. Maximal recovery may take several years.

XII. Peripheral Nerve Tumors

A. Neuroma—not a neoplasm:

1. Inflammatory mass consisting of tangled axons, Schwann cells, and fibroblasts following injury.

2. Usually painful and rubbery.

B. Benign nerve sheath tumor.

1. Schwannoma:

a. Firm, encapsulated, benign tumors growing eccentrically on the nerve with an epineurium capsule.

b. Occur intracranially and along the spinal cord at the root entry zone of sensory nerves, in the head and neck, posterior mediastinum, retroperitoneum, and flexor surface of the extremities.

c. Treatment—surgical resection when symptomatic, usually with excellent results.

2. Neurofibroma:

   a. Fusiform, unencapsulated, benign tumors infiltrating the width of the nerve.

   b. Cannot be completely removed without sacrificing the nerve.

   c. No reliable way to determine preoperatively whether the tumor is a schwannoma or a neurofibroma.

C. Malignant peripheral nerve sheath tumor (MPNST):

   1. Unlike a benign tumor, usually painful, rapidly enlarging mass, and frequently causes motor deficit.

   2. 50% of patients have neurofibromatosis I (NF-1). 25% have had prior radiation.

   3. Imaging—frequently masses with irregular borders/enhancement or necrosis.

   4. Cases suspected of MPNST, consider percutaneous or limited open biopsy.

   5. Treatment—wide resection and radiation, occasionally chemotherapy.

   6. Survival 50% at 5 years.

D. Syndromes:

   1. NF-1—well-known stigmata. Neurofibromas (often plexiform); 5–10% of patients may develop MPNST.

   2. NF-2–bilateral acoustic neuromas, peripheral schwannomas.

   3. Schwannomatosis—schwannomas affecting peripheral nerves and occasionally cranial nerves (not vestibular nerves).

E. Mass behind knee:

   1. Obtain image.

   2. Popliteal artery aneurysm.

   3. Ganglion (Baker–extraneural) cyst from knee joint may affect peroneal or tibial nerve behind knee; or intraneural ganglion cyst arising from superior tibiofibular joint.

   4. Nerve sheath tumor—positive Tinel sign, able to be moved side-to-side, but not the length of the nerve, rarely with motor deficit unless malignant.

XIII. Neuropathic Pain

A. Pain may follow nerve injury.

B. Pain may be due to nerve compression/irritation; or injury (neuroma-in-continuity or stump neuroma).

C. Examples of painful neuromas—superficial radial nerve near wrist, sural nerve near ankle.

   1. Evaluation:

      a. History—previous trauma?

   2. Examination—presence of percussion tenderness over the site of a nerve? Near scar?

    3. EMG/NCS.

    4. Imaging.

    5. Nerve block (diagnostic).

D. Management:

    1. Medical (and a tincture of time after injury; nerve pain may recover as function improves).

    2. Nonoperative (avoidance of activities, splinting, therapeutic blocks).

    3. Operative.

    4. When pain is related to a functioning nerve, neurolysis can be considered.

    5. When pain is related to a non-functioning nerve, neurolysis or nerve reconstruction can be considered.

    6. When pain is related to a painful nerve stump, sharp, re-resection of the proximal end of the nerve deep, within a muscle, and away from a joint may be helpful.

    7. Note a stump neuroma will always form after cutting a nerve. The goal of surgery for stump neuromas is to convert a painful neuroma to a painless neuroma.

Helpful Hints

1. GRAND THERAPIST is another useful mnemonic for peripheral neuropathies—Guillain–Barré syndrome, renal disease, alcoholism, nutrition (B_{12} deficiency), diabetes, trauma, genetics, endocrine system-based, entrapment, radiation, amyloid, porphyria, infection, sarcoid, toxin (lead), paraneoplastic syndrome, and psychiatric issues.

2. ROBERT TAYLOR DRINKS COLD BEER is a useful mnemonic for brachial plexus anatomy—roots/nerves, trunks, divisions, cords, then branches.

14 Critical Care and Neuroanesthesia

I. Shock

A. Hypovolemic—usually a 30% decrease in blood volume before impaired organ perfusion.

B. Cardiogenic—due to impaired cardiac pumping.

C. Septic—due to lowered peripheral vascular resistance, usually associated with gram-negative rods.

D. Neurogenic—due to decreased sympathetic output causing lowered peripheral vascular resistance, with blood pooling in veins after a spinal cord injury.

II. Adrenal Insufficiency

A. Low adrenocorticotropic hormone (ACTH)—can usually be replaced with just glucocorticoid (dexamethasone).

B. Primary adrenal insufficiency (Addison disease)—must be treated with mineral and glucocorticoids (hydrocortisone or prednisone). Patients on steroids for >2 weeks must be tapered off over 2 weeks.

C. Symptomatic adrenal insufficiency—includes fatigue, hypotension, hypoglycemia, hyponatremia, hyperkalemia, and hyperthermia.

III. Hypothyroidism

A. Signs/symptoms—usually fatigue, coarse hair, cold intolerance, constipation, and possibly neurologic impairment.

B. Myxedema coma—includes hypotension, bradycardia, hypothermia, hyponatremia, and hypoglycemia with 50% mortality. T_3 is the active form of the hormone.

IV. Syndrome of Inappropriate Antidiuretic Hormone (SIADH)

A. Normovolemia—serum osmolarity (Osm) < 280, urine Osm > serum Osm, serum Na^+ < 135 mEq/L, and urine Na^+ > 50 mEq/L.

B. Urine output—usually low (~40–60 mL/h).

C. Urine Na^+—usually close to 50 mEq/L.

D. Treatment—fluid restriction 1 L/d, NaCl 3% 30 mL intravenously (IV) every hour (q1h) × 3 and Lasix to reach 125–130 mEq/L. Avoid rapid correction more than 1 mEq/L/h to avoid central pontine myelinolysis. Consider adding demeclocycline 300 mg orally (PO) q8h or lithium 300 mg PO q8h to cause nephrogenic diabetes insipidus (DI) in refractory cases.

V. Cerebral Salt Wasting

A. Hypovolemia—with loss of free water and Na⁺.

B. Decreased weight and central venous pressure (CVP).

C. Urine output—usually high (>100 mL/h).

D. Urine Na⁺—usually around 130 mEq/L.

E. Treatment—0.9% normal saline (NS) boluses.

VI. Diabetes Insipidus

A. Urine output— >300 mL/h × 3, specific gravity <1.005.

B. Urine Na⁺— <10 mEq/L, serum Na⁺ >145. Watch to differentiate from normal postoperative diuresis that maintains a normal serum Na⁺.

C. Treatment—fluid replacement of half NS and desmopressin acetate (DDAVP) 0.1–0.2 μg IV q8h. Long-term care may require intranasal DDAVP 10–40 μg twice a day.

VII. Transfusion Reactions

A. Hemolytic—caused by ABO blood incompatibility:

  1. Signs/symptoms—lumbar pain, disseminated intravascular coagulopathy (DIC), and shock.

  2. Treatment—stop the transfusion and diurese with mannitol and fluids.

B. Allergic—caused by antibodies to plasma proteins:

  1. Signs/symptoms—hives.

  2. Treatment—Diphenhydramine. The transfusion usually does not need to be stopped.

C. Febrile—caused by antibodies to donor white blood cells (WBCs):
  1. Signs/symptoms—fever.

  2. Treatment—Paracetamol. The transfusion usually does not need to be stopped. Send off blood for analysis to rule out hemolysis.

VIII. Anaphylaxis

A. Treatment—epinephrine 1:1000 0.5 mL subcutaneously (SQ), Diphenhydramine 50 mg intramuscularly (IM), and Dexamethasone 10 mg IV.

IX. Deep Vein Thrombosis

A. Prevent with thromboembolic deterrent (TED) hose, sequential compression devices, and heparin SQ 5000 mg twice a day or Lovenox 30 mg SQ twice a day.

B. Rule out pulmonary embolus with ventilation–perfusion (V/Q) scan, spiral computed tomography (CT), or pulmonary angiogram.

C. Treatment—Anticoagulation or Greenfield inferior vena cava filter.

X. Warfarin

A. Weaning off for surgery:
1. Patients with a mechanical heart valve—stop the Warfarin for 2 days then admit to the hospital for heparin.
2. Patients with atrial fibrillation—stop the Warfarin 5 days before surgery. It is usually safe to resume heparin 5 days after a craniotomy.

XI. Preop Analgesia

A. Dexamethasone 10 mg IV, Ketorolac 30 mg IV, and Bupivacaine 0.5% SQ and IM.

XII. Preintubation Treatment

A. Denitrogenation with 100% oxygen (O_2) for 5 minutes; atropine to decrease the vagal cardiac response and secretions; lidocaine 100 mg IV to decrease pharyngeal reactivity and intracranial pressure (ICP).

XIII. Competitive Muscle Blockade

A. Reverse from pancuronium with neostigmine and atropine or glycopyrrolate.

XIV. Evoked Potential Monitoring

A. Avoid inhalation agents; nitrous oxide and narcotics preferred. Short-acting muscle relaxants are okay, but not benzodiazepines or barbiturates.

B. Turn off nitrous oxide 10 minutes before dural closure to avoid tension pneumocephalus.

XV. Malignant Hyperthermia

A. Hypermetabolic state of skeletal muscle due to an idiopathic block of calcium reentry into the sarcoplasmic reticulum causing increased O_2 consumption.

B. 50% of patients have had normal anesthesia.

C. Increased incidence with halothane and succinylcholine.

D. Temperature may increase to 44°C (113°F) at 1° per 5 minutes.

E.   Watch for increased pCO_2, decreased pO_2, tachycardia, disseminated intravascular coagulation (DIC), acidosis, rigid limbs, increased creatine kinase (CK), and ultimately hypotension and death.

F.   Patients are normally hypothermic with anesthesia.

G.   Treatment—Stop the anesthesia; change the tubing; administer dantrolene sodium and 100% O_2; lower the core temperature with cool IV fluids; perform wound, nasogastric, and rectal irrigation; administer bicarbonate to decrease acidosis, and insulin and glucose to decrease K^+.

H.   Test preop with a muscle biopsy to see if it contracts to halothane or caffeine.

I.   Watch for masseter spasm after injection of succinylcholine during the case.

Helpful Hints

1.   Calculating fluid restriction: (urine Na + urine K)/plasma Na = solute ratio (SR). If SR > 1, restrict to < 500 mL/d, if SR = 1, 500–700 mL/d, if SR < 1, 1 L/d.

2.   Calculating water deficit: Total body water = (140)(0.6)(wt in kg)/serum Na. Free water deficit = 0.6 (wt in kg) – TBW.

Case 40

A 50-year-old man presents postop day (POD) 10 from successful clip ligation of a ruptured broad neck anterior communicating artery aneurysm. Past medical history is significant for hypertension, coronary artery bypass surgery (CABG) with saphenous vein grafts, chronic hyponatremia, and peripheral vascular disease (PVD). Examination changed from neurologically intact to alert, disoriented ×3, otherwise intact. Arterial blood gases (ABGs) showed increased Aa gradient. Electrocardiogram (ECG) showed tachycardia and ST-T changes. Stat head CT revealed stable ventriculomegaly.

Case 41

A 50-year-old woman presents POD 10 after complete resection of a brain tumor (preop image shown) with new-onset generalized tonic-clonic (GTC) seizure. Past medical history is significant for meningioma, peptic ulcers, gastroesophageal reflux disease (GERD), and irritable bowel syndrome (IBS). Examination revealed she was neurologically intact, but drowsy with Glasgow Coma Scale (GCS) = 13 after receiving Lorazepam.

Na = 128 mEq/L, serum osmolality = 225 mOsm/L, urine sodium 50 mEq/L, urine: serum osmolality ratio = 2:1, blood urea nitrogen (BUN) = 12 mg/dL, creatinine = 1.1 mg/dL (**Fig. 14.1**).

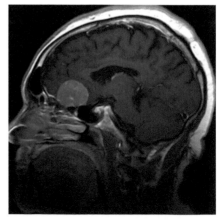

Fig. 14.1

Case 42

A 52-year-old man presents with marked lethargy on POD 7 after resection of a recurrent prolactinoma. Past medical history is significant for 1 year of bromocriptine before the tumor became unresponsive to therapy, chronic obstructive pulmonary disease (COPD) on steroids, and PVD. Examination revealed marked lethargy; the patient opened eyes to painful stimuli only, was nonverbal, and localized but did not follow commands symmetrically. Brainstem reflexes were intact (**Fig. 14.2**).

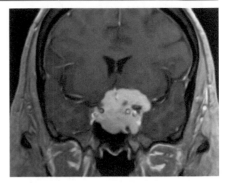

Fig. 14.2

15 Neurology

I. Seizure Disorders

A. Evaluation—electrolytes (hypoglycemia, hyponatremia, hypocalcemia), complete blood cell count (CBC), computed tomography (CT), lumbar puncture (LP), toxicology screen, arterial blood gases (ABGs), and electroencephalogram (EEG).

B. Traumatic:
1. Definition—early is <1 week after injury and late is >1 week.
2. Treatment—prophylactic anticonvulsants are used for only 1 week after traumatic hemorrhage if no seizure. Use for 3 weeks to 3 months if there is a cortical lesion; then perform EEG before tapering off over 2–4 weeks.

C. Status epilepticus:
1. Signs/symptoms—continuous seizures for >30 minutes or intermittent without a conscious interval; neurons may be damaged after 20 minutes of firing continuously.
2. Treatment—Lorazepam 0.1 mg/kg over 2 minutes (or Diazepam 0.2 mg/kg) and simultaneously load with Phenytoin 20 mg/kg intravenously (IV) or phenobarbital 20 mg/kg IV (100 mg/min).
3. If unsuccessful, consider general anesthesia [always use ABCs (airway, breathing, circulation)]; send for electrolytes, glucose, and ABG.
4. If unsuccessful, consider giving 50 mL of D50 or thiamine 100 mg IV.

D. Tonic-clonic seizures:
1. Treatment—Phenytoin, Carbamazepine, or phenobarbital.

E. Absence seizures:
1. Treatment—ethosuximide or valproic acid.

F. Partial complex seizures:
1. Treatment—Carbamazepine or Phenytoin.

G. Antiepileptic drug side effects:
1. Phenytoin—nystagmus, ataxia, rash, gingival hypertrophy.
2. Carbamazepine—ataxia, syndrome of inappropriate antidiuretic hormone (SIADH), leukopenia, hepatitis (stop if γ-glutamyl transferase [GGT] 2× normal).
3. Levetiracetam—thrombocytopenia.

H. Pregnancy:
1. Folic acid—use in the first trimester to decrease birth defects.
2. Anticonvulsants—increase the risk of congenital malformations; however, persistent seizures carry a higher risk.

I. Surgery—consider in a patient who has failed 1 year of multidrug therapy.
1. Evaluation:
   a. Magnetic resonance imaging (MRI)—look for cortical dysplasia, tumor, or mesial temporal sclerosis.

b. Video EEG.

c. Positron emission tomography (PET) scan—Localized hypometabolism ipsilateral to seizure focus in the postictal phase.

d. Wada test—assess dominant hemisphere language and memory function with large resection—intracarotid Amytal injection and angiogram to see cross-flow from dominant hemisphere; patient should have a flaccid arm for 5 minutes.

e. Surgically implanted subdural surface grids—may be used to locate a focus. Avoid intraop benzodiazepines and barbiturates; use only narcotics and droperidol. Stimulate the cortex with 60 Hz frequency and 1 V for 2 msec. Taper the anticonvulsants preop and treat intraop seizures with phenobarbital 130 mg IV.

After resections, continue anticonvulsants 2-year postoperative. 50% of patients become seizure-free, and 80% have decreased frequency after surgery.

2. Resections:

a. Anterior temporal lobe—for mesial temporal sclerosis or local lesion.

b. Spare the superior temporal gyrus.

c. Incise the middle temporal gyrus to the temporal horn of the lateral ventricle; dissect over the hippocampus to incisura and choroidal fissure.

d. Stay subpial to preserve posterior cerebral artery (PCA) branches.

e. Resect 5 cm on the dominant side and 7 cm on the nondominant side.

f. Risks—Vessel injury, Meyer loop injury (contralateral pie-in-sky field cut), and 3rd nerve injury near tentorium.

3. Amygdalohippocampectomy.

4. Discrete lesionectomy—cortical migration, tumor, or arteriovenous malformation (AVM).

J. Disconnections—if seizures involve both hemispheres or are from an eloquent location.

1. Corpus callosotomy—for drop attacks (atonic seizures):

a. There is a 70% improvement in seizures.

b. Cut only the anterior one-third of the corpus callosum to avoid disconnection syndrome (left tactile anomia and dyspraxia, right olfactory anomia and hand spatial problems, decreased spontaneous speech, and incontinence).

c. Don't cut the anterior commissure.

d. Consider Wada test for left-handed patients to avoid language and behavioral problems.

2. Functional hemispherectomy—80% of patients improve:

a. Leave the basal ganglia intact.

3. Subpial transections—for partial complex seizures in eloquent cortex:

a. Cut every 5 mm to interrupt horizontal spread and leave vertical columns intact.

K. Vagal nerve stimulator—can decrease seizure frequency, but does not eliminate seizures; implant on the left side.

II. EEG Monitoring

A. Helpful in the diagnosis of Creutzfeldt–Jakob disease (CJD) and subacute sclerosing panencephalitis (SSPE).

B. Can determine burst suppression with barbiturates when used for cerebral ischemia.

C. Intraop reversal of somatosensory evoked potential (SSEP) wave helps localize the motor–sensory strip junction.

   1. An evoked potential decrease in amplitude of 50% or an increase in latency of 10% is considered significant, though there is much debate over how useful this is in surgery with tumor resection.

III. Dementia

A. Treatable causes (20%)—medications, alcohol (ETOH), heavy metals, central nervous system (CNS) infection, hyperthyroidism, hypothyroidism, hyperglycemia, hypoglycemia, decreased parathyroid hormone (PTH), hypopituitarism, hyponatremia, Cushing disease, Wilson disease, uremia, porphyria, hydrocephalus, chronic subdural hematoma, tumor, hypertension (HTN), deficiency of vitamin B_1 and B_{12} or folate.

B. Untreatable causes (80%)—Alzheimer disease (50%), multi-infarct dementia (15%), Pick disease, progressive supranuclear palsy (PSNP; Steele–Richardson–Olszewski syndrome), Parkinson disease, Huntington chorea, multiple sclerosis (MS), systemic lupus erythematosus (SLE), sarcoid, progressive multifocal leukoencephalopathy (PML), and CJD.

C. Evaluation—CBC (infection or B_{12}/folate deficiency with mean corpuscular volume [MCV] >100); electrolytes (glucose, Na+, blood, urea, nitrogen [BUN]); thyroid; B_{12}; folate; urine toxicity screen; electrocardiogram (ECG; AFIB with lacunes); chest X-ray (CXR), CT, LP, Venereal Disease Research Laboratory (VDRL).

IV. Wernicke Encephalopathy

A. Cause—Thiamin deficiency, usually in alcoholics.

B. Signs/symptoms—Confusion, conjugate gaze and lateral rectus palsies, nystagmus, and gait ataxia.

C. Evaluation—MRI may detect inflammation and necrosis of the mamillary bodies, periventricular thalamus and hypothalamus, periaqueductal gray, floor of the fourth ventricle, and superior cerebellar vermis.

D. Treatment—Thiamine 100 mg IV followed by daily supplements and a normal diet.

E. Korsakoff psychosis—A more chronic disorder with short-term memory loss and learning difficulties.

V. Creutzfeldt–Jakob Disease

A. Cause—Prion or slow virus.

B. Signs/symptoms—Dementia, ataxia, visual loss, and myoclonus.

C. Evaluation—MRI (hyperintense on T2 in basal ganglia), LP (rule out syphilis, may see increased protein), EEG (periodic spikes), and biopsy (spongiform encephalitis with decreased cells and no inflammation, stain for protease-resistant protein).

D. Treatment—No treatment; death usually within 1 year.

E. Precaution—Sterilize biopsy equipment with steam and sodium hydroxide.

VI. Progressive Supranuclear Palsy (PSNP; Steele–Richardson–Olszewski Syndrome)

A. Cause—unknown, possibly autoimmune.

B. Signs/symptoms—progressive deterioration in intellect, speech, vision, gait, voluntary eye control, and pseudobulbar palsy. Most patients are 50- to 60-year-old males.

C. Evaluation—mainly clinical. MRI may show atrophy of the midbrain, superior colliculus, and subthalamic nuclei.

D. Treatment—none.

VII. Parkinsonism

A. Cause—substantia nigra pars compacta degeneration producing decreased dopamine and increased acetylcholine (ACh)

B. Signs/symptoms—pill-roll tremor, cogwheel rigidity, bradykinesia, shuffle gait, and masked face

C. Secondary parkinsonism—olivopontocerebellar degeneration, Shy-Drager syndrome (autonomic dysfunction with orthostatic hypotension), progressive SNP (impaired vertical gaze, dysarthria, dysphagia, axial dystonia, emotional lability, survival 6 years), medically induced (Haloperidol, Prochlorperazine, Metoclopramide), lacunes, and trauma.

D. Treatments.

1. Dopamine agents—Sinemet with levodopa and carbidopa:

    a. Dopamine does not cross the blood–brain barrier (BBB) but L-dopa does.

    b. Carbidopa (currently the most effective agent) inhibits peripheral decarboxylation of L-dopa and is best for bradykinesia, but less effective for tremor.

    c. The major side effect is dyskinesia.

2. Dopamine agonists—bromocriptine (Parlodel).

3. Increase dopamine levels—Eldepryl (monoamine oxidase B [MAO-B] inhibitor) and amantadine (dopamine agonist; inhibits reuptake).

4. Anticholinesterase—Diphenhydramine (rarely used).

5. Pallidotomy—radiofrequency (RF) lesion or stimulator to GPi or subthalamus:

    a. Success rates—dyskinesia 90%, bradykinesia 85%, rigidity 75%, tremor 57%.

    b. Also improves on/off symptoms.

    c. Complications—visual field cut 3%, hemiparesis, dysarthria 8%, and speech and cognitive decline if bilateral lesions created.

6. Thalamotomy—RF or stimulator to ventral intermediate thalamic nucleus (VIM) most effective for tremor.

VIII. Acute Disseminated Encephalomyelitis

A. Cause—Autoimmune, usually after a viral illness or vaccination.

B. Signs/symptoms—Monophasic deterioration with variable deficits that may include altered mentation, weakness, sensory loss, etc.

C. Evaluation—MRI with hyperintense T2 plaque.

D. Treatment—Steroids.

IX. Multiple Sclerosis

A. Cause—Demyelination of white matter tracts in the CNS (especially periventricular).

B. Signs/symptoms—Optic neuritis 50%, internuclear ophthalmoplegia (almost always indicates MS), motor, sensory, and genitourinary.

C. Evaluation—two attacks in different places at different times, cerebrospinal fluid (CSF) oligoclonal bands of immunoglobulin G (IgG) with normal serum IgG, and protein <100, and MRI plaques (94% specific).

D. Treatment—Interferon beta-1b (Betaseron) injections decrease frequency of attacks by 30%; steroids are of unproven benefit.

X. Amyotrophic Lateral Sclerosis

A. Cause—degeneration of α motor neurons in the spinal cord and brainstem as well as corticospinal tracts.

B. Signs/symptoms:
1. Upper and lower motor neuron dysfunction.
2. No cognitive, sensory, or autonomic dysfunction.
3. Extraocular muscles and urinary sphincter usually spared.
4. Tongue fasciculations common.
5. Often lower motor neuron weakness in the legs with a normal MRI.

C. Evaluation—clinical and electromyogram (EMG; fibrillations).

D. Survival—4 years.

E. Treatment:
1. Riluzole can be administered, slows disease progression in some patients by reducing glutamate in the brain. Oral formulation.
2. Edaravone, now FDA approved, shows reduction in decline of daily function; given via IV infusion.

XI. Subacute Combined Systems Disease

A. Cause—vitamin B_{12} deficiency, usually with malnutrition or pernicious anemia.

B. Signs/symptoms—upper and lower motor neuron dysfunction (also may have peripheral neuropathy), impaired bilateral vibratory and touch sensation, and rarely mental or visual deterioration.

C. Evaluation:

1. CBC to evaluate for macrocytic anemia (MCV >100) and hypersegmented poly-morphonuclear neutrophils (PMNs).

2. MRI may reveal cervical and thoracic posterior and lateral column demyelination.

3. Other tests include B_{12} assay and serum methylmalonic acid and homocysteine.

4. Shilling test is used to evaluate for pernicious anemia.

D. Treatment—B_{12} injections. Folic acid may correct anemia, but may worsen neuro-logic symptoms.

XII. Friedreich Ataxia

A. Cause—autosomal recessive from chromosome 9.

B. Signs/symptoms:

1. Gait ataxia, upper limb motor and sensory loss, and speech disturbances.

2. Degeneration of axons and myelin in the posterior columns, corticospinal tracts, and spinocerebellar tracts.

3. Degeneration of the cerebellum and brainstem nuclei.

4. Motor neurons usually spared.

5. Patients tend to have high-arched feet and pes cavus.

C. Evaluation—clinical and MRI with cerebellar and spinal degeneration.

D. Treatment—none. Patients are usually nonambulatory 5years after onset (before 20 years of age) and die by mid-30s.

XIII. Acute Transverse Myelitis

A. Cause—cell mediated immunity to CNS by infection, trauma, tumor, or toxin.

B. Signs/symptoms—varied deficits, peaks at 2 days.

C. Evaluation—usually hyperintensity on T2-weighted MRI.

D. Treatment—Steroids (unclear benefit); 50% of patients have a good recovery.

XIV. Guillain–Barré Syndrome

A. Cause—possibly an antibody to peripheral myelin causing focal segmental demye-lination with acute peripheral neuropathy.

B. Signs/symptoms:

1. Usually symmetric weakness, more proximal than distal.

2. Little sensory involvement.

3. Possible involvement of cranial nerves (CNs).

4. Possible autonomic dysfunction.

5. Onset 3 days to 5 weeks after an upper respiratory infection, surgery, or immu-nization. Symptoms peak by 4 weeks with recovery over a few weeks after progression stops.

C.   Evaluation—CSF with increased protein and normal cells; nerve conduction velocity (NCV) with prolonged latencies.

D.   Treatment—plasmapheresis, steroids (not proven helpful), and antibodies (unclear benefit).

E.   Differentiate from:

1.   Acute intermittent porphyria—normal CSF protein, abdominal cramps, urine with δ-aminolevulinic acid.

2.   Lead poisoning—wrist drop, may be asymmetrical.

3.   Botulism—descending symmetrical bulbar paresis often with dilated pupils; normal NCV:

a.   Cause—presynaptic impairment of ACh release.

b.   Treatment—supportive by managing airway and circulation until toxin leaves system. Antitoxin may be used.

XV. Myasthenia Gravis

A.   Cause—antibodies to nicotinic ACh-receptors on muscles.

B.   Signs/symptoms—intermittently weak (at end of day) with diplopia and ptosis in young females and older males.

C.   Evaluation—CXR (15% have thymoma), collagen panel (other autoimmune diseases common), Tensilon test (edrophonium IV or neostigmine improves symptoms), EMG (decreased muscle action potential with repetitive nerve stimulation), and anti-ACh-receptor assay.

D.   Treatment—anticholinesterase (pyridostigmine, consider decreasing muscarinic side effects with atropine), thymectomy (helps 80% of patients even without thymoma; there is frequent hyperplasia), plasma-pheresis, azathioprine (immunosuppressant), and steroids.

XVI. Eaton–Lambert (Myasthenic) Syndrome

A.   Cause—antibodies to the presynaptic neuromuscular junction preventing ACh release.

B.   Signs/symptoms—symmetrical proximal pelvis and shoulder girdle weakness that improves with repetitive activity of the muscles; possible autonomic dysfunction.

C.   Evaluation—search for primary neoplasm, especially pulmonary oat cell. Only 50% of patients have a known cancer at the time of diagnosis. EMG with incremental response.

D.   Treatment—steroids and azathioprine (immunosuppression).

XVII. Paraneoplastic Syndrome

A.   Cause—unknown, possibly autoimmune (anti-Yo, anti-Hu, etc.).

B.   Signs/symptoms—variable with different parts of CNS and PNS involved; may be acute or subacute and may be purely motor or sensory.

C. Evaluation—search for occult malignancy with CXR, etc.; CSF to search for cytology and IgG.

D. Treatment—steroids.

XVIII. Meningeal Carcinomatosis

A. Cause—meningeal seeding by tumor cells.

B. Signs/symptoms—headache, multiple cranial neuropathies, cerebrovascular assident (CVA), variable symptoms.

C. Evaluation—MRI with thickened enhancing leptomeninges; CSF with elevated protein and cells.

D. Treatment—steroids, but prognosis dismal.

XIX. Polymyositis

A. Cause—autoimmune attack on muscles.

B. Signs/symptoms—proximal symmetrical muscle weakness sparing ocular movements.

C. Evaluation—elevated creatine kinase (CK) and EMG with fibrillations. Rule out steroid myopathy, myasthenia gravis, hypothyroidism, and hyperparathyroidism.

D. Treatment—steroids.

XX. Steroid Myopathy—Usually Symmetrical Proximal Lower Extremity Weakness that Resolves after Steroid Discontinued

XXI. Epidural Lipomatosis

A. Cause—accumulation of epidural fat compressing the thoracic or lumbar thecal sac, usually related to steroids or obesity.

B. Signs/symptoms—back pain, lower extremity weakness, spasticity, sensory loss, and urinary retention or incontinence.

C. Evaluation—MRI.

D. Treatment—discontinue steroids, weight loss, and rarely laminectomy with resection of adipose tissue.

XXII. Neurosarcoid

A. Cause—unknown.

B. Signs/symptoms—cranial neuropathy, hydrocephalus.

C. Evaluation—elevated serum angiotensin-converting enzyme (SACE) level 85%, CXR (hilar nodes), and skin biopsy with noncaseating granulomas.

D. Treatment—steroids; usually slow recovery.

XXIII. Fibromuscular Dysplasia

A. Cause—unknown, but possibly a congenital medial defect.

B. Signs/symptoms—headache, vertigo, transient ischemic attacks (TIAs); increased incidence of aneurysm (30%), tumor, and dissection.

C. Evaluation:
   1. Angiogram.
   2. Second most common cause of internal carotid artery (ICA) stenosis.
   3. 80% of cases are bilateral.
   4. Most common site is the renal artery, followed by the cervical ICA.

D. Treatment—ASA, angioplasty, and resection with reconstruction (difficult).

XXIV. Syncope—Transient Loss of Consciousness due to Decreased Cerebral Blood Flow

A. Causes:
   1. Circulatory failure:
      a. Impaired vasoconstriction (vasovagal response, postural hypotension, and primary autonomic insufficiency).
      b. Hypovolemia.
      c. Decreased venous return (Valsalva maneuver, coughing, straining).
      d. Decreased cardiac output (dysrhythmia or obstructive).
   2. Altered substrate delivery:
      a. Hypoxia.
      b. Anemia.
      c. Hypoglycemia.
   3. Emotional disturbance.

B. Signs/symptoms:
   1. Seizures causing sudden loss of consciousness.
   2. No prodrome, headache, or skin pallor changes.
   3. Syncopal episodes lack a postictal phase.

XXV. Headaches

A. Differential—Hemorrhage, pseudotumor cerebri, meningitis, venous sinus thrombosis, tumor, migraine, sinus disease, ear disease, dental disease, Tolosa-Hunt syndrome.

B. Innervation—there is no C1 sensory innervation:
   1. Greater occipital nerve—from C2/3 dorsal rami; provides sensation to the area rostral and medial behind the ear.
   2. Lesser occipital nerve—from C2 ventral ramus; provides sensation to the area caudal and lateral behind the ear.
   3. Posterior head—neck junction—innervated by the supraclavicular nerve from the C3/4/5 ventral and dorsal rami.

C. Migraine:

1. Common—unilateral throbbing headache, nausea, vomiting, photophobia, and sometimes no aura of deficit.

2. Classic—includes an aura of focal deficit <24 hour.

3. Complicated—deficit may last up to 30 days.

4. Migraine equivalent—focal deficit without headache:

   a. Treatment (acute episode)—Prochlorperazine 10 mg IV, Ketorolac 30 mg IV, sumatriptan subcutaneously (SQ), caffeine/ergot 100 mg/1 mg 2 orally (PO). Ergots and triptans are vasoconstrictors.

   b. Prophylaxis—β-blockers (avoid in asthmatics), calcium-channel blockers, methysergide (serotonin agonist), control of HTN, and avoidance of oral contraceptive pills.

5. Other—there is frequently a family history of migraines. Children may present with an acute confusional state.

D. Cluster headaches—unilateral oculofrontal or oculotemporal headaches with ipsilateral conjunctival injection, nasal congestion, rhinorrhea, lacrimation, partial Horner syndrome, agitation, and flushing (autonomic); usually in males and last 30–90 minutes per day (at similar times) for 4–12 weeks with many months of remission:

1. Treatment (acute episode)—100% O_2, ergotamines, sumatriptan, steroids, or radiofrequency sphenopalatine ganglion lesion.

2. Prophylaxis—lithium 300 mg PO three times daily and methysergide.

E. Pseudotumor cerebri (benign intracranial hypotension)—increased intracranial pressure (ICP) and papilledema without a mass lesion and with a normal CT/MRI. Usually self-limited, though may cause blindness by optic atrophy. Occur most often in overweight females:

1. Evaluation—MRI (there may be slit ventricles), LP (ICP > 20 cm water), visual fields (enlarged blind spot and constricted visual fields), CBC, and collagen panel; be sure to rule out venous sinus thrombosis, sarcoid, and lupus erythematosus.

2. Treatment—weight loss, diuretics (acetazolamide or Lasix), steroids, lumboperitoneal shunt (for headaches), or optic nerve sheath fenestration (for visual deterioration).

F. Spontaneous intracranial hypotension—positional headaches exacerbated by standing:

1. Cause—possibly by a tear in a nerve root sleeve.

2. Signs/symptoms—postural headache exacerbated by standing

3. Evaluation—MRI demonstrates meningeal enhancement. Consider myelography to locate leak.

4. Treatment—bedrest, hydration, Fioricet, nonsteroidal anti-inflammatory drug (NSAIDs), and blood patch; similar to post-LP headaches and should be treated in a similar manner.

XXVI. Temporal Arteritis

A. Cause—autoimmune disease.

B. Signs/symptoms—headache, eye pain, visual loss (papilledema or optic atrophy, permanent blindness in 7%), jaw claudication.

C. Evaluation—elevated erythrocyte sedimentation rate (ESR) and C-reactive protein (CRP) (50% have polymyalgia rheumatica with elevated CK) and biopsy (granulomatous skip lesions on external carotid artery [ECA] branches and ophthalmic arteries).

D. Treatment—steroids.

XXVII. Trigeminal Neuralgia

A. Rule out—atypical facial pain, V1 zoster, dental and orbital problems, temporal arteritis, and tumor.

B. Etiology—possibly due to ephaptic transmission of action potential.

C. Signs/symptoms—lancinating, paroxysmal, sharp, electric, facial pain in a trigeminal distribution.

D. Evaluation—extraocular movements, facial sensation, corneal reflexes, jaw opening (pterygoid) and closing (masseter).

E. Treatment:

1. Pharmacologic—Carbamazepine 200 mg three times a day (up to 1600 mg/d, may cause confusion and lethargy, low white blood count [WBC; keep >3000], SIADH, and elevated liver enzymes], baclofen, Gabapentin, and Amitriptyline. Narcotics are usually not effective.

2. Surgical:

   a. Destructive techniques—includes percutaneous balloon gangliolysis; (Fig. 15.1a, b), and glycerol or radiofrequency rhizotomy. The needle for percutaneous techniques is inserted 1 cm from the angle of the mouth, tunneled under the skin inside the cheek, aimed toward the foramen ovale under fluoroscopic guidance along the midpupillary line, and angled toward the zygoma 2 cm from the tragus. The needle should extend to the clivus–petrous ridge on lateral X-ray. Gamma knife radiosurgery is a new option that requires 2–6 weeks for improvement in pain. All of the procedures create new numbness as a trade-off for pain relief.

   b. Nondestructive technique—microvascular decompression. A vessel (usually by the superior cerebellar artery) compressing the trigeminal nerve is felt to cause emphatic transmission of painful impulses. A small retrosigmoid craniotomy is performed and the vessel is dissected off the nerve which is then insulated with a Teflon pattie. A rare complication is hearing loss; so be sure the patient has contralateral hearing preoperatively. This technique is not usually useful for trigeminal neuralgia related to MS.

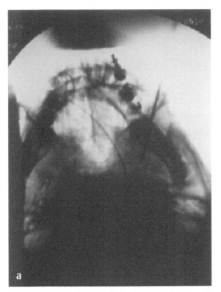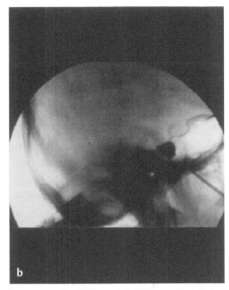

Fig. 15.1 **(a)** Submental skull X-ray with needle in foramen ovale. **(b)** Lateral skull X-ray with inflated balloon showing characteristic "pear" shape. (Source: Citow JS. Neurosurgery Oral Board Review. 1st ed. New York, NY: Thieme Medical Publishers; 2003: 23, Fig. 3.1A, B.)

XXVIII. Glossopharyngeal Neuralgia

A. Signs/symptoms—lancinating pain into the posterior throat or ear; afferent fibers from the carotid body to the dorsal X brainstem nucleus may cause the heart to stop with the pain.

B. Treatment:

   1. Pharmacologic—similar to that for trigeminal neuralgia.

   2. Surgical—consists of craniotomy for microvascular decompression (posterior inferior cerebellar artery [PICA]) or sectioning CNs IX (above the arachnoid fold) and X (only upper two rootlets).

XXIX. Transient Global Amnesia

A. Cause—may be related to migraine or vasospasm.

B. Signs/symptoms—impaired recent and present memory in middle-aged persons; no other symptoms, benign course, seldom recurs.

XXX. Malignant Neuroleptic Syndrome

A. Causes:

   1. Blockage of dopamine receptors in the basal ganglia and hypothalamus after treatment with phenothiazines (Prochlorperazine or Chlorpromazine) or Haloperidol.

   2. Possible dysfunction of the muscular sarcoplasmic reticulum.

   3. Possible autosomal dominance inheritance.

B.   Signs/symptoms—stupor, hyperthermia, hypotension, and rigidity.

C.   Evaluation—hyperkalemia, myoglobinuria (may cause renal failure), elevated CK.

D.   Treatment—bromocriptine (for CNS) and dantrolene (for muscles).

XXXI. Coma

A.   Evaluation—electrolytes, CBC, ABG, urine toxicity screen, CT, LP (if CT normal):

1.   Oculovestibular reflex (cold calorics)—do if the tympanic membrane is intact with head of bed (HOB) at 30 degrees. Irrigate 100 mL of ice water in one ear. In an awake patient there should be slow deviation ipsilaterally and the fast nystagmus component contralaterally (cold opposite and warm same [COWS]). In a comatose patient with a normal brainstem, there should be conjugate ipsilateral deviation but no nystagmus because this requires cortical input.

B.   Treatment—consider glucose D50 25 mL, thiamine 100 mg, Naloxone, and Flumazenil. Dilated pupils are usually due to a structural cause, anoxia, or anticholinesterases. Pupils may be dilated with botulism, though the patient is usually awake. Pupils tend to be small with narcotics and pontine lesions.

XXXII. Brain Death

A.   Signs/symptoms—pupils fixed and dilated, absent corneal reflexes, oculocephalic reflexes (Doll's eyes), oculovestibular reflexes, gag flexes, and no movement of the body to a painful stimulus (the lower extremities may still have spinal-mediated withdrawal).

B.   Evaluation.

1.   Apnea test:

a.   Requires pCO_2 > 60 mm Hg without initiation of a breath.

b.   Start with 15 minutes of 100% O_2 and pCO_2 40.

c.   Use passive O_2 6 L/min during the test and wait 6–12 minutes while maintaining the pO_2 > 80.

2.   Contributing factors to eliminate:

a.   Temperature > 32.2°C (90°F).

b.   No intoxication.

c.   Normal O_2.

d.   Systolic blood pressure (SBP) > 90.

3.   Re-examination—usually in 12 hours. For patients 1 year (1 day), 2 months (2 days), neonates (7 days).

4.   Confirmation—usually not required. Consider EEG, cerebral blood flow (CBF; radionucleotide angiography), or test with atropine 1 mg (shouldn't affect heart rate because there will be no vagal tone).

XXXIII. Brainstem and Cortical Syndromes

A. Weber syndrome—CN III deficit with contralateral hemiplegia.

B. Benedikt syndrome—Weber's plus red nucleus lesion (ataxia and tremor of upper extremity).

C. Millard-Gubler syndrome—CNs VI and VII deficit with contralateral hemiplegia.

D. Parinaud syndrome.

  1. Signs/symptoms:

    a. Decreased convergence, accommodation, and upward gaze (setting sun sign, supranuclear dysfunction) with normal vertical Doll's eyes.

    b. Possible lid retraction, usually caused by a pineal or quadrigeminal plate tumor or elevated ICP with the third ventricle pushing down upon the tectum.

    c. Differential diagnosis of impaired ocular motility also includes Guillain–Barré syndrome, myasthenia gravis, botulism, Wernicke encephalopathy, and hypothyroidism.

E. Foster–Kennedy syndrome—anosmia, ipsilateral optic atrophy, and contralateral papilledema, usually caused by an olfactory groove meningioma.

F. Dominant parietal lobe lesion—Gerstmann syndrome with acalculia, agraphia (without alexia), right/left confusion, and finger agnosia.

G. Nondominant parietal lobe lesion—dressing apraxia and neglect (may be from either side).

H. Cortical sensory syndrome—decreased two-point discrimination, agraphesthesia (draw a number on the palm), and astereognosis (identify a coin in the hand).

I. Alexia without agraphia—usually by a left PCA stroke.

J. Prosopagnosia—due to a lesion in the bilateral or right medial parieto-occipital area.

XXXIV. Superior Vermian Atrophy

A. Trauma, Phenytoin, ethyl alcohol (ETOH).

XXXV. Posterior Column Degeneration

A. Subacute combined systems disease (SCSD; B_{12} deficiency), tabes dorsalis, Freidrich ataxia.

XXXVI. Atonic Bladder

A. Use Bethanechol to increase ACh. Evaluate with cystometrogram.

XXXVII. Spastic Bladder (Hyperreflexic Detrusor)

A. Use Ditropan to decrease ACh.

XXXVIII. Reversible Posterior Leukoencephalopathy

A. Demyelination of occipital lobes related to immunosuppression (cyclosporin), HTN, eclampsia. Usually resolves when the offending agent is withdrawn.

XXXIX. Selective Vulnerability to Hypoxia

A. Hippocampus (CA1,3), parieto-occipital cortex (layers 3,5), Purkinje cells, outer caudate, and putamen. Likely due to elevated glutamate levels.

XL. Ophthalmology

A. Monocular blindness—consider amaurosis fugax, optic neuritis, retinal detachment.

B. Optic neuritis—usually seen with MS (especially if bilateral) and sarcoid.

1. Signs/symptoms:

a. Early stage—may appear as papilledema (blurred disk margins).

b. Later stage—may appear as optic atrophy (bright white optic disk with clean margins).

C. Diabetic third nerve palsy (vasculitic/ischemic)—pupil sparing and painful.

D. Compressive third nerve palsy—pupil dilated early and painless.

E. Horner syndrome—ptosis, miosis, and anhidrosis:

1. Sympathetic input to the head is through the superior cervical ganglion.

2. Spontaneous causes—arterial dissection and tumor.

F. Internuclear ophthalmoplegia:

1. Cause—Medial longitudinal fasciculus dysfunction.

2. Signs/symptoms—Contralateral medial rectus fails to move the eye medially to maintain conjugate gaze with the ipsilateral 6th nerve action (other third nerve function is normal).

3. Frequently associated with MS (especially if bilateral) or CVA.

G. Sixth nerve palsy:

1. Causes—elevated ICP, diabetes, cavernous sinus lesion, or Dorello canal inflammation.

2. Gradenigo syndrome—apical petrositis with sixth nerve palsy, V1- distribution retro-orbital pain, and a draining ear (due to infection).

H. Painful ophthalmoplegia:

1. Cause—often mucormycosis or diabetes.

2. Tolosa-Hunt syndrome—granulomatous inflammation of the cavernous sinus and superior orbital fissure.

I. Painless ophthalmoplegia—consider myasthenia gravis.

J. Raeder's paratrigeminal neuralgia—partial Horner syndrome (no anhidrosis) with numbness in the trigeminal distribution.

K. Syphilis—causes near-light dissociation; pupil accommodates but does not react.

XLI. Otology

A. Meniere disease (endolymphatic hydrops):

1. Signs/symptoms—vertigo (5–30-min episodes), emesis, tinnitus, and low-frequency hearing loss.

2. Evaluation—electronystagmography, audiogram, and MRI.

3. Treatment—salt restriction, diuretics, Diazepam, Antivert, avoidance of caffeine, eighth nerve sectioning, and shunting of the endolymphatic sac.

4. Rule out benign positional vertigo, vestibular schwannoma, and vestibular neuronitis.

B. Hearing loss—use Rinne test to differentiate conductive versus sensorineural hearing.

C. Tinnitus—consider glomus jugulare, dural arteriovenous fistula (AVF), and cavernous-carotid fistula.

XLII. Facial Nerve Syndromes

A. Facial palsy:

1. Causes—usually due to Bell's palsy, trauma, zoster, or tumor.

2. Treatment—repair with a direct anastomosis of XII, XI, or IX to VII.

B. Bell's palsy:

1. Cause—probably caused by a virus (usually herpes simplex virus [HSV], occasionally by Lyme disease).

2. Treatment—steroids and eye protection (gold weight or tarsorrhaphy).

3. Spontaneous recovery occurs in 80% (10% only partial); improvement begins in 3 weeks.

C. Branches of the facial nerve (from proximal to distal)—to geniculate ganglion (lacrimation), stapedial (hyperacusis), chorda tympani (salivation, taste), and facial motor.

D. Decreased facial sensation—consider hypocalcemia.

Helpful Hints

1. There is always a case of status epilepticus on oral board examination.

2. Know handedness and memory location before temporal lobectomy.

3. Don't confuse dementia with delusional state.

4. There is always a case of MS on oral board examination.

5. Amyotrophic lateral sclerosis (ALS) = progressive upper motor neurons (UMN) + lower motor neurons (LMN) signs, no sensory loss.

6. Guillain–Barré syndrome = acute symmetric proximal weakness, autonomic dysfunction.

7. Myasthenia gravis = weakness at end of day.

8. Causes of loss of consciousness—low blood flow (BF), hypoxia, hypoglycemia, seizure, drugs, high ICP.

Case 43

A 32-year-old woman presents with chronic headaches. Past medical history is significant for temporary visual disturbance 1 year earlier, multiple miscarriages, and obesity. Examination was normal.

Case 44

A 45-year-old man presents with gradual difficulty over the past year standing up from a chair. Past medical history is significant for smoking. Examination revealed ⅘ motor strength and mild atrophy in leg extensors, mild leg spasticity, and jerky tongue.

Case 45

A 45-year-old man presents with sudden difficulty over the past 2 days standing up from a chair, diplopia. Past medical history is significant for smoking, appendectomy 2 weeks ago followed by enteritis. Examination revealed ⅗ motor strength in hip extensors and areflexia.

Case Vignettes

Category 1: General Cases

Case No. 1

You are called to the emergency department (ED) to evaluate a 35-year-old male who was involved in a motor vehicle accident as an unrestrained driver at highway speeds. He was not thrown from the vehicle, but was noted to be unconscious at the scene and there was a prolonged extraction. He was subsequently intubated and paralyzed out of concern for airway protection. En route he received another dose of vecuronium prior to presentation to the ED.

Response

Initial examination and vital signs? Any other injuries?

The patient is intubated on assist control (AC) mode with 40% fraction of inspired oxygen (FiO$_2$) and 5 of positive end expiratory pressure (PEEP). Vital signs are stable and there is no evidence of any other injury except a laceration and large hematoma of the left parietal scalp. The neurologic examination is confounded by his paralytic, and he is currently a Glasgow Coma Scale (GCS) of 3t. His left pupil is 4 mm and reactive, his right pupil is 6 mm and sluggish.

Response

Advise to hold any further paralytics, raise the head of the bed to 30 degrees. Maintain normal blood pressure. Consider temporarily over-breathing the ventilator to an end-tidal carbon dioxide (CO$_2$) 25 to 30 mm Hg and administer 1 gm/kg of mannitol to lower likely elevated intracranial pressure. Obtain STAT head CT.

Head CT is shown in the figure.

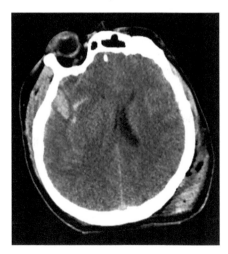

Further Reading

Greenberg MS. ICP management protocol: quick reference summary. In: Handbook of Neurosurgery, 8th ed. New York, NY: Thieme; 2016

Response

The patient's head computed tomography (CT) demonstrates a right frontotemporal contusion as well as right hemispheric edema causing a midline shift from right to left. This likely represents a contrecoup injury and the midline shift may explain his pupillary asymmetry and depressed examination. The patient should be taken to the operating room for immediate decompressive hemicraniectomy and placement of an external ventricular drain to both monitor intracranial pressure (ICP) as well as provide for cerebrospinal fluid (CSF) diversion if required. (Examinee should explain the planned procedure step by step.) The patient should be started on an antiepileptic regimen postoperatively.

Further Reading

Rey-Dios R, Esposito DP. Decompressive craniectomy for intracranial hypertension and stroke, including bone flap storage in abdominal fat layer. In: Ullman J, Rsksin B, eds. Atlas of Emergency Neurosurgery. New York, NY: Thieme; 2015:53–72

The patient recovers from the operation well. Postoperative intracranial pressure (ICP) is in the normal range. Over the next week, his examination improves and he is extubated. He follows commands bilaterally with some weakness on the left. He is minimally verbal but improving. On postoperative day 10 he appears worsened to nursing, with decreased function of his left upper extremity and now is non-verbal. His flap is very depressed and sunken.

Response

The patient likely has sinking skin flap syndrome or "syndrome of the trephined" and atmospheric pressure is causing the skin flap to sink and put pressure on the brain. He should undergo cranioplasty with or without shunt placement (depending on ventricular size and other markers of hydrocephalus).

Further Readings

Ullman JS. Replacement of cranial bone flap. In: Ullman J, Raksin P, eds. Atlas of Emergency Neurosurgery. New York, NY: Thieme; 2015:412–423
Sabbagh AJ, et al. Decompressive craniectomy. In: Nader R, Gragnaniello C, Berta S et al. eds. Neurosurgery Tricks of the Trade. Cranial. 1st ed. New York, NY: Thieme; 2014:505–511

Potential Other Complications

Misplaced ventriculostomy, hemorrhage due to torn sinus, cervical injury/plexus injury due to operating room (OR) positioning. Single hypertensive or hypoglycemic episode is associated with worse outcomes. Postoperative hygroma/hydrocephalus; contralateral subdural/epidural hematoma.

Case No. 2

You are asked to evaluate an 8- year-old woman in the emergency department (ED) who suffered a fall earlier in the day that was witnessed by family, who called emergency medical services (EMS). She reports "my right leg just gave out." She also states that she hit her head 3 days ago when opening a cupboard, and has had a headache since then. Her daughter is with her in the ED and states that she feels like the patient is having some trouble getting words out.

Response

What are the patient's vital signs and neurological examination reveal? Any use of anticoagulants and/or other significant medical conditions?

The patient's vitals are stable and she is awake, alert and oriented to person, place and time, but she states that the year is 1918. She can name three objects and repeat. On physical examination she has full strength of her left hemibody but has an appreciable pronator drift of the right upper extremity with corresponding weakness in a pyramidal distribution. She has 3/5 strength of the right hip flexors. She takes 81 mg of aspirin daily for heart health and has no other significant comorbidities.

Response

The patient should undergo head CT and basic labs should be obtained.

Basic laboratory tests are within normal limits and head CT is shown below.

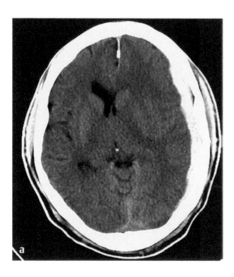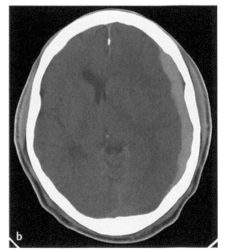

Response

The patient's head CT demonstrates a large, left-sided panhemispheric acute subdural hematoma with corresponding ventricular effacement and midline shift from left to right. This mass lesion explains her symptoms and meets criteria for surgical evacuation. Given her aspirin use, administration of platelets prior to the operating room (OR) can be considered. (Examinee should explain the planned procedure step by step.)

Further Reading

Timmons SD. Surgery for epidural and subdural hematomas. In: Ullman JS, Raksin P, eds. Atlas of Emergency Neurosurgery. New York, NY: Thieme; 2015:2–15

The patient tolerates the procedure well and recovers well in the postanesthesia care unit. The morning after surgery she is noted to be difficult to arouse, but after persistence she wakes up, however, she is very confused, alert to person only, and has clearly worsened right hemibody weakness. STAT head CT is negative for recurrence or new lesion. What is the cause?

Response

The patient may be experiencing focal or general seizures emanating from the irritated brain in the surgical bed. Spot electroencephalogram (EEG) should be considered, and administration or increase in automated external defibrillators (AEDs) should occur. Seizure prophylaxis can be used for 7 days in cases of epidural or subdural hematoma requiring surgery. Evidence of persistent seizure activity after evacuation may prompt longer duration of AED treatment.

Further Reading

Timmons SD. Extra-axial hematomas In: Loftus C, ed. Neurosurgical Emergencies. 3rd Edition. New York, NY: Thieme; 2017:60–71

Potential Other Complications

Infection, cerebrospinal fluid (CSF) leak, venous stroke, cardiac arrhythmias, hematoma recurrence.

Case No. 3

A 54-year-old man is referred to your clinic by a local neurologist after he was found to have the following lesion on magnetic resonance imaging (MRI). He initially presented to his primary care physician with headaches for several months. After failure of medical therapy the MRI was performed. On examination he reports a right hemispheric headache, but is otherwise neurologically intact. The local neurologist placed him on dexamethasone. He has no odd habits or history of drug use. There are no signs or symptoms suggestive of metastatic disease.

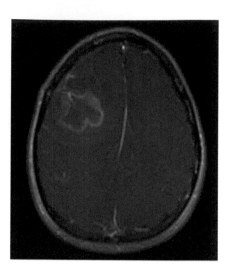

Response

The MRI scan demonstrates a ring-enhancing mass lesion within the right frontal lobe with corresponding vasogenic edema and mild right to left midline shift. While the differential can include glioblastoma, metastatic lesion, or abscess, this lesion is most likely to be a glioblastoma. Given the location, resection of the mass is feasible, and the patient should be scheduled for resection. Given its anterior and right frontal location, intraoperative mapping is not likely required. Intraoperative administration of dexamethasone and AED with postoperative MRI within 48 hours. (Examinee should explain the planned procedure step by step.)

Further Reading

Hassaneen W, Sawaya R. Glioma resection. In: Nader R, Gragnaniellло C, Berta S et al. eds. Neurosurgery Tricks of the Trade. Cranial. 1st ed. New York, NY: Thieme; 2014:62–65

You perform a complete resection of the mass and intraoperative pathology confirms high-grade glioma. The patient is recovered in the operating room (OR), but is noted to not able to move the left hemibody when the anesthetic is wearing off. The plegia continues into the postanesthesia care unit. On your examination there is increased tone on the left hemibody. You order a STAT head CT which demonstrates a resection cavity filled with

Response

The patient is likely experiencing a postoperative supplementary motor area (SMA) syndrome. Since the tumor is anterior in the frontal lobe, extensive resection could lead to a postoperative SMA. Importantly, the patient's tone is increased on the left, which suggests SMA, compared to flaccid paralysis, as may be seen in cases of damage to primary motor cortex. Rehabilitation should be consulted, and the patient should be counseled that recovery is expected usually over the ensuing days to weeks.

Further Reading

Gunel JM, Piepmeier JM. Perioperative management. In: Bernstein M, Berger M, eds. Neuro-Oncology: The Essentials. 3rd ed. New York, NY: Thieme; 2015:105–113
Warnick RE, Petr MJ. Complications of surgery. In: Bernstein M, Berger M, eds. Neuro-Oncology: The Essentials. 3rd ed. New York, NY: Thieme; 2015:167–177

Potential Other Complications

Postoperative hematoma; postoperative seizures, deep vein thrombosis/pulmonary embolism (DVT/PE), brain edema, pneumocephalus, meningitis, myocardial infarction, pneumonia.

Case No. 4

The neurology service asks you to perform a biopsy on a patient they are concerned has inflammatory neurodegeneration. They state that the patient has been NPO since midnight and are wondering when you have an availability to perform the biopsy?

Response

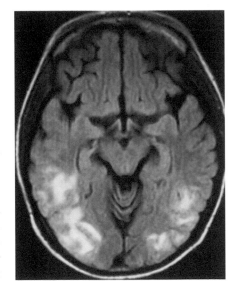

What is the patient's history, vital signs, and examination? Any Imaging?

The patient is a 63-year-old man on immunosuppressives for a kidney transplant who initially presented 3 days ago with confusion and subsequently developed evidence of seizure activity. He is currently controlled on 500 mg bid levetiracetam (Keppra), but his condition has been worsening since admission. He is now only oriented to person, but not place or time, and he had a breakthrough seizure yesterday requiring administration of IV lorazepam (Ativan) due to persistent seizure activity. He moves all four extremities spontaneously, but interestingly he does not appear to blink to threat, and does not track the examiner. Blood pressure has been elevated and difficult to control. It is currently 173/91. MRI is shown in the image.

Response

The patient's symptoms and imaging are suggestive of posterior reversible encephalopathy syndrome, or PRES. The elevated systolic blood pressure and predominately posterior parietal/occipital involvement are highly suggestive of this process. Blood pressure should be lowered to normal levels for the patient, immunosuppressive held if possible, and seizures should be controlled aggressively. This is believed to be a disorder of autoregulation. Supportive care should be continued until resolution, and the patient should remain in the ICU for monitoring of neurologic status during initial management. Biopsy is not indicated for this patient at this time.

Further Reading

Robinson TM, Stippler M. Posterior reversible encephalopathy syndrome. In: Harbaugh R, Shaffrey C, Couldwell W et al. eds. Neurosurgery Knowledge Update. A Comprehensive Review. 1st ed. New York, NY: Thieme; 2015:850–852

Intravenous antihypertensives are initiated and the blood pressure is lowered. When you are examining the patient yourself, he is noted to have a generalized, tonic-clonic seizure. It is persistent, and you have given a dose of 1 mg of Ativan with no effect. The seizure has persisted now for 5 minutes, what are the next steps?

Response

During the initial phase of status epilepticus, the patient should be evaluated for ABCs, intubating if required, and obtaining IV access if not present. After 5 minutes of activity, a benzodiazepine should be used. IV lorazepam (Ativan) can be used up to 0.1 mg/kg/dose (max 4 mg/dose, may repeat once). IM midazolam (Versed) 10 mg single dose and IV diazepam (Valium) up to 0.2 mg/kg/dose (max 10 mg, may repeat once). If no effect and seizures continue at 20 minutes, second-line therapy should be administered, either fosphenytoin (Cerebyx) (20 mg/kg bolus), Levetiracetam (Keppra) (60 mg/kg bolus) or valproic acid (40 mg/kg bolus). If still no effect and seizures last to 30 minutes, anesthetic agents should be used. Midazolam (Versed) (0.2 mg/kg bolus followed by infusion at 0.1–2.9 mg/kg/h), or propofol (1–2 mg/kg IV push, followed by 33 µg/kg/min infusion). Last-line therapy is pentobarbital (loading dose 5 mg/kg IV and maintenance dose of 1–5 mg/kg/h).

Further Reading

Fu AX, Hirsch LJ. Status epilepticus. In: Loftus C, ed. Neurosurgical Emergencies. 3rd ed. New York, NY: Thieme; 2017:164–173

Potential Other Complications

Hemorrhage, ischemic stroke, pneumonia.

Case No. 5

A patient comes to your clinic complaining of persistent headaches. When she is lying down her headaches improve substantially, however, when she sits up or stands for any length of time her headaches return. She does not have any other neurologic complaints at this time and her vital signs/examinations are within normal limits.

Response

The patient has symptoms consistent with positional headaches, and in this case, potential low pressure syndrome. An imaging study of the brain is indicated, either CT scan or MRI.

MRI Scan is shown in the photograph.

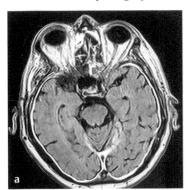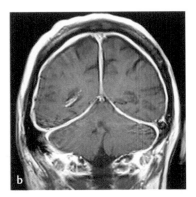

Response

The MRI scan demonstrates pachymeningeal enhancement and general sagging of the brain consistent with, and classic for a low pressure syndrome. There is no evidence of a causative lesion on this scan. Further imaging of the spine should be performed to evaluate for potential source of CSF leak.

Spine Imaging is shown in the photograph.

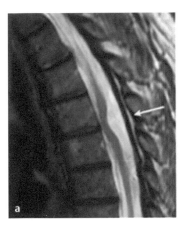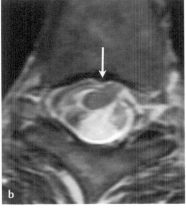

Response

The thoracic MRI demonstrates evidence of kinking of the spinal cord ventrally. On axial MRI the spinal cord is seen herniating through a ventral dural defect. With this degree of herniation, a patient would likely exhibit signs or symptoms of spinal cord pathology. In cases without herniation, a ventral dural defect can be challenging to evaluate. Cine MRI or CT myelography can be helpful. If a mild leak is suspected, bed rest and/or caffeine can be utilized. Epidural blood patches may have some efficacy. If a defect is seen, the patient should undergo intradural exploration at that level and closure of the defect. The dentate ligament can be cut to allow for access to the ventral space and defect closure. (Examinee should explain the planned procedure step by step.)

Further Reading

Greenberg MS. Hydrocephalus and cerebrospinal fluid. In: Handbook of Neurosurgery, 8th ed. New York, NY: Thieme; 2016:389–391

Conservative measures fail and the patient undergoes an intradural exploration and closure of a ventral dural defect. The patient's symptoms improve on postoperative day 1. On postoperative day 2 the patient develops her previous symptoms again and the nurse noticed some serosanguinous drainage from the incision.

Response

The return of symptoms are concerning for either continued drainage through the ventral defect, or development of a pseudomeningocele in the surgical cavity allowing egress of spinal fluid and return of symptoms. An image of the surgical cavity should be obtained.

A thoracic MRI is obtained and a large pseudomeningocele is demonstrated. The patient is taken back to the OR for drainage of the pseudomeningocele and closure of the dura.

Potential Other Complications

Persistent ventral leak, subdural hematoma, hygroma.

Case No. 6

You are evaluating a 73-year-old man who reports symptoms of low back and bilateral leg pain that have been bothering him for 6 months. He reports low back pain for "decades" but states that the onset of leg pain is more recent. The pain radiates from his lower back to the mid-thigh bilaterally, and is worsened when he goes for walks with his wife. He feels as though his legs are weaker recently. The pain is 75% leg, 25% back. His wife states that they take frequent sitting breaks during their walks to relieve his pain. He has seen his primary care provider and physical therapy has been ineffective to this point.

Response

His symptoms are concerning for pseudoclaudication, potentially due to lumbar spinal stenosis. He should undergo imaging including standing X-rays as well as a lumbar MRI. What is his examination?

His examination is notable for potential bilateral hip flexor weakness, although it is somewhat pain- limited. He has evidence of a distal peripheral neuropathy in a stocking distribution. His reflexes are normal and Hoffman sign is negative. X-rays demonstrated no bony defects. MRI is shown in the in the images.

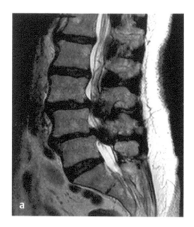 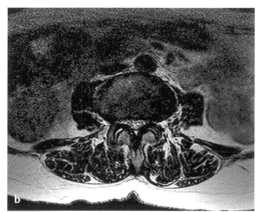

Response

This MRI demonstrates L3–4 and L4–5 spinal stenosis, which explains his presentation, and examination. Normal reflexes decrease the likelihood of coexistent cervical stenosis/myelopathy, but this should be considered. This patient should undergo nonoperative physical therapy trials and could consider epidural steroid injections for initial relief.

The patient receives an epidural steroid injection at L3–4 and undergoes 6 weeks of physical therapy. The steroid injection was immensely helpful, but the pain has returned. Physical therapy has not yielded any further improvement.

Response

The patient should be cleared medically for a surgery, and should undergo a lumbar decompression targeting L3–4 and L4–5. (Examinee should explain the planned procedure step by step.)

Further Reading

Jalabe CC, Berbeo Calderon ME, Diaz R, et al. Lumbar epidural steroid injections. In: Nader R, Gragnanielllo C, Berta S et al. eds. Neurosurgery Tricks of the Trade. Spine and Peripheral Nerves. 1st ed. New York, NY: Thieme; 2014:338–340

Gragnanielllo C, Nader R. Lumbar laminectomy and laminotomy. In: Nader R, Gragnaniellllo C, Berta S et al. eds. Neurosurgery Tricks of the Trade. Spine and Peripheral Nerves. 1st ed. New York, NY: Thieme; 2014:110–113

The patient undergoes a standard L3–4, L4–5 laminectomy where severe spinal stenosis was observed. The patient is doing well immediately postop, and the Foley catheter has been removed. During the evening, the nurse calls, reporting a severe worsening of the patient's pain, and that while he was initially voiding spontaneously, she had to perform straight catheterization due to a high volume on post-void residual scanning. The patient told her that he had no sensation during the catheterization, which was new.

Response

This patient has new severe pain, urinary retention, and saddle anesthesia, all symptoms concerning for cauda equina syndrome, especially in a patient who just underwent a lumbar laminectomy. This likely represents an epidural hematoma in the operative bed, and the patient should either go for STAT imaging, or directly to the OR for exploration of the surgical bed. Time is critical, so if imaging will cause any significant delay, proceeding directly to the OR is warranted.

Further Reading

Gragnaniello C, Albanese R, Chau AMT, et al. Cauda equina syndrome. In: Nader R, Gragnaniellllo C, Berta S et al. eds. Neurosurgery Tricks of the Trade. Spine and Peripheral Nerves. 1st ed. New York, NY: Thieme; 2014:394–398

The patient is taken to the OR and the wound is explored. A large hematoma is found compressing the spinal canal. After removal of the hematoma, a bleeding epidural vein is discovered and cauterized. The patient recovers well.

Potential Other Complications

Durotomy, iatrogenic damage to the pars.

Case No. 7

You are asked to consult on a 52-year-old woman who underwent a screening CT angiogram (due to a family history of two sisters and mother who suffered a ruptured intracranial aneurysm). She was told she has an irregularity of a blood vessel on the right side of her brain. Unfortunately she did not bring her previous imaging to this consult.

Response

It sounds like the patient has a significant family history of intracranial aneurysms, is she a smoker and/or does she have hypertension? Given the likely presence of an aneurysm on the prior CT angiogram, she should undergo a conventional diagnostic cerebral angiogram (required imaging varies among providers, as some will treat with

CT or MR angiogram only, while others will obtain formal cerebral angiogram). What is her examination?

The patient has been treated for hypertension for as long as she can remember, and she has a 30 pack-year history of smoking, although she says she is trying to quit. On examination she has no focal deficits. She underwent a conventional angiogram and the results are shown in the image on next page. The radiologist compared these images to the previous CTA and reports that over the past 6 months the aneurysm has increased in size by approximately 3 mm. The endovascular team could not adequately access the aneurysm for coiling or stenting.

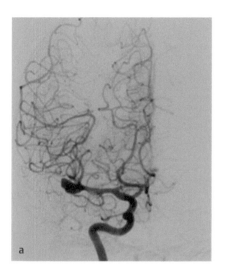

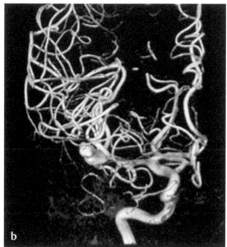

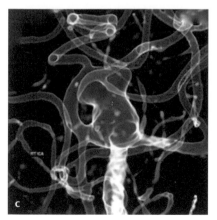

Response

The angiogram demonstrates an irregularly shaped aneurysm of the right MCA bifurcation with a recent history of growth in a hypertensive smoker with a family history of ruptured aneurysms. This is a high-risk aneurysm that likely does not fall into the standard ISUIA natural history. It should undergo treatment. Given the difficulty with endovascular approaches, a standard craniotomy and aneurysm clipping should be performed. (Examinee should explain the planned procedure step by step.)

Further Readings

Lawton M. Pterional approach. In: Seven Aneurysms. Tenets and Techniques for Clipping. 1st ed. New York, NY: Thieme; 2011:29–31
Lawton M. Middle cerebral artery aneurysms. In: Seven Aneurysms. Tenets and Techniques for Clipping. 1st ed. New York, NY: Thieme; 2011:65–93

The patient undergoes a right-sided craniotomy for clipping of the aneurysm. The Sylvian fissure is split and the aneurysm dome is identified. While mobilizing the aneurysm in an attempt to achieve better visualization of the proximal M1 segment and lenticulostriate perforators, the operative field suddenly fills with pulsatile, arterial blood.

Response

The aneurysm has ruptured, and anesthesia should be notified of the potential for significant blood loss. Two large-bore suctions should be utilized in an attempt to decrease the volume of blood in the surgical cavity and to help identify the source of bleeding. If the source can be identified, a suction and cottonoid patty should be used in an attempt to divert the bleeding while proximal control is obtained. A temporary clip should be placed across the M1 segment proximal to the aneurysm. Given the difficulty in this maneuver, it is possible that a lenticulostriate perforating vessel is captured by the temporary clip, and a timer should be considered. It is likely that a proximal clip will decrease the rate of blood egress but not completely eliminate it due to arterial backflow. A temporary clip should be placed across the aneurysm neck and the M1 clip should be removed, restoring normal flow. The temporary clip can be inspected to ensure no other vessels have been occluded by the clip. Now the aneurysm can be permanently clipped.

Further Reading

Lawton M. Intraoperative rupture. In: Seven Aneurysms. Tenets and Techniques for Clipping. 1st ed. New York, NY: Thieme; 2011:25–26

Case No. 8

You are consulted by the inpatient neurology service regarding an 8- year-old man who was admitted to their service after experiencing the onset of mild dysarthria and a left pronator drift, although these seem to have improved since admission. He further reports an episode approximately 1 month ago where he suddenly lost vision in his right eye, but his vision returned after a brief period of time. He has a history of hypertension and takes aspirin 81 mg daily.

Response

The patient's symptoms are concerning for a right hemispheric TIA, and a prior instance of right amaurosis fugax, both suggestive of potential extracranial carotid atherosclerotic disease. If there is no concern for cardioembolic phenomena, the carotid arteries should be imaged to evaluate for stenosis.

As a part of his initial workup, he underwent an MRI of the brain (which demonstrated no areas of restricted diffusion) as well as MRA of the neck, which is shown in the image given on next page.

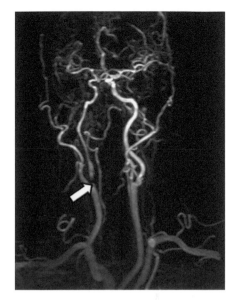

Response

The MRA demonstrates critical stenosis of the right internal carotid artery at the level of the bifurcation. While the specific degree of stenosis is not reported, it is clearly greater than 50%, and in this 84 year-old man with hypertension, this symptomatic carotid stenosis should be treated based on NASCET criteria. Surgery or carotid angioplasty and stenting could be considered based on patient and lesion characteristics. (Examinee should explain the planned procedure step by step.) Remember the appropriate steps for releasing clamps at the end of the procedure to make sure all emboli and air are flushed into the external carotid and not the internal carotid.

Further Reading

Ackerman P, Loftus C. Symptomatic extracranial carotid artery stenosis. In: Harbaugh R, Shaffrey C, Couldwell W, et al. eds. Neurosurgery Knowledge Update. A Comprehensive Review. 1st ed. New York, NY: Thieme; 2015:94–98

You elect to perform a right carotid endarterectomy, and you have cross-clamped the common carotid artery. After your arteriotomy, your monitoring technician informs you that there are decreased responses from the right hemisphere compared to the left.

Response

The patient may not have an intact circle of Willis, or the flow from the contralateral hemisphere is not strong enough to perfuse the right hemisphere. This patient will likely require an intraoperative, common-to-internal carotid artery shunt. Flow is then restored to the right hemisphere through the shunt while the plaque removal proceeds around the shunt. The patch is sewn in around the shunt, which is not removed until the very end, when the carotid is cross-clamped again and the final suture repair occurs.

Further Reading

Mukherjee D, Kfoury E. Carotid endarterectomy: vascular surgery perspective > surgical technique. In: Sekhar L, Fessler R eds. Atlas of Neurosurgical Techniques: Brain, Volume 1. 2nd ed. New York, NY: Thieme; 2016:598–600

Potential Other Complications

Hypoglossal nerve injury, spinal accessory nerve injury, postoperative hematoma, postoperative carotid occlusion, myocardial infarction.

Further Reading

Howington JU. Carotid endarterectomy: decision analysis and surgical technique > complications of carotid endarterectomy. In: Bendok B, Naidech A, Walker M, et al. eds. Hemorrhagic and Ischemic Stroke. Medical, Imaging, Surgical and Interventional Approaches. 1st ed. New York, NY: Thieme; 2012:221–233

Case No. 9

You are evaluating a 27-year-old man in the emergency department. He appears disheveled, and is clearly very confused and agitated. He is febrile to 39°C and tachycardic to 115. He moves all four extremities spontaneously but does not follow commands due to agitation. As you are attempting to continue the examination he becomes unresponsive and starts to have a generalized seizure.

Response

The patient is having a seizure and initial management should focus on ABCs. He had a concerning neurologic status before the seizure, and now warrants airway protection. He should be intubated and given IV lorazepam (Ativan) in an attempt to break the seizure. IV access should be obtained and basic labs as well as blood cultures should be sent. As soon as deemed safe, imaging of the brain, CT or MRI should be obtained.

The patient is intubated, 2 mg lorazepam (Ativan) is administered, and the seizure stops. IV access is present and lab values demonstrate normal hemoglobin, a significant leukocytosis, but otherwise normal electrolyte levels, including glucose. Sedation with propofol is started and he is taken for MRI of the brain, which is shown in the image on next page.

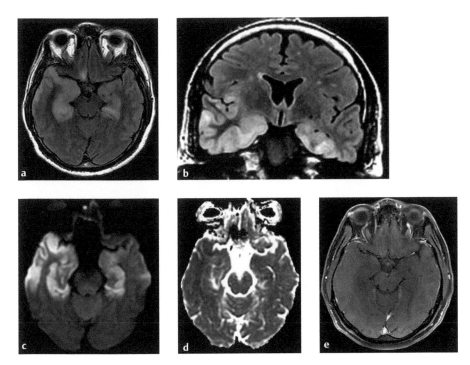

Response

The patient's MRI demonstrates hyperintensities of the bilateral temporal lobes, very concerning for herpes encephalitis, and the patient's presentation would fit this diagnosis. He should immediately be started on acyclovir (30 mg/kg/d divided over Q8h doses). Cerebrospinal fluid (CSF) should be sampled via lumbar puncture (up to three times as false-negatives can occur). The herpes simplex virus (HSV) polymerase chain reaction (PCR) can take a couple of days or up to 2 weeks to return positive.

Further Reading

Greenberg M. Other nonbacterial infections > herpes simplex encephalitis. In: Handbook of Neurosurgery. 8th ed. New York, NY: Thieme; 2016:364–366

The patient was started on acyclovir and a lumbar puncture (LP) was performed. There was a monocytosis of the CSF, but initial LP was negative for HSV. A second LP was performed 3 days later which showed a mild decrease in the monocytosis, but the HSV PCR returned positive. The patient remained in a comatose state for the 12 days despite adequate treatment with acyclovir. A tracheostomy was performed and supportive care was continued. On hospital day 13 the nurse noted that the patient has been coughing regularly and appears agitated. Oxygen saturation has decreased, and the nurse has had to increase the oxygen via tracheostomy mask. A chest X-ray (CXR) is obtained which is negative for consolidation.

Response

The patient has been comatose and immobile for 13 days and is at high risk for development of a deep venous thrombosis (DVT) and/or pulmonary embolism (PE). Given the coughing, decreased O_2 saturation and CXR negative for pneumonia, CT angiogram PE protocol should be ordered to evaluate the lungs for PE. Given the pulmonary symptoms, the pretest probability is already high, and CTA should be performed rather than simple lower extremity Doppler ultrasound, which will likely demonstrate DVTs.

CT angiogram of the lungs demonstrates a segmental filling defect consistent with PE.

Response

If the patient does not have any extreme contraindications, heparin should be administered. During heparin administration, platelets should be monitored to identify heparin–induced thrombocytopenia (HIT) if it occurs. The vascular medicine team can be consulted regarding potential long-term treatment options. Given that herpes encephalitis can lead to hemorrhagic destruction of the temporal lobes, repeat imaging should be performed to confirm stability of intracranial pathology prior to and perhaps during heparin administration.

Further Reading

Pineo G, Hamilton M. Venous thromboembolism (DVT and PE): diagnosis and treatment. In: Hamilton M, Golfinos J, Pineo G, et al. eds. Handbook of Bleeding and Coagulation for Neurosurgery. 1st ed. New York, NY: Thieme; 2015:117–152

Potential Other Complications

Intracranial hemorrhage, hydrocephalus, ventilator-associated pneumonia, meningitis, rates of false-negative on biopsy/CSF studies.

Case No. 10

A 1- year-old girl is brought to your office by her mother with intermittent headaches that have been occurring over the past year. They seem to be worsened by coughing, which she reports her daughter has been doing more frequently while eating lately. After a few bites of food she will start coughing and in turn develop a significant headache, becoming very irritable. The headache is also brought on by extension of her neck.

Response

The patient has symptoms that are potentially referable to the craniocervical junction, and given her specific symptoms, a Chiari malformation may be present. She should undergo MRI of the cervical spine extending into the supratentorial space to evaluate for Chiari malformation. A complete neurologic exam should also be performed.

On examination she demonstrates mild hyperreflexia but preserved strength throughout. There are no sensory abnormalities. She has slight, left-sided uvular deviation but otherwise no cranial nerve abnormalities. There is no papilledema. She undergoes MRI of the cervical spine which is shown in the image.

Response

This T2-sagittal MRI demonstrates a Chiari I malformation with cerebellar tonsillar herniation through the foramen magnum. The herniation is clearly more than 5 mm and more importantly is symptomatic, so she should undergo surgical decompression. She would be offered a suboccipital craniotomy/craniectomy with decompression of the posterior fossa and removal

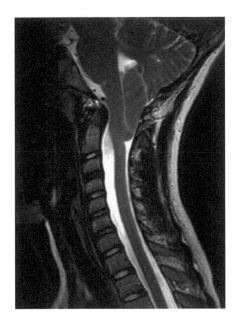

of the C1 lamina. While a syrinx is not present in this case, it may be in others. Often, simple treatment of the Chiari malformation will lead to resolution of the syrinx without direct treatment of the syrinx itself. Given the degree of tonsillar herniation, a duraplasty with tonsillar reduction could be considered. (Examinee should explain the planned procedure step by step.)

Further Reading

Hickman Z, Feldstein N. The Chiari I malformation. In: Cohen A, ed. Pediatric Neurosurgery: Tricks of the Trade. 1st ed. New York, NY: Thieme; 2016:210–221

The patient tolerates the procedure well and postoperatively her symptoms abate. She is discharged on postoperative day 2 and returns home. You receive a call on postoperative day 4 from her mother who states that her headaches have returned and are fairly severe. She seems very irritable and has worsening of her pain when she bends her head forward. She has a temperature of 39°C.

Response

These symptoms are concerning for ether infectious meningitis or aseptic meningitis. The patient should return and be evaluated in the emergency department, including imaging and CSF sampling (protein, glucose, cell count, and culture).

The patient returns, imaging is normal and she is febrile with a mild peripheral leukocytosis, irritable with headache and has mild meningismus. A lumbar puncture (LP) is performed which demonstrates a normal cell count, mildly elevated protein, normal glucose and the initial Gram stain is negative for the presence of any bacteria, culture is pending.

Response

The patient should be admitted to the hospital for monitoring, and started on broad-spectrum antibiotics (vancomycin and cefepime for example). Given the reassuring CSF studies, this is most likely to be aseptic meningitis from the duraplasty performed, and her symptoms should resolve over time, and may benefit from low-dose administration of dexamethasone.

The patient's CSF remains negative, and low-dose dexamethasone improved her symptoms dramatically. Antibiotics are stopped as infection is ruled out. She normalizes after 2 days and is discharged home.

Potential Other Complications

Hydrocephalus, meningitis, pseudomeningocele, superficial siderosis, symptom recurrence from inadequate decompression, vertebral artery injury, sinus injury, air embolism.

Category 2: Neurology Mimics

Case No. 1

Central Nervous System (CNS) Lymphoma

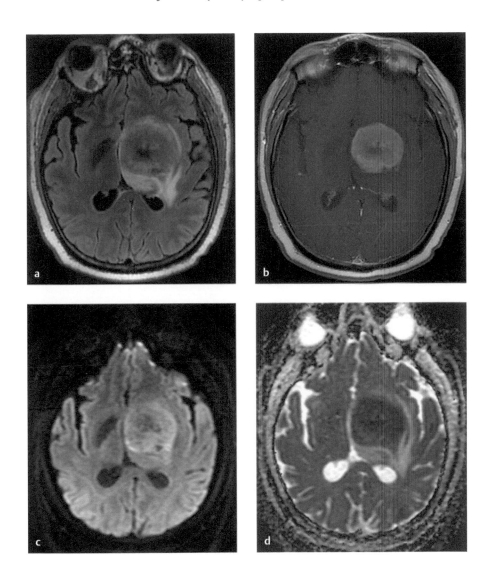

Primary central nervous system (CNS) lymphoma can be mistaken for other CNS neoplasms that require gross total resection; however, CNS lymphoma is sensitive to chemotherapy and radiation. Images of CNS lymphoma presentations are shown. If there are odd features for a given mass lesion, lymphoma should be considered, and a biopsy performed to provide tissue diagnosis. If lymphoma is discovered on intraoperative pathology, the resection should be stopped as there is not significant evidence that gross total resection provides superior outcomes to chemotherapy and radiation.

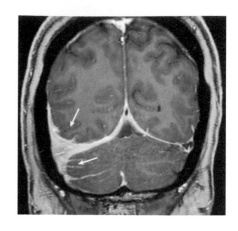

Further Reading

Tsyvkin E, DeAngelis L. Primary central nervous system lymphoma. In: Bernstein M, Berger M eds. Neuro-oncology: The Essentials. 3rd ed. New York, NY: Thieme; 2015:439–450

Case No. 2

Eagle Syndrome

Eagle syndrome is characterized by pain in the distribution of the glossopharyngeal nerve (ear, neck, pharynx, and tongue) caused by compression of cranial nerve (CN) IX by an elongated styloid process (as shown in the image). Symptoms are often worsened by turning the neck. This can be a key distinguishing factor between glossopharyngeal neuralgia and Eagle syndrome. Conservative management is recommended, but if severe, the patient could undergo resection of the styloid process.

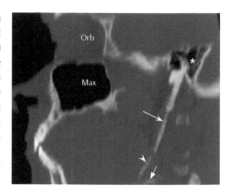

Further Reading

Binder D, Sonne D, Fischbein N. Glossopharyngeal nerve > glossopharyngeal nerve: pathologic images. Cranial Nerves: Anatomy, Pathology, Imaging. 1st ed. New York, NY: Thieme; 2010:151–157

Di Ieva A, Lee J, Cusimano M. Clinical and neurologic findings in skull base pathology > Skull base syndromes. In: Handbook of Skull Base Surgery. 1st ed. New York, NY: Thieme; 2016:183–185

Case No. 3

Meniere disease

Meniere disease causes attacks of violent vertigo with associated tinnitus and hearing loss. One of the keys to diagnosis is that the patient will report tinnitus that sounds like "escaping steam." Attacks can last from minutes to hours and from several times per year to several times per week. Differential diagnosis includes benign paroxysmal positional vertigo (BPPV), vertebrobasilar insufficiency, and vestibular schwannoma. Thought to be due to abnormal regulation of endolymphatic fluid, leading to increased volume and pressure within the endolymph. Imaging will be negative. Treatment entails reduction of salt intake and diuretics. Surgical treatment is rare but can involve endolymphatic shunting, corticosteroid application, and even selective vestibular neurectomy.

Further Reading

Greenberg M. Neurotology > Meniere disease. In: Handbook of Neurosurgery. 8th ed. New York, NY: Thieme; 2016:573–576

Case No. 4

Dementia with Lewy Body Disease

Patients who develop dementia with Lewy bodies have several distinguishing features to help differentiate between Alzheimer dementia (AD) and Parkinsonism with dementia. Patients who develop dementia with Lewy bodies often have the onset of dementia initially, followed by Parkinsonian symptoms (rigidity, bradykinesia, slow shuffling gate) that develop later. This distinguishes the patient from AD, where Parkinsonian features are not present. In Parkinsonism with dementia, the Parkinsonian features occur first, followed by dementia onset at least 12 months later. Another common differentiating feature is visual hallucinations and depression. On imaging, there will be a lack of temporal lobe atrophy (as compared to AD). There is no current medical therapy targeted to dementia with Lewy bodies, however, cholinesterase inhibitors may have some effect on neuropsychiatric and cognitive symptoms.

Further Reading

Capizzano A, Moritani T. Dementia with Lewy body disease. In: Kanekar S, ed. Imaging of Neurodegenerative Disorders. 1st ed. New York, NY: Thieme; 2016:150–156

Case No. 5

Neuromyelitis Optica

Neuromyelitis optica (NMO) is a demyelinating condition that involves three or more levels within the spine and also presents with visual symptoms from optic neuritis. This condition is mediated by antibodies against the aquaporin-4 protein. It is important to think of NMO whenever there is longitudinal edema within the spinal cord present on imaging (as shown in the image). There is rarely brain involvement in this condition. Any patient with these findings on imaging, but also with visual symptoms should undergo workup for demyelinating disease prior to any cervical spine intervention.

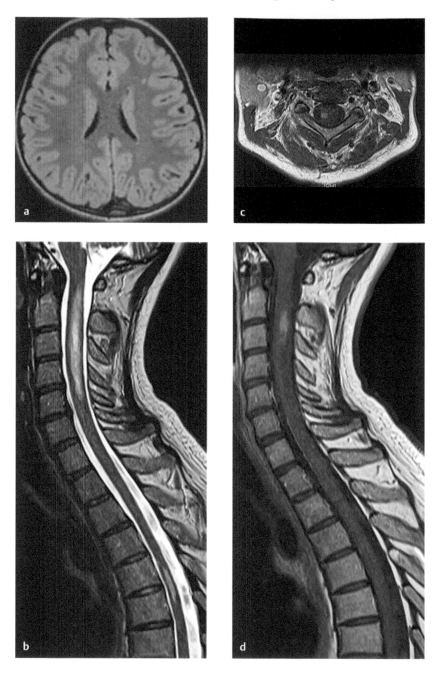

Further Reading

Choudhri A. Infection and inflammation > inflammatory processes. In: Pediatric Neuroradiology. Clinical Practice Essentials. 1st ed. New York, NY: Thieme; 2017:86–88

Case No. 6

Indications/Contraindications for IV tPA

The initial study of IV tPA use during acute ischemic stroke demonstrated a favorable outcome odds ratio of 2.81 with administration at 90 minutes, and 1.55 with administration by 180 minutes. There is a risk of hemorrhage of roughly 6%, but nearly 30% of patients will be symptom-free at 3 months with IV thrombolysis. More recently, the time window has been extended to 4.5 hours since the patient was last seen normal or symptom onset. It is important to understand the contraindications for IV TPA administration.

Contraindications

- Stroke/serious head injury within 3 months.
- Evidence of intracranial hemorrhage or established computed tomography (CT) hypodensity > one-third of middle carotid artery (MCA) territory.
- Active internal bleeding or evidence of arteriovenous malformation (AVM), aneurysm, or certain neoplasms.
- Heparin or warfarin administration with activated partial thromboplastin time (aPTT) elevation or international normalized ratio (INR) >1.7 within past 48 hours.
- Platelet count below 100,000, blood glucose below 50 mg/dL.
- Persistent hypertension despite treatment (systolic blood pressure [SBP] >185, diastolic blood pressure [DBP] >110).
- Arterial puncture at noncompressible site within past 7 days.

Further Reading

Jones M, Schneck M, Ashley W Jr, et al. Chemical thrombolysis and mechanical thrombectomy for acute Ischemic stroke. In: Loftus C, ed. Neurosurgical Emergencies. 3rd ed. New York, NY: Thieme; 2018:106–114

Case No. 7

Eosinophilic Granuloma: Vertebra Plana (Flattened Vertebral Body)

Eosinophilic granuloma of the spine is benign, but destructive lesions that affect the pediatric population most frequently. They present with localized pain and occasionally with neurologic symptoms due to local compression or irritation. The subsequent vertebra plana (as shown in the image) can lead to spinal deformity and further symptoms.

They should not be mistaken for an aggressive spinal tumor. The lesions themselves contain histiocytes, and if lesions are found in other regions, the patient may have histiocytosis X or Hand-Schuller-Christian disease. Intervention for these patients should only be undertaken for neurologic deficit or progressive deformity. Patients without symptoms can likely be observed and/or braced.

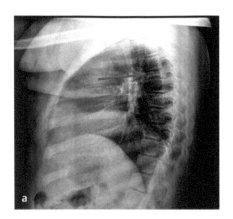
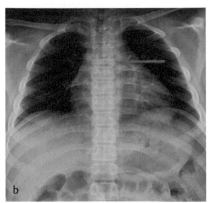
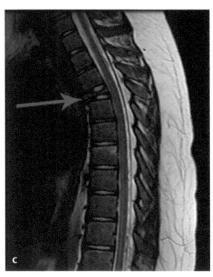

Further Reading

Harter D, Weiner H. Spine tumors. In: Albright A, Pollack I, Adelson P eds. Principles and Practice of Pediatric Neurosurgery. 3rd ed. New York, NY: Thieme; 2015:614–625

Case No. 8

Acute Inflammatory Demyelinating Polyradiculoneuropathy (AIDP or Guillain–Barré Syndrome)

Acute inflammatory demyelinating polyradiculoneuropathy (AIDP) or Guillain–Barré syndrome is characterized by ascending, symmetric motor weakness with areflexia and preservation of sensation. Weakness may begin in proximal leg muscles (differs from classic neuropathies that often begin distally) and ascend to involve the upper extremities and cranial nerves in up to 50% of patients over time. Dysautonomia is common (70%) and vital sign changes can be rapid. This condition has multiple causes, but oftentimes a previous viral or bacterial infection (campylobacter jejuni classically) precede the symptoms. Cerebrospinal fluid (CSF) demonstrates albuminocytologic disassociation (elevated protein with normal or low white cell count). Treatment involves plasma exchange or intravenous immunoglobulin (IVIG) and observation. The most concerning symptoms are respiratory compromise and ventilator failure, which can occur in up to 30% of patients. They should be admitted to the neuro intensive care unit (ICU) and respiratory function testing (forced vital capacity and negative inspiratory force) should be performed every 2 to 6 hours. It is important to understand the indications for intubation in these patients.

Indications

* Steadily declining NIF and/or vital capacity (VC)
* Negative inspiratory force (NIF) worse than -20 cm H_2O
* VC less than 10 to 15 mL/kg

Case No. 9

Prion Disease: Avoid Biopsy without Proper Precautions

Creutzfeldt–Jakob disease (CJD) is a prion-mediate neurodegenerative condition that is fatal and highly contagious. Patients often present with mutism, myoclonus, and rapid cognitive decline. CSF can be sent to check for 14–3-3 protein which is very sensitive and specific for CJD. Electroencephalogram (EEG) will demonstrate periodic sharp waves, and this finding has a sensitivity of 67% and specificity of 86%. Magnetic resonance imaging (MRI) can have a classic appearance with restricted diffusion throughout the cortex, as shown in the image. You will be asked to perform biopsy on this patient, but it is important to note that any equipment used during a biopsy procedure must be quarantined and undergo substantial decontamination may be required. The protein is highly contagious and is not removed with standard autoclave treatments, making reuse of the equipment a risk for contamination of future patients.

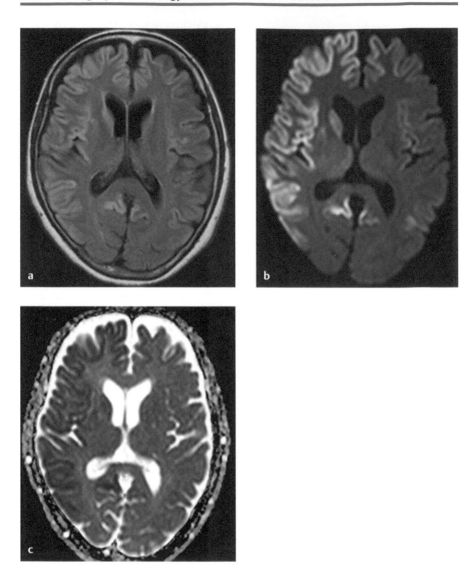

Further Reading

Baruah D, Mohan S, Wang S. Diffusion tensor imaging in neurodegenerative disorders > Human prion disease. In: Kanekar S, ed. Imaging of Neurodegenerative Disorders. 1st ed. New York, NY: Thieme; 2016:44

Case No. 10

Bell's Palsy

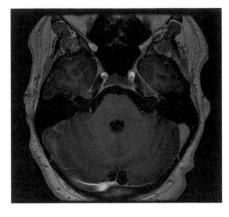

Bell's Palsy is a cause of unilateral facial nerve weakness that begins over 2 to 3 days and may last for up to 6 weeks. It is often preceded by an upper respiratory tract infection, and patients report facial weakness as well as a sensation of fullness in the ear. The causative agent is thought to be herpes simplex virus, and nearly 75% of patients will have an excellent outcome with spontaneous resolution. It is important to determine which patients may benefit from further treatment. MRI can demonstrate asymmetric enhancement of the facial nerve (as shown in the image). Steroids, including prednisone (1 mg/kg initially followed by taper), have been used if the patient can tolerate steroid-induced side effects. It is not certain if steroids provide substantial benefit for a condition that does spontaneously abate. Electroneurography (EnoG) of the facial nerve can be used to help determine which patients may require invasive treatment, including surgical decompression. If there is complete paralysis on examination, no voluntary potentials demonstrated on EnoG, and response degradation more than 90%, decompression of the facial nerve via a middle fossa approach can be considered.

Further Reading

Adunka O, Buchman C. Disease-specific diagnostics and medical management > Disorders of the facial nerve. In: Otology, Neurotology, and Lateral Skull Base Surgery. An Illustrated Handbook. 1st ed. Stuttgart: Thieme; 2011:216–223

Category 3: Spine

Case No. 1

A patient is sent to you for evaluation of persistent back pain and progressive weakness of both lower extremities. She is 34 years old and has no history of back problems. Her primary care provider obtained basic X-rays which were normal, had her complete a short trial of physical therapy which did not help, and sent her to you for further evaluation due to progressive weakness.

Response

The patient should undergo a complete neurologic examination to better document her weakness as well as any sensory abnormalities. Given the weakness, further imaging, preferably magnetic resonance imaging (MRI) of the lumbar spine should be performed.

On examination the patient has preserved distal strength, but there is appreciable weakness (4-) in bilateral hip flexors. Reflexes are normal, and there are noticeable sensory abnormalities in the S2–4 regions. Lumbar spine MRI is shown in the image.

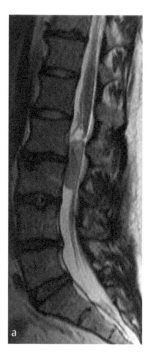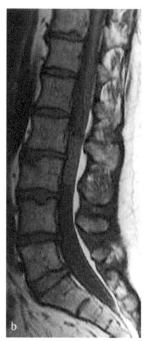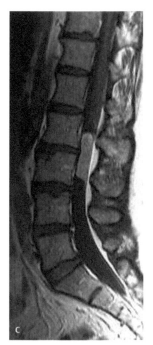

Response

The imaging of the lumbar spine demonstrates an enhancing mass lesion associated with the conus medullaris. It appears to be well-circumscribed and may be associated with the filum terminale. This lesion is likely to be a myxopapillary ependymoma. The patient should undergo intradural exploration and resection of this lesion. It will be important during surgery to completely identify the entirety of the tumor as well as its proximal and distal connection points to the filum. Attempts should be made to completely excise the tumor without violating the capsule if at all possible. Local recurrence rates after surgery increase significantly if the tumor capsule is violated. Care should be taken to avoid injuring any nerve roots in the region, as they could be draped around the tumor. Intraoperative monitoring could be considered as an aid for surgery. (Examinee should explain the planned procedure step by step.)

The patient is taken to surgery for tumor resection and intraoperative pathology is consistent with myxopapillary ependymoma. The distal attachment is easily identified and transected. The tumor is progressively removed toward its proximal attachment. At the conus, it is apparent that the tumor does not easily peel off the conus itself. Despite several maneuvers, no easily identifiable plane can be generated between the conus and the tumor capsule.

Response

While complete excision of the tumor with its attachments to the filum without violating the capsule can be curative, in this case, aggressively attempting to re-sect the portion that is adherent to the conus medullaris could lead to significant postoperative morbidity, as any violation of the conus can cause severe, permanent deficits. The tumor should be completely excised, but the adherent portion should be left in place if it cannot be safely removed. Attempts to destroy the tumor tissue with a bipolar cautery could be considered if the damage doesn't transfer to the normal conus tissue. Leaving the adherent portion will likely lead to higher rates of local recurrence, but this could be treated with repeat surgery or radiation. It is not worth giving the patient permanent deficits from conus injury to achieve a complete excision.

Further Reading

Tubbs RS, Oakes WJ. Resection of cauda equina ependymomas. In: Fessler R, Sekhar L, eds. Atlas of Neurosurgical Techniques. Spine and Peripheral Nerves. 2nd ed. New York, NY: Thieme; 2016:707–710

Potential Other Complications

Capsule violation, encasement of nerve roots, deep venous thrombosis (DVT), wound infection.

Case No. 2

You are consulted by the medicine inpatient team regarding a 42-year-old man who was admitted to their service after progressively worsening back pain, but no other neurologic deficits on detailed examination. He has a history of intravenous (IV) drug use and was found to be bacteremic with Staphylococcus aureus growing from his blood cultures. Given his back pain, the primary team obtained an MRI of the lumbar spine which is shown in the image. They have consulted you based on the findings.

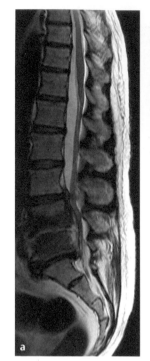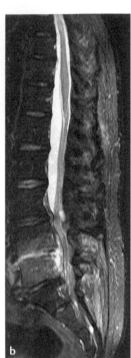

Response

This patient appears to have diskitis/osteomyelitis of the L4/L5 vertebral bodies with an associated epidural abscess. The primary team has identified a likely causative organism and IV antibiotics should be administered, targeted to the identified organism. The epidural abscess is concerning, given that it appears to be compressing the thecal sac; however, currently the patient does not have any neurologic deficits, and observation/antibiotics should be the initial management. Nearly 75% of these cases may resolve with immobilization (bracing) and targeted antibiotics. Serial erythrocyte sedimentation rate/C-reactive proteins (ESR/CRPs) can be used to track progress of the infection/treatment.

Further Reading

Hofstetter C, Wang M. Infections of the spine. In: Harbaugh R, Shaffrey C, Couldwell W, et al. eds. Neurosurgery Knowledge Update. A Comprehensive Review. 1st ed. New York, NY: Thieme; 2015:608–614

Varthi AG, Long W III, Toy J, et al. Infction > Pyogenic vertebral osteomyelitis and diskitis. In: Baaj A, Mummaneni P, Uribe J, et al. eds. Handbook of Spine Surgery. 2nd ed. New York, NY: Thieme; 2016:156–158

The patient is started on IV vancomycin and a brace is utilized. Four days later, the medicine team calls again stating that the nurse noticed this morning the patient was retaining urine and appeared to have weakness in his left leg. Specifically, he couldn't raise it off the bed against gravity. They obtained another MRI which showed slight worsening of the epidural abscess.

Response

The new neurologic deficit is worrisome for ongoing compression of the neural elements by the epidural abscess despite antibiotic treatment. The patient should be scheduled for surgical decompression of the epidural phlegmon. Likely a L3–5 laminectomy and decompression will suffice, ensuring the thecal sac is circumferentially decompressed; however, ventral exploration could be performed during the procedure by gentle retraction of the dura to better access the ventral component of the epidural abscess for removal. The wound should be debrided and washed out as well. (Examinee should explain the planned procedure step by step.)

The patient is taken to surgery and an L3–5 decompressive laminectomy is performed successfully. Significant compression of the thecal sac is encountered. When the thecal sac is being slightly retracted to remove ventral phlegmon, a brisk cerebrospinal fluid (CSF) leak is observed.

Response

The CSF leak should be completely identified and repaired primarily. Abscess tissue should be sent for culture to ensure all potential causative organisms are identified. With an intraoperative CSF leak in an infected spine, the chance of the patient developing meningitis has increased. Therefore the patient should be closely observed after surgery for any signs or symptoms of neurologic decline that might be suggestive of meningitis. Prior to patient discharge from the hospital, obtaining CSF for labs/culture via a safe venue (not likely through lumbar puncture in this patient) could be considered to ensure adequate treatment of any potential meningitis.

Potential Other Complications

Instability on flexion/extension films, abscess recurrence.

Case No. 3

You are called to the emergency department (ED) to evaluate a 37-year-old woman who was involved in a motor vehicle collision at highway speeds. She is awake but mildly sedated in the trauma bay, and she is not moving any of her extremities. She is in a cervical collar and a computed tomography (CT) scan is obtained and shown in the image.

Response

The patient's CT scan demonstrates a fracture dislocation of the cervical spine at C3/4. Based on the CT, there is obvious compression of the spinal cord. The patient should be stabilized, remain in the cervical collar, and a complete, detailed American Spinal Injury Association (ASIA) examination should occur. The primary team could begin increasing the mean arterial pressure (MAP) in an attempt to improve spinal cord perfusion, and the elevation of MAPs should continue for 7 days.

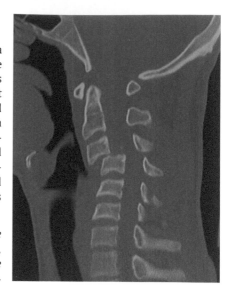

MAPs are increased and on examination the patient has no movement of the extremities, however, sensation is preserved from the shoulders down. There is no bulbocavernosus reflex appreciable.

Response

The patient currently has an ASIA B spinal cord injury; however, there may still be an element of spinal shock given the lack of bulbocavernosus reflex. Steroids could be considered, and are used at some institutions, however, current guidelines recommend against the use of high-dose methylprednisolone in these cases. Next steps in management should focus on removing pressure from the spinal cord. In this case, the patient is awake and has an examination that can be followed, so closed, cervical traction should be performed. Gardner-Wells tongs are applied and weights are added sequentially, using serial X-rays, in an attempt to reduce the fracture. Detailed examination should occur after each set of weights are applied. If there is evidence of disc space distraction at non-involved levels, the most recent weight should be removed as the traction weight is likely too high. (Examinee should explain the planned procedure step by step.)

Further Reading

Vadalà G, Russo F, Denaro V. Closed cervical traction reduction techniques. In: Vaccaro A, Albert T, eds. Spine Surgery: Tricks of the Trade. 3rd ed. New York, NY: Thieme; 2016;376–379

The patient is placed in tongs and successfully reduced with 40 lbs of traction.

Response

The patient should remain in traction until a stabilization procedure can be performed. The patient will need anterior stabilization that can be performed via a C3–4 ACDF; however, given the degree of dislocation, a combined anterior-posterior approach could be considered. (Examinee should explain the planned procedure step by step.)

Further Reading

Dhall S, Resnick DK. Cervicothoracic spine fracture dislocation injuries. In: Harbaugh R, Shaffrey C, Couldwell W, et al. eds. Neurosurgery Knowledge Update. A Comprehensive Review. 1st ed. New York, NY: Thieme; 2015:504–506

The patient is taken initially for a C3–4 ACDF which is performed without difficulty. Under the same anesthetic, the patient is flipped and a posterior decompression and fusion is performed. When you are placing the left C3 lateral mass screw, after tapping the screw tract, you see substantial, bright red blood coming from the screw tract. It is clearly arterial and under high pressure.

Response

It is likely that a vertebral artery injury has occurred with the tap. Anesthesia should be notified of the injury and the potential for significant blood less as well as vertebrobasilar ischemia. Attempts should be made to control the bleeding if possible, but only with large hemostatic agents that are not able to embolize within the vessel. Tamponade through the screw tract may require placement of the lateral mass screw into the bleeding tract. When the hemorrhage is controlled, the patient should immediately be taken to angiography for evaluation. Depending on severity of the injury and control of hemorrhage, treatment could include simple antiplatelet therapy up to vessel sacrifice.

Potential Other Complications

Worsened examination during traction, large posterior disc fragment, inability to reduce with traction.

Case No. 4

You are asked to evaluate a 33-year-old woman who has been admitted to the neurology service after experiencing a 2-month history of worsening spastic paresis of both lower extremities, and now bladder incontinence. She was initially walking but is now wheelchair-dependent. The neurology team has obtained CSF which is negative. MRI demonstrates some expansion of the conus medullaris with T2 hyperintensities throughout the cord.

Response

The patient has slowly progressive lower extremity symptoms and newer onset bladder incontinence. In the setting of T2 hyperintensities within the conus, a vascular malformation of the spinal cord should be considered. The patient's presentation is consistent with the "Foix Alajouanine" syndrome associated with vascular malformations. The patient should undergo some form of vascular imaging, either MR angiogram or conventional spinal angiogram where individual levels are injected.

The patient undergoes a conventional spinal angiogram and the left T10 intercostal branch injection is shown in the image. The previous MRI is also shown.

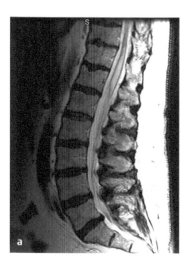 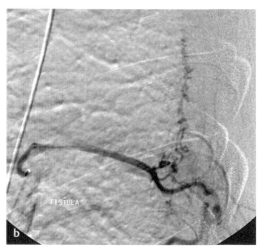

Response

The MRI demonstrates T2 hyperintensities of the conus and flow voids. The angiogram demonstrates a fistulous connection between the intercostal branch and the intradural spinal veins. This appears to be a Type I spinal AVM (spinal dural arteriovenous fistula). This type of spinal cord AVM is best treated with surgical disconnection. The patient should be scheduled for surgery with intradural exploration and disconnection of the fistulous connection. Intraoperative monitoring should be considered prior to coagulation/disconnection. (Examinee should explain the planned procedure step by step.)

Further Reading

Kalani MA, Karim SA, Soltys SG, et al. Radiosurgery for spinal arteriovenous malformations > Endovascular and surgical management of spinal arteriovenous malformations. In: Spetzler R, Kalani M, Nakaji P, eds. Neurovascular Surgery. 2nd ed. New York, NY: Thieme; 2015:958

The patient is taken to the operating room and a T10 laminectomy is performed. A potential feeding vessel is identified in the left T10 foramen. There is an obvious intradural connection to the venous abnormalities. A temporary clip is placed on the believed arterial feeder. Approximately 30 seconds later, intraoperative monitoring reports that somatosensory evoked potentials (SSEPs) remain stable, but motor waveforms have diminished significantly.

Response

It is likely that the temporary clip has captured the radiculomedullary artery feeding the anterior spinal artery, in this case the artery of Adamkiewicz. If the clip is left in place, the patient will likely have an anterior spinal cord infarct. The temporary clip should be removed and return of motor responses should be confirmed. The clip should be placed in a more distal position along the vessel, and it could be used intradurally just to ensure that the proposed region of disconnection does not lead to an anterior spinal artery syndrome. Intraoperative indocyanine green (ICG) can also be used to ensure that there is no flow into the abnormal veins. When a safe area of disconnection is identified, bipolar cautery can be used to permanently disconnect the fistulous connection.

Further Reading

Nelson PK, Shapiro M. Spinal vascular anatomy > Developmental aspects: the grid-like pattern of the vertebrospinal arterial arrangement. In: Spetzler R, Kalani M, Nakaji P, eds. Neurovascular Surgery. 2nd ed. New York, NY: Thieme; 2015:89–103

Potential Other Complications

Persistent fistulous connection, spinal cord infarct, persistent icg filling after disconnection, hemorrhage.

Case No. 5

A 58-year-old man comes to your spine clinic complaining of severe back and leg pain. He says he has had back pain for many years, but it has gotten progressively worse over the past 3 months. His leg pain is in the back of both legs, and seems to worsen as he stands for longer periods of time. His pain is 80% back and 20% leg. He has started using a walker to lean on when ambulating, and feels like he is "tipping forward."

Response

The patient has symptoms concerning for spinal stenosis, but the majority of his pain is located in his back. It is also concerning that he feels as though he is tipping forward. Initially he should undergo a physical examination, as well as imaging which should include MR of the lumbar spine. Standing and flexion/extension X-rays could be considered if there is concern for spondylolisthesis or global imbalance of the spine.

On examination, the patient is full strength in bilateral lower extremities. X-rays demonstrate loss of lumbar lordosis, but no movement on flexion/extension images. MRI of the lumbar spine is shown in the image.

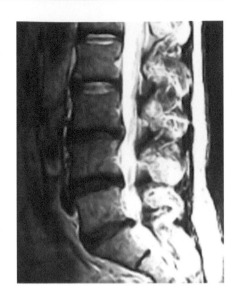

Response

The MRI demonstrates multilevel lumbar stenosis and a loss of lordosis. The stenosis present could explain some of the back and leg pain; however, the loss of lordosis is concerning for a larger problem, namely a sagittal imbalance that may need to be addressed. Long-cassette X-rays should be obtained so a sagittal vertical axis (SVA) can be calculated.

Long cassette (36 inch) X-rays are obtained and shown in the image. SVA is found to be +8 cm.

Response

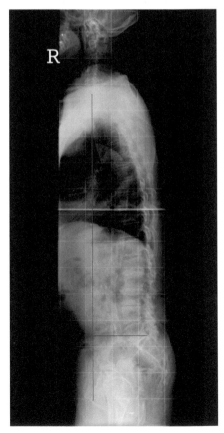

The long cassette X-rays confirm a significantly positive SVA, suggestive of sagittal imbalance. The sagittal imbalance explains both his back and leg pain, and studies have demonstrated that outcomes are better in patients who have an SVA less than +5 cm. This patient needs a procedure that will relieve the lumbar stenosis, but also one that addresses the sagittal imbalance. There are multiple techniques to address the imbalance, but a deformity procedure will likely be required. The loss of lumbar lordosis can be addressed by multiple techniques, including multiple Smith-Peterson osteotomies, a pedicle subtraction osteotomy or even a vertebral column resection if necessary. A long segment, thoracolumbar fusion will be required. In many cases, an L5 transforaminal lumbar interbody fusion (TLIF) is performed to support the lumbosacral junction, and pelvic fixation is utilized. The patient will need to be optimized for such a large surgery, and intraoperative monitoring should be utilized for any deformity correction maneuvers. (Examinee should explain the planned procedure step by step.)

Further Reading

La Marca F, Park P, Valdivia JM. Pedicle subtraction osteotomy/Smith-Petersen osteotomy. In: Baaj A, Mummaneni P, Uribe J, et al. eds. Handbook of Spine Surgery. 2nd ed. New York, NY: Thieme; 2016:351–355

Cheung K, Cheung J. Decision making in adult deformity surgery: decompression versus short or long fusion. In: Vialle L, ed. AOSpine Masters Series, Volume 4: Adult Spinal Deformities. 1st ed. New York, NY: Thieme; 2015:12–27

The patient is taken to the operating room for a long segment thoracolumbar fusion with pelvic fixation and deformity correction. An L3 pedicle subtraction osteotomy is completed. During closure of the osteotomy, the intraoperative monitoring technician alerts the team that the SSEP waveforms have dropped out and the motor evoked potentials have decreased by 75%.

Response

With a significant monitoring change, the first maneuver is to make sure that all monitoring leads are correctly connected and there are no areas of interference in the monitoring setup. If it is confirmed that there are no abnormalities in the system, a surgical cause is likely. In the case of deformity correction, whatever maneuvers precipitated the loss in monitoring should be reversed. In this case, the closure of the osteotomy should be reversed, as this may have caused cord compression at some location. Areas of potential compression should be evaluated and further decompression should be performed if necessary. After the causative maneuver is reversed, observation for return of potentials should be performed. If potentials remain depressed, MAPs can be elevated and further decompression/exploration of potential compression sites should be performed. A last option is to perform an intraoperative wakeup test to determine if monitoring abnormalities correlate with physical examination.

Further Reading

Kadam A, Millhouse PW, Behrend C, et al. Effective use of neuromonitoring during spinal deformity surgery. In: Vaccaro A, Albert T, eds. Spine Surgery: Tricks of the Trade. 3rd ed. New York, NY: Thieme; 2016:292–295

Potential Other Complications

Proximal junctional kyphosis (PJK), hardware failure, blood loss, screw misplacement.

Case No. 6

A 62-year-old woman comes to your clinic with a complaint of bilateral hand weakness that has been progressively worsening over the past 2 months. She also has neck pain that she reports has "probably been there for a year or so." She is having trouble with her hands, specifically noticing difficulty with tasks such as buttoning her shirt and holding her coffee cup.

Response

The patient has symptoms potentially referable to cervical spine pathology. A complete neurologic examination should be performed, and likely the patient will require imaging of her cervical spine, including an MRI. Plain X-rays could be considered, but the MRI will be necessary due to her neurologic symptoms.

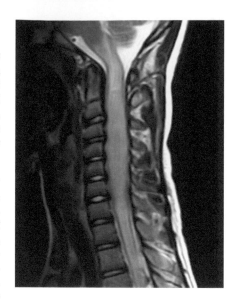

On examination, the patient has 4+ strength in the right deltoid and biceps, 4- in the right triceps, finger flexors, and intrinsics. On the left, the patient has full strength of the left deltoid, 4- in the left biceps and triceps, and 4+ strength in the left finger flexors and intrinsics. There is patchy sensory loss throughout both upper extremities that does not seem to follow a specific nerve distribution. Hoffman sign is positive bilaterally. MRI of the cervical spine is shown in the image.

Response

The patient has multilevel motor weakness and sensory loss, as well as a positive Hoffman sign. The MRI demonstrates a likely intradural, intramedullary spinal cord tumor of the cervical spine. There is significant spinal cord expansion as well as T2 hyperintensities above and below the lesion. The length of the lesion explains the multilevel neurologic findings. While an inflammatory lesion is possible, the cord expansion is more suggestive of a tumor. Inflammatory lesions should be included on the differential and ruled out if possible. In order to determine the underlying pathology and help guide treatment, tissue should be obtained. This patient should be taken to the operating room for intradural exploration and cervical spinal cord biopsy. (Examinee should explain the planned procedure step by step.)

Further Reading

Park P, Farley CW, LaMarca F. Intradural spinal tumors. In: Harbaugh R, Shaffrey C, Couldwell W, et al. eds. Neurosurgery Knowledge Update. A Comprehensive Review. 1st ed. New York, NY: Thieme; 2015:603–607

A biopsy is taken and the intraoperative pathology is consistent with astrocytoma. No further resection is performed. The wound is closed and the patient initially recovers well from the procedure. On the morning after surgery, the patient has significant weakness of the left hemibody. Her left arm is clearly worse, and now her left leg is weak as well. She appears less responsive than she was after surgery.

Response

The new weakness and mental status changes are concerning, especially after a spinal cord biopsy was obtained. However, the weakness is new overnight, and also involves the leg. This finding associated with mental status changes is consistent with intracranial pathology. STAT imaging of the head should be obtained.

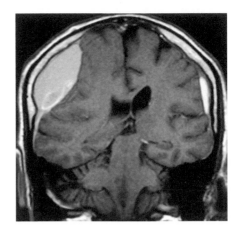

An MRI is performed and the results are shown in the image.

Response

The MRI demonstrates bilateral subdural hematomas, with an obvious compressive subdural on the right side. These subdural hematomas could have been caused by CSF loss during open biopsy. It should be confirmed that there isn't a continued spinal fluid leak, but the right-sided subdural hematoma will need to be removed as it is symptomatic for this patient.

Potential Other Complications

Worsened weakness after biopsy, infection prior to radiation, CSF leak/pseudomeningocele, persistent bleeding from biopsy site.

Case No. 7

A 52- year-old man comes to your clinic with complaints of back and right leg pain. The pain is more severe when he is up and walking, and is relieved when he sits down and leans forward. His right leg pain goes down the lateral aspect of his knee to the top of his foot and big toe. His pain is 50% back and 50% leg. He also reports left leg symptoms, but the right is more severe. If he stands and walks far enough, both legs become very painful.

Response

The patient has symptoms concerning for lumbar spine pathology. A complete physical examination and appropriate imaging should be obtained. Imaging such as MRI of the lumbar spine and X-rays could be considered to evaluate alignment and mobility.

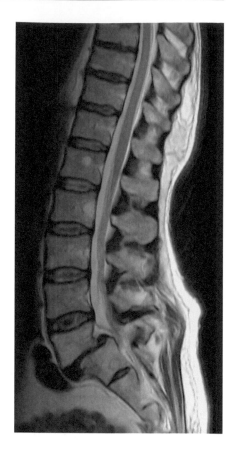

On examination, the patient has some pain-limited weakness of the right hip flexors, but strength is intact with the exception of 4- strength of the right ankle dorsiflexion and big toe extension. There are mild sensory abnormalities in an L5 distribution on the right as well as decreased hip abduction strength (4/5) as well. The left leg is full strength and has no evidence of sensory abnormalities. X-rays are still pending. MRI was obtained and is shown in the image.

Response

The patient has a grade II spondylolisthesis of L5-S1, and there is likely corresponding stenosis and foraminal compression. The findings on MRI explain the patient's back and leg pain, and likely requires treatment. Motion on flexion/extension X-rays would further promote the need of operative intervention. While it is controversial in the literature, a mobile spondylolisthesis with back pain and radiculopathy is likely a good candidate for decompression and fusion. There are multiple techniques for performing a fusion in this case, but a posterior decompression and posterolateral fusion with an interbody graft would be a reasonable option to treat this patient's current symptoms and stop the progression of the spondylolisthesis. Others may consider minimally invasive bilateral decompression alone in an attempt to preserve the posterior tension band and avoid a fusion. (Examinee should explain the planned procedure step by step.)

Further Reading

Matheus V, Francis T. Transforaminal and posterior lumbar interbody fusion. In: Vaccaro A, Albert T, eds. Spine Surgery: Tricks of the Trade. 3rd ed. New York, NY: Thieme; 2016: 144–149

An H, Singh K. Lumbar spondylolisthesis. In: Synopsis of Spine Surgery. 3rd ed. New York, NY: Thieme; 2016:210–220

The patient is taken to the operating room and a posterior decompression and fusion with a right-sided TLIF at L5–S1. The procedure goes as planned and the patient initially recovers well. The evening of surgery, the patient had not yet ambulated, but reports improvement in his right leg pain. The morning after surgery, the patient is mobilized, and in the afternoon, nursing calls to report that the patient has a severe, shooting pain in his right leg, which is similar to the pain from before surgery, perhaps even worse. It is relieved somewhat when he sits in the chair, but is quite severe when he is up and walking.

Response

The patient has had a recurrence of his radiculopathy. In some cases this can be due to nerve irritation from mobilization during the TLIF; however, this patient's leg pain was initially better after surgery. The recurrence is concerning for new compression of the nerve. A steroid dose pack could be considered, but the timeframe of the recurrence suggests a possible structural cause. Imaging (CT scan) should be obtained to better evaluate the right L5 foramen as well as the instrumentation.

A CT scan is performed and all hardware/instrumentation is properly placed. The L5 foramen looks to be compressed by bone fragments coming from the disc space.

Response

It is likely that bone graft backed out of the disc space and entered the right L5 foramen, compressing the nerve and causing the recurrent radiculopathy. Unfortunately, this patient will likely require a reoperation to clean out the foramen and remove any compressive bone fragments.

Potential Other Complications

TLIF too anterior, Cage kick out, endplate violation, graft subsidence, nerve root injury, pedicle screw pullout during reduction.

Case No. 8

A 60-year-old man comes to your clinic with mid-scapular back pain, some difficulty standing from a seated position, and trouble with his hands. This has been going on for several months and has been getting progressively worse over that time frame. He feels unstable on his feet and has had particular difficulty buttoning his shirt in the morning.

Response

The patient has symptoms that could be due to myelopathy, and the mid-scapular back pain as well as hand symptoms suggests that the cervical spine could be a causative region. He should undergo a detailed neurologic examination as well as imaging, including MRI of the cervical spine.

On examination, the patient is full strength in bilateral upper extremities with the exception of 4- grip strength in the right hand, and 4/5 grip strength in the left hand. He is 4- in both hip flexors, but is otherwise intact on motor examination of the lower extremities. He has clonus at the ankle bilaterally, as well as Hoffman sign bilaterally. MRI results are shown in the image.

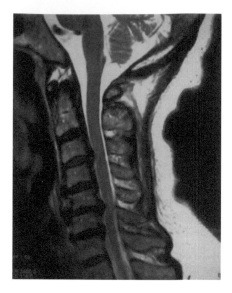

Response

The patient has multilevel cervical spondylosis as well as a loss of lordosis. There are multiple disc bulges, the most notable at C5–6, which appears to cause canal stenosis and loss of T2 signal around the cord at that level. The T2 hypointense, contiguous thickening of the posterior longitudinal ligament on the MRI is concerning for the possibility of ossification of the posterior longitudinal ligament. If this is found, it will alter surgical decision-making for this patient. A CT scan of the cervical spine should be obtained to determine if ossification of the posterior longitudinal ligament (OPLL) is present.

A CT scan is obtained and is shown in the image.

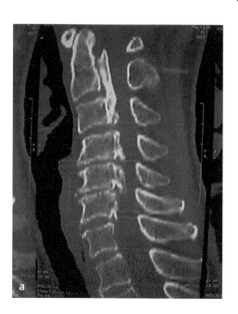

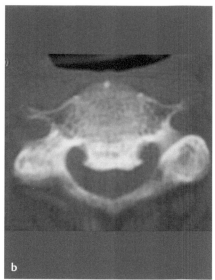

Response

The CT scan confirms ossification of the posterior longitudinal ligament in this patient. This makes an anterior approach via a standard anterior cervical discectomy and fusion (ACDF) difficult and potentially dangerous as there can be adherence to and erosion of the ventral dura. It remains an option, but care must be taken during the anterior approach to avoid risk of CSF leak or cord injury. The patient will require a decompressive surgery, but this can be performed via a posterior approach. The need for fusion depends on the length of decompression, cervical parameters as well as other factors. Laminoplasty could be considered as well. (Examinee should explain the planned procedure step by step.)

Further Reading

Mokhtar S, Gragnaniello C, Nader R, et al. Surgical management of cervical ossification of posterior longitudinal ligament®. In: Nader R, Berta S, Gragnanielllo C, et al. eds. Neurosurgery Tricks of the Trade. Spine and Peripheral Nerves. 1st ed. New York, NY: Thieme; 2014:383–387

The patient is taken to surgery for a posterior cervical decompression. There are no complications during surgery and the areas of stenosis are successfully decompressed. The patient recovers well initially but continues to have hand weakness the evening of surgery. The next morning on examination, you notice substantial deltoid weakness (3/5) bilaterally.

Response

Unfortunately the patient has likely experienced a postoperative C5 palsy. The etiology is poorly understood, but may be due to several factors, including dorsal cord drift and nerve stretching, heat transfer from the drill or irritation from surgical instruments. Imaging should be obtained to rule out other causes, but if negative, a C5 palsy is likely. Observation and physical therapy should be initiated as many C5 palsies recover, but the recovery period lasts months.

Further Reading

Shridharani S, Rowan FA. Cervical laminectomy with and without fusion. In: Baaj A, Mummaneni P, Uribe J, et al. eds. Handbook of Spine Surgery. 2nd ed. New York, NY: Thieme; 2016:295–301

Potential Other Complications

Durotomy, vertebral artery injury, monitoring change, instrument slip into cord.

Case No. 9

You are asked to see a 44-year-old woman who has been experiencing a fairly rapid neu-rologic decline over the past 2 weeks. She was initially walking without issue, but is now in your office in a wheelchair. She has severe mid to lower back pain (points to roughly the thoracolumbar junction) that has worsened over the past week. She states that she is in a wheelchair because her "legs get very tired and weak walking short distances." The weakness has gotten worse as well. She states that over the past day or two she has had some difficulty with urinary incontinence.

Response

The patient's symptoms are very con-cerning, and they are clearly worsening. There seems to be an element of myelop-athy; however, cauda equina syndrome should be highly considered based on these symptoms. She should undergo complete physical examination as well as MRI of the thoracolumbar spine.

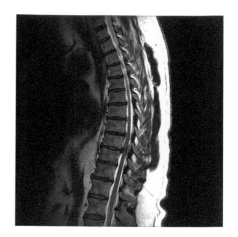

On examination the patient has 3/5 strength in bilateral hip flexors, 4-/5 strength in knee extension bilaterally, and the distal exam-ination is normal. She appears to have a sensory level at T8, although the loss below this level is patchy. She has several-beat clo-nus of the ankles bilaterally, but no Hoffman sign. The upper extremities are normal. MRI of the thoracic spine is shown in the image.

Response

The patient has a large disc herniation in the lower thoracic spine that is clearly com-pressing the cord at that level. This finding explains her decline as well as her symp-toms. She should undergo surgery as soon as feasible to avoid any further progression of her neurologic deficits as well as to give her the best chance of recovery. This disc can be approached via several techniques, including lateral thoracotomy, posterior cos-totransversectomy/transpedicular approach. A midline posterior approach should not be utilized due to the risk of further deterioration from cord manipulation. Attention should be paid toward accurate identification of the correct level in the thoracic spine as it can be difficult to identify intraoperatively. Adjuncts, such as gold seed pedicle placement by interventional radiology could be considered. Overall, there are several techniques that can be used to access the disc, but cord displacement should be avoided if at all possible. (Examinee should explain the planned procedure step by step.)

Further Reading

Benglis D Jr, Fessler R, Haid R Jr. Transpedicular thoracic diskectomy. In: Fessler R, Sekhar L, eds. Atlas of Neurosurgical Techniques. Spine and Peripheral Nerves. 2nd ed. New York, NY: Thieme; 2016:455–460

The patient is taken to the operating room the next day for a costotransversectomy and disc removal. The case is completed and the disc protrusion is completely removed. The patient's pain is improved postoperatively. The morning after surgery, the nurse notifies you that the patient has been coughing more than normal, and O2 saturations are 91%, she is starting the patient in nasal cannula oxygen.

Response

The new oxygen requirement is concerning, given that she was not having this issue in the immediate postoperative period. A chest X-ray should be obtained.

A chest X-ray is obtained and shown in the image.

Response

The patient has a pneumothorax, likely from an unidentified violation of the pleura during the surgical approach. Thoracic surgery should be consulted for assistance managing the pneumothorax, which will likely require placement of a pigtail catheter.

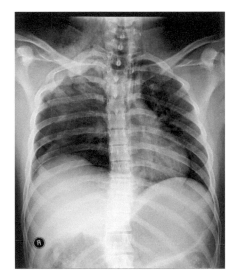

Potential Other Complications

Durotomy, neurologic worsening, calcified disc, spinal cord infarct.

Case No. 10

You are called to the emergency department to evaluate a 55-year-old man who was just involved in high-speed motor vehicle collision. He was a restrained driver and has an obvious right humeral fracture. He complains of severe mid to lower back pain. After the trauma team has completed their primary and secondary surveys, it is determined that the patient has pain-limited weakness of the right upper extremity, but is otherwise full strength in all four extremities.

Response

The patient should remain in spine pre-cautions and a CT scan of the entire spine should be performed.

The patient is taken to the CT scanner and a single slice of the sagittal reconstruction is shown in the image.

Response

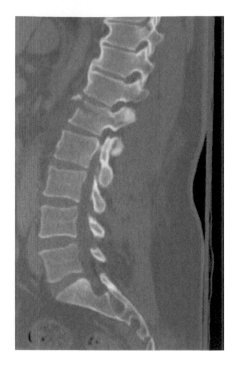

The patient has a fracture of the L1 vertebral body that involves all three columns. It originates in the anterior cortex, and travels through the pedicle into the posterior elements. This would be considered a flexion/distraction injury, and is consistent with a "bony Chance fracture." It is unstable owing to all three columns being involved in the fracture. The patient should remain on spine precautions until operative intervention can be performed. The fracture is located at the thoracolumbar junction, so a longer fusion construct should be considered, likely 2 to 3 levels above and 2 to 3 levels below the injury level. (Examinee should explain the planned procedure step by step.)

Further Reading

Vialle L, Vialle E, Guasque J, et al. Short or long posterior fusion: determining the extent of fixation. In: Vialle L, ed. AOSpine Masters Series, Volume 6: Thoracolumbar Spine Trauma. 1st ed. New York, NY: Thieme; 2016:85–96

The patient was taken to the operating room for fixation of the fracture via a long segment fusion. He tolerated the procedure well and was neurologically stable after the procedure. He was ambulating on postop day 1 and obtained X-rays. On postop day 3 he was working with physical therapist who reported that he had the onset of significant back pain and felt the need to lean forward and rest on support while standing. His therapy session was stopped prematurely due to pain and he has remained in bed since the pain started.

Response

The new onset pain could be due to hardware failure or other mechanical abnormalities associated with the construct. Initial management of the new symptom should involve imaging. An X-ray of the region could be obtained quickly to evaluate the hardware.

A standing X-ray was obtained and is shown in the image. The initial postoperative X-ray is demonstrated on the left, and the postoperative day 3 post symptom is demonstrated on the right.

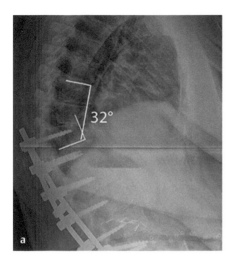 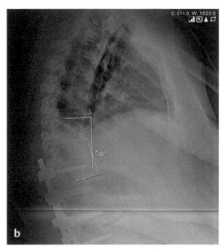

Response

The patient has evidence of early proximal junctional kyphosis and probable screw back out at the top of the construct. The patient will require an early reoperation with significant extension of fusion superiorly to treat the PJK.

Further Reading

Kim H, Iyer S, Shaffrey C Sr. Junctional issues following adult deformity surgery. In: Vialle L, ed. AOSpine Masters Series, Volume 4: Adult Spinal Deformities. 1st ed. New York, NY: Thieme; 2015:106–111

Potential Other Complications

Misplaced pedicle screw, hardware failure, wound infection.

Category 4: Vascular

Case No. 1

A 19-year-old man is referred to your clinic from a local neurologist for evaluation of "eye symptoms." His history includes a recent all-terrain vehicle (ATV) accident approximately 3 months ago where he hit his head, but did not seek medical attention. He believes he lost consciousness during the accident. His post-concussive symptom resolved, but he has noticed the onset of redness of his eye, and feels that his eye is "swollen." He has had worsening retro-orbital pain since the accident.

Response

The patient has suffered significant head trauma for which he did not undergo evaluation. He should have a thorough physical examination followed by vascular-focused imaging. Given the trauma history, a traumatic vascular lesion is possible and a head computed tomography (CT) with computed tomography angiogram (CTA) or conventional angiography is warranted.

On examination, the patient is neurologically intact with the exception of right-sided chemosis, mild proptosis, mildly decreased visual acuity, and an orbital bruit is appreciated. He undergoes a CT scan of the head and conventional cerebral angiography.

Response

The patient's head CT demonstrates evidence of skull base fractures from his trauma, and the lateral angiogram demonstrates a carotid cavernous (CC) fistula with drainage through the superior ophthalmic vein. This lesion accounts for his symptoms due to vascular outflow obstruction, and if left untreated could lead to blindness in the eye. With a history of trauma, it is most likely that this represents a direct CC fistula

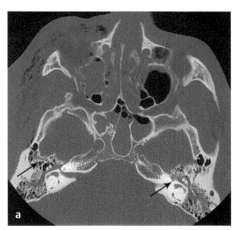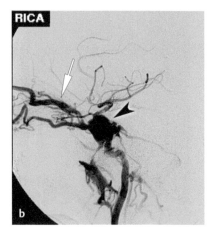

rather than an indirect, and it is important to determine the difference between these two. (Direct fistula occurs with injury to wall of the carotid, while indirect fistula occurs when a smaller vessel branching from the carotid is injured.) Indirect CC fistulas can spontaneously resolve within several months, but direct CC fistulas should be promptly treated due to higher risk of neurologic injury. When considering endovascular approaches, a direct CC fistula can often be treated via a transarterial route, while an indirect is often treated via a transvenous route, although approaches vary among providers. There is a risk of reflux of embolic material into the internal carotid artery (ICA) during treatment. Coiling of the cavernous sinus via endovascular approach is recommended. (Examinee should explain the planned procedure step by step.)

Further Reading

Park MS, Sanborn MR, McDougall CG, et al. Carotid cavernous fistulas. In: Harbaugh R, Shaffrey C, Couldwell W, et al. eds. Neurosurgery Knowledge Update. A Comprehensive Review. 1st ed. New York, NY: Thieme; 2015:187–192

The endovascular team identified the lesion as a direct CC fistula and it was coiled via a transarterial approach. After the coils were deployed, filling of the superior ophthalmic vein during the arterial phase was eliminated. The patient otherwise tolerated the procedure well. Several hours after the procedure, the patient reports to the floor nurse that he is having blurred vision. He sees double images in the horizontal plane.

Response

It is likely that the patient is experiencing irritation of the abducens nerve in the cavernous sinus as it and the carotid artery are the two free floating structures within the cavernous sinus. The coil mass and inflammation caused by thrombosis are likely irritating the abducens nerve and leading to a mild palsy. The patient should be monitored and a short course of steroids could be considered. It is likely to resolve over time.

Further Reading

Levitt MR, Morton RP, Ghodke B. Carotid cavernous fistula > Potential complications and avoidance. In: Sekhar L, Fessler R, eds. Atlas of Neurosurgical Techniques: Brain, Volume 1. 2nd ed. New York, NY: Thieme; 2015:550

Potential Other Complications

Embolic reflux into ICA, retrograde cortical venous drainage, indirect CC fistula, residual fistula.

Case No. 2

A 42-year-old male smoker with hypertension presents to your clinic for evaluation of what he states as a "brain aneurysm on the top of my head." He says it was found on a brain magnetic resonance imaging (MRI) after he had been worked up for recent refractory headaches. He had one headache approximately 3 days ago that was very severe, and he states that it was the worst headache he has ever experienced. He has since recovered with no other symptoms.

Response

The patient has a concerning presentation in the setting of a potential intracranial aneurysm. His more recent severe headache may be representative of a sentinel headache if an aneurysm is present. He should undergo a physical examination, dedicated vascular imaging (preferably a conventional angiogram), and a lumbar puncture with evaluation for xanthochromia could be considered to rule out a prior subarachnoid hemorrhage.

On physical examination the patient is neurointact with no focal deficits. A lumbar puncture is performed and there is no evidence of xanthochromia. Cerebrospinal fluid (CSF) studies are within normal limits. He undergoes a conventional cerebral angiogram and the results are shown in the image.

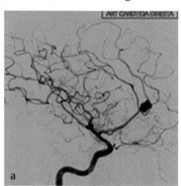
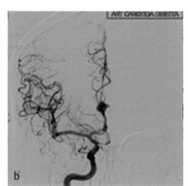
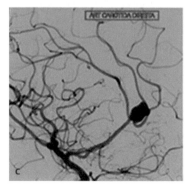

Response

The conventional angiogram demonstrates a large, pericallosal aneurysm at the branch point between A2 and the callosal marginal/pericallosal artery takeoff. It has multiple excrescences, and has an irregular shape that is concerning. Even with negative CSF, the previous sudden headache is concerning for a sentinel headache, or at least could represent aneurysmal growth. He is a smoker with hypertension and his risk of rupture is elevated. This aneurysm should be treated endovascularly if possible, but if not, he should undergo surgical clipping via an interhemispheric approach. (Examinee should explain the planned procedure step by step.)

Further Reading

Lawton M. Pericallosal artery aneurysms. In: Seven Aneurysms. Tenets and Techniques for Clipping. 1st ed. New York, NY: Thieme; 2011:147–163

The endovascular team states that they are not able to coil the aneurysm, so he is taken to the operating room for surgical clipping. During the procedure, you have achieved adequate proximal control and have only minimally mobilized the aneurysm. You are working on distal control and to obtain a better view, you elect to relocate your retractor. When you retract, you see sudden, brisk arterial bleeding coming from the callosal marginal artery, which has clearly been damaged.

Response

Anesthesia should be notified of arterial bleeding, but not from the aneurysm. Large bore suctions should be used to control the surgical field, and a cottonoid patty should be placed over the bleeding segment while the extent of injury is inspected. Given that this vessel supplies interhemispheric motor cortex controlling the contralateral leg, repair should be pursued if possible to avoid an ischemic insult leading to postoperative deficit. A temporary clip can be applied proximal to the vessel injury which should allow for further inspection. If possible, direct repair of the vessel could be attempted utilizing 9-0 or 10-0 monofilament suture under the operative microscope. If this is too difficult, a muscle pledget could be used to help with the repair. The surgeon should be aware that muscle tissue exposed to the lumen would have a high chance of thrombosis, and while it can help with the repair, a primary repair is likely better. Other options include clip grafts and/or cotton-assisted repair. A proximal temporary clip is applied and the vessel is repaired directly using a micro suture. The aneurysm is clipped and postoperative angiogram demonstrates aneurysm occlusion and good distal flow through the callosal marginal artery.

Potential Other Complications

Aneurysm rupture, sinus injury, residual aneurysm, seizures, leg weakness, cortical vein injury.

Case No. 3

You are asked to see a 33-year-old woman currently on the cardiology service who has developed altered mental status prompting a head CT which demonstrated a potential vascular irregularity. No further studies have been performed.

Response

What is the patient's history and examination? Why is she currently admitted to the cardiology service?

The patient has a history of intravenous (IV) drug use and has been found to have vegetation on the mitral valve. She is currently on broad-spectrum antibiotics, and blood cultures are pending. She is febrile, and confused, but otherwise demonstrates no focal deficits on examination. Her confusion prompted the head CT. The read from radiology is suggestive of a vascular irregularity, but the radiologist cannot clarify further based on those images alone.

Response

Given a history of IV drug use and a concern for left-heart bacterial endocarditis in the setting of a potential vascular irregularity on brain imaging, the concern for mycotic aneurysm in this patient is high. She should undergo conventional cerebral angiography to better identify and localize any intracranial vascular lesions, and antibiotics should be continued.

She has a conventional angiogram performed and the results are shown in the image.

Response

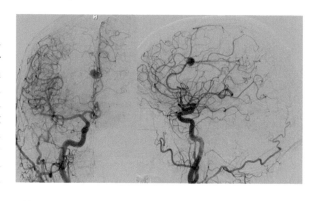

The angiogram demonstrates a distal anterior circulation aneurysm. In the setting of bacterial endocarditis, this has a high likelihood of being a mycotic aneurysm. In many cases mycotic aneurysms can be treated via antibiotic administration and monitoring. The fragile nature of the aneurysm wall can make attempts at open surgical clipping difficult and dangerous. At this time she should be closely monitored with follow-up imaging and continuation of antibiotics selected toward whatever organism is identified.

The patient continues antibiotics, and they are tailored to target Staphylococcus aureus, the causative organism. A repeat angiogram 2 days later demonstrates interval stability. The next day, nursing reports a sudden change in mental status, and significant weakness of the left leg.

Response

These new findings are concerning for aneurysmal rupture, and a STAT head CT should be performed.

A head CT is shown in the image.

Response

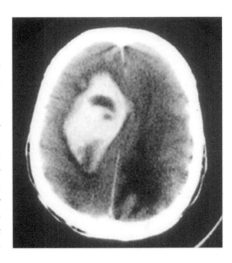

The aneurysm has ruptured and there is an intracerebral hematoma, potentially with active bleeding. The patient should be intubated and measures should be taken to decrease intracranial pressure (ICP). There are two treatment options, open surgery or endovascular parent vessel sacrifice. Open surgery will be challenging due to a large acute hematoma and potential difficulty of identifying and controlling the source of the bleeding. Immediate endovascular access and parent vessel sacrifice to stop the bleeding via either liquid embolic agents or coils should be considered. Surgical decompression may still be required to relieve mass effect, either with a large craniectomy, or with a more focused, port-based clot removal, but the bleeding should be stopped immediately. (Examinee should explain the planned procedure step by step.)

The patient is taken for emergent endovascular parent vessel sacrifice using onyx. The bleeding is stopped and the hematoma did not expand further.

Further Reading

Walcott BP, Ogilvy CS. Cerebral aneurysms: to clip or coil? > Mycotic aneurysms. In: Spetzler R, Kalani M, Nakaji P, eds. Neurovascular Surgery. 2nd ed. New York, NY: Thieme; 2015:781–782

Potential Other Complications

Aneurysm growth on antibiotics, meningitis, sepsis.

Case No. 4

An 86-year-old man is brought to the emergency department by his wife, who reports that he has developed left arm weakness and trouble speaking. He was last seen normal approximately 2.5 hours ago when she left the house to run errands. He has a history of atrial fibrillation and hypertension.

Response

It appears based on the patient's presentation that he is having an acute ischemic stroke. Given that he is 2.5 hours since onset of symptom, he should undergo thorough evaluation by the on-call neurologist as well as CT/perfusion imaging. He should be considered for IV-tPA administration if eligible.

The patient is seen by neurology and has a National Institutes of Health Stroke Scale (NIHSS) of 20 (significantly elevated). His imaging results are shown in the image. Ultimately he receives IV-tPA within 20 minutes of initial evaluation. The IV-tPA fails to improve his symptoms, and he continues to score a 20 on the NIHSS.

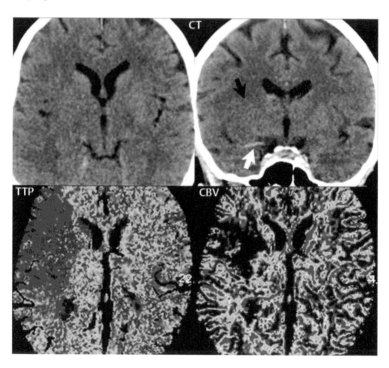

Response

The imaging demonstrates some blurring of the lentiform nuclei as well as a hyper-dense right middle cerebral artery (MCA) sign and perfusion mismatch. Given the lack of improvement in his examination after IV-tPA administration, he should be considered for mechanical thrombectomy by the endovascular team. (Examinee should explain the planned procedure step by step.)

Further Reading

Elad I. Levy and Maxim Mokin. Endovascular revascularization for acute stroke. In: Harbaugh R, Shaffrey C, Couldwell W, et al. eds. Neurosurgery Knowledge Update. A Comprehensive Review. 1st ed. New York, NY: Thieme; 2015:208–212

Taussky P, Tawk RG, Miller DA, et al. Current endovascular treatment of acute ischemic stroke. In: Spetzler R, Kalani M, Nakaji P, eds. Neurovascular Surgery. 2nd ed. New York, NY: Thieme; 2015:351–359

The patient is taken emergently to the endovascular suite where access is gained and an occlusive right MCA thrombus is demonstrated. A stent retriever is utilized and the thrombus is successfully removed with good evidence of blood flow to the right MCA after the procedure. An hour after the procedure, the patient's left-sided weakness has recovered substantially and the dysarthria has improved. Six hours later you are called by nursing after the patient acutely becomes unresponsive. The nurse called a code, and the critical care team is evaluating the patient and planning to intubate.

Response

The sudden onset of symptoms in the setting of a recently treated stroke is very concerning for reperfusion hemorrhage. Given the large perfusion mismatch on preprocedure CT, the patient could have a very large hemorrhage that is life-threatening. The patient should be evaluated immediately and intubated if the critical care team is concerned about airway protection. Blood pressure should be controlled and the patient should undergo STAT imaging via head CT.

The critical care team intubates and sedates the patient and the head CT is shown in the image.

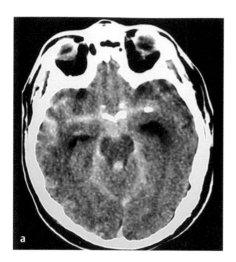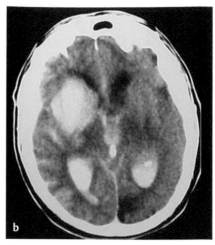

Response

The head CT demonstrates a large right-sided likely reperfusion hemorrhage with intraventricular extension and subsequent hydrocephalus. Reperfusion hemorrhage can occur in 1 to 10% of cases. Unfortunately this is a severe injury that may be catastrophic. Supportive care should continue and external ventricular drainage should be considered and discussed with family members.

Further Reading

Kurre W. Intracranial stenoses. In: Jansen O, Brückmann H, eds. Interventional Stroke Therapy. 1st ed. New York, NY: Thieme; 2013:167–177

Potential Other Complications

Difficult access, femoral pseudoaneurysm/hematoma, retroperitoneal hematoma, incomplete thrombectomy, arterial perforation/dissection.

Case No. 5

You are asked to evaluate a 25-year-old man who has had two episodes of sudden right-sided facial weakness, horizontal double vision, and left hemibody weakness. These episodes occurred 2 months ago and 1 year ago. He was evaluated and told he had a brainstem mass by an outside physician.

Response

The patient's symptoms are referable to the brainstem and the sudden onset nature suggests vascular lesion. This is most likely to be a cavernous malformation, but other vascular abnormalities are also possible. The outside imaging should be evaluated or reordered, and the patient should have a thorough physical examination.

On examination the patient has mild left upper extremity pronator drift, but full strength in the left lower extremity. There are no appreciable cranial nerve (CN) deficits on examination. The MRI was repeated and is shown in the image.

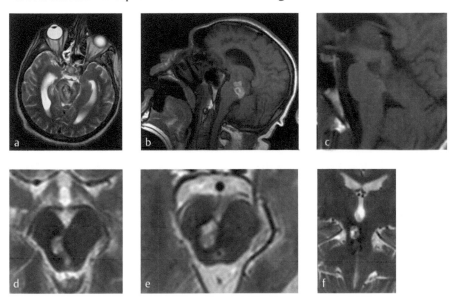

Response

The MRI demonstrates evidence of a cavernous malformation in the pontomesencephalic region on the right side. This lesion is large, has some evidence of edema and represents the causative lesion for the patient's symptoms. The MRI also demonstrates increased ventricular size in the temporal horns, and the patient may have associated hydrocephalus from mass effect. Consideration should be given to CSF diversion if symptomatic. In regards to the cavernous malformation, the patient has largely recovered from the last hemorrhage, but two recent hemorrhages are concerning for an early recurrent hemorrhage in the near future. Surgically resecting the malformation now would come with significant risk of neurologic deficit, while waiting for another hemorrhage could risk severe complications of the subsequent hemorrhage. The data vary on the best timing for resection, and surgical decision-making should be tailored to the specific patient.

Further Reading

Abla AA, Kalani M, Spetzler R. Surgery for brainstem cavernous malformations. In: Spetzler R, Kalani M, Nakaji P, eds. Neurovascular Surgery. 2nd ed. New York, NY: Thieme; 2015: 436–447

The patient is adamant on undergoing a surgical resection and is willing to accept the associated risk of postoperative neurologic deficit. The idea of simply waiting until the next devastating bleed is too much for him to handle. He would like surgery as soon as possible. You take him to surgery via your preferred approach, and when you expose the brainstem in the region you expected to find the lesion coming to the pial surface, you see nothing but normal brainstem. What are the safe entry zones to the brainstem?

Response

In regards to approach, and easy method is to place a point on the middle of the malformation, and another on the portion that is closest to the pial surface, or the portion that is closest to noneloquent structures. The connection of these two lines can help direct the best surgical route to the malformation. If no portion is observable on the pial surface, the malformation at the pontomesencephalic junction can be approached via the peri-trigeminal safe zone. This region is located between the trigeminal nerve and the facial nerve. This should provide access to the malformation and allow resection with minimal displacement of critical brainstem structures. Intraoperative ultrasound could be considered to aid in localization. It should be noted that after a hemorrhage, distortion and compression of the brainstem can make previously safe entry zones no longer safe as critical structures are displaced by the malformation. Resection should focus on the surface of the malformation itself, attempting to minimize any damage to surrounding brainstem tissue. If a developmental venous anomaly is encountered, it should be preserved, as the developmental venous anomaly (DVA) can be draining normal tissue. Resection could lead to ischemic stroke of the surrounding tissue. (Examinee should explain the planned procedure step by step.)

Further Reading

Spetzler R, Kalani M, Nakaji P, et al. Safe Entry Zones. In: Color Atlas of Brainstem Surgery. 1st ed. New York, NY: Thieme; 2017:85–102

Potential Other Complications

Radiosurgery associated edema, venous infarct from DVA resection, postoperative neurological deficits.

Case No. 6

You are consulted in the emergency department to see a 25-year-old woman who experienced a sudden onset headache followed by confusion and altered mental status. The emergency department physician notifies you that she is getting progressively more somnolent and they are concerned that she will not be able to protect her airway. She is spontaneously moving her right side, but has very sluggish movements on the left.

Response

The patient should be intubated if there is concern for her airway. Access should be obtained and the patient should undergo STAT imaging as soon as she is stabilized.

The patient is intubated and sedated, subsequently taken for head CT, which is shown in the image.

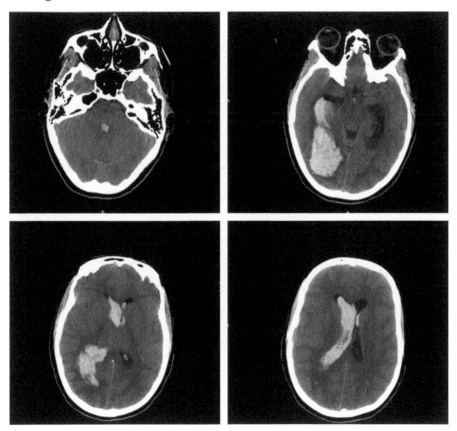

Response

The patient has suffered a right parieto-occipital hemorrhage with intraventricular extension and hydrocephalus. Blood pressure should be maintained below 140 mm Hg. Due to her being intubated and sedated, no examination can currently be performed, and the radiographic hydrocephalus should warrant external ventricular drain (EVD) placement. Also, given her age and location of the hemorrhage, it is less likely that this hemorrhage represents a hypertensive hemorrhage (which are more common in the basal ganglia in older patients), and there could be an underlying vascular malformation. After her hydrocephalus is treated, she should undergo vascular imaging, either a CT angiogram or conventional cerebral angiogram.

An EVD is placed and the CSF is under pressure. The patient undergoes a conventional cerebral angiogram and a single lateral image is shown in the image. The report states a nidus of 3.5 cm.

Response

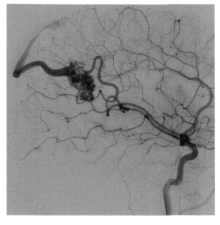

The lateral digital subtraction angiogram demonstrates a distal right MCA arteriovenous malformation. It has superficial venous drainage and is likely a grade III arteriovenous malformations (AVM), given that the nidus is 3.5 cm, the AVM appears to be close to eloquent motor cortex with superficial drainage. There do not appear to be any associated feeding aneurysms, which can be associated with a higher risk of rupture. Regardless, the patient could be considered for embolization; however, a surgical approach will allow for decompression of the hematoma as well as resection of the AVM. If it is thought that the hematoma is obstructing the venous outflow tract, the AVM should be resected promptly, to avoid a devastating rebleed. (Examinee should explain the planned procedure step by step.)

Further Reading

Puffer R, Lanzino G. Hemorrhage from arteriovenous malformations and its management. In: Dumont A, Lanzino G, Sheehan J, eds. Brain Arteriovenous Malformations and Arteriovenous Fistulas. 1st ed. New York, NY: Thieme; 2018:154–158

Lawton M. Parieto-occipital arteriovenous malformations. In: Seven AVMs. Tenets and Techniques for Resection. 1st ed. New York, NY: Thieme; 2014:115–150

The patient is taken to the operating room for clot decompression and AVM resection. The AVM resection is difficult, but no further bleeding is encountered. The patient recovers from the procedure, and on postop day 1, she undergoes a conventional angiogram to evaluate the AVM. The results are shown in the image.

Response

The postoperative angiogram demonstrates a residual nidus of the AVM. Residual AVM has a similar rate of bleeding as an untreated AVM, and this patient should undergo repeat resection as soon as possible in order to completely resect the residual AVM. Other options include endovascular management, or stereotactic radiosurgery, however, SRS would require a much longer interval to complete exclusion with risk of hemorrhage during that interval. Repeat surgical resection should be performed.

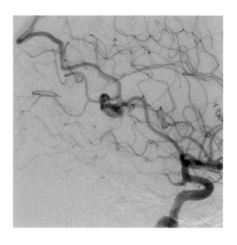

Further Reading

Lawton M. Arteriovenous malformation resection > Residual AVM. In: Seven AVMs. Tenets and Techniques for Resection. 1st ed. New York, NY: Thieme; 2014:35

Potential Other Complications

Intraoperative rupture and presence of pedicle aneurysm.

Case No. 7

A 68-year-old man presents to your clinic with a 3-month history of pulsatile tinnitus and a recent seizure that he says started with funny shapes in the left side of his vision and progressed to mild shaking of the left hand. It stopped spontaneously. He has been seen by his primary care provider and subsequently by a neurologist who put him on 500 mg of levetiracetam twice daily. He has not had any further seizure activity, but still reports pulsatile tinnitus. His examination is otherwise normal. He brings a CT scan and MRI performed at an outside institution that show no parenchymal abnormalities, but the radiologist's comments on the right-sided transverse sinus saying there is a mild irregularity/enlargement, but no further comment could be made based on imaging modality.

Response

The patient has symptoms that may be consistent with a vascular malformation of some type, especially with pulsatile tinnitus. Vascular imaging should be obtained, most likely a conventional cerebral angiogram. With pulsatile tinnitus and an irregularity associated with the transverse sinus, a full diagnostic angiogram would be preferred, with selective injection of the external carotid arteries as well.

The patient undergoes a conventional diagnostic cerebral angiogram and a single, lateral view is shown in the image.

Response

This lateral digital subtraction angiogram is a selective external carotid artery injection that demonstrates early venous filling during the arterial phase, and is highly suggestive of a dural arteriovenous fistula. In this case the dural arteriovenous fistula (dAVF) feeds into the transverse sinus, and does appear to have some leptomeningeal venous reflux, making it a Cognard IIa+b classification, and at higher risk of rupture. The leptomeningeal reflux likely also explains his seizures, while the dAVF itself could

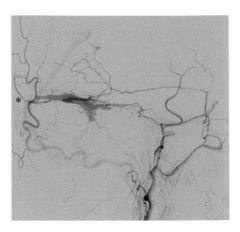

cause pulsatile tinnitus. There also appears to be a feeding branch from the occipital artery. This dAVF should be treated due to elevated risk of rupture with leptomeningeal reflux and neurological symptoms. The posterior branch of the middle meningeal artery appears to have a straight path to the nidus and would be a likely candidate for superselective catheterization and embolization with an agent such as Onyx. Transvenous and/or open surgical resection are also possible treatment modalities for this fistula. (Examinee should explain the planned procedure step by step.)

Further Readings

Dannenbaum MJ, Schuette AJ, Case DB, et al. Cranial dural arteriovenous fistulas. In: Spetzler R, Kalani M, Nakaji P, eds. Neurovascular Surgery. 2nd ed. New York, NY: Thieme; 2015:833–842

Boccardi E, Valvassori L. Endovascular treatment of dural arteriovenous fistulas of the brain. In: Dumont A, Lanzino G, Sheehan J, eds. Brain Arteriovenous Malformations and Arteriovenous Fistulas. 1st ed. New York, NY: Thieme; 2018:185–193

The patient is taken back to the endovascular suite and superselective catheterization of the posterior branch of the middle meningeal artery is performed, and Onyx is delivered to the nidus, demonstrating complete occlusion of the dAVF. What should the endovascular surgeon be aware of when using embolic agents such as Onyx or nBCA?

Response

There is a risk when using liquid embolic agents that the embolic material can reflux into unwanted local arteries and cause ischemia. When catheterizing the external carotid arteries, care should be taken to avoid reflux as branches can be supplying the CNs, or form an anastomosis with an intracranial artery. The ascending pharyngeal artery can have a branch that feeds CNs X, XI, and XII as well as form an anastomosis with the vertebral artery, the posterior auricular artery can give off a stylomastoid branch that supplies CN VII. Further, embolic agents could travel into a cortical vein receiving reflux and cause a venous stroke. Careful monitoring of the flow of embolic agents is required when treating a dAVF via endovascular techniques.

Further Reading

Grand W, Hopkins L, Siddiqui A, et al. External carotid artery. In: Vasculature of the Brain and Cranial Base. Variations in Clinical Anatomy. 2nd ed. New York, NY: Thieme; 2016:21–42
Boccardi E, Valvassori L. Endovascular treatment of dural arteriovenous fistulas of the brain. In: Dumont A, Lanzino G, Sheehan J, eds. Brain Arteriovenous Malformations and Arteriovenous Fistulas. 1st ed. New York, NY: Thieme; 2018:185–193

Potential Other Complications

Wedged (stuck) distal catheter, residual nidus after Onyx, Intraprocedural rupture.

Case No. 8

You are consulted by the neurology stroke service regarding a 72-year-old woman who is currently on dual-antiplatelet therapy for recent coronary stenting procedures who is now hospitalized after having several episodes of dizziness and one episode of syncope that seem to happen "all of the sudden" and are not associated with any specific activity. She has undergone cardiac evaluation and it is negative for signs of cardiogenic syncope. She also reports to you that occasionally if she turns her head she will get dizzy and feels like she might "pass out." An MRI performed by the neurology team is negative for areas of restricted diffusion. Her examination is neurologically intact during your visit.

Response

The patient has a history consistent with coronary atherosclerotic disease, and her current symptoms are concerning for vertebrobasilar insufficiency with transient ischemic attacks (TIAs). She should undergo a diagnostic cerebral angiogram to look for areas of stenosis.

She undergoes a conventional diagnostic cerebral angiogram. The anterior circulation is normal, and the injection through the dominant right vertebral artery is shown in the image.

Response

This lateral digital subtraction angiography (DSA) image via a right vertebral artery injection demonstrates critical stenosis of the vertebral artery. Given that her left vertebral artery is dominant, it is likely that she has vertebrobasilar insufficiency leading to her brainstem TIAs. She is already on dual-antiplatelet therapy, but her medications should be optimized if possible. Given the multiple TIAs despite therapy, endovascular management via balloon angioplasty and stenting could be considered. (Examinee should explain the planned procedure step by step.)

The patient is scheduled for an angioplasty and stenting procedure. The angioplasty of the critical stenosis is successfully achieved, and a stent is placed across the area of stenosis with good wall approximation. The post-placement injection demonstrates significantly improved flow through the vertebrobasilar system compared to the pre-placement injection. Before the catheter is removed, one more injection is performed, and the images are shown in the images.

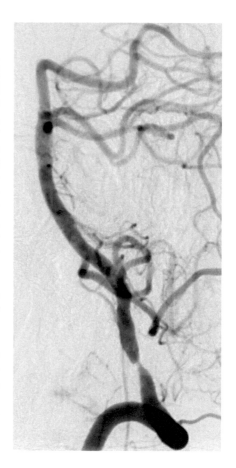

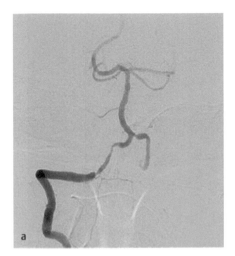

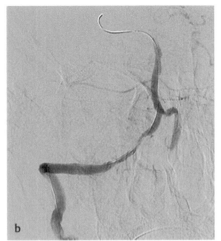

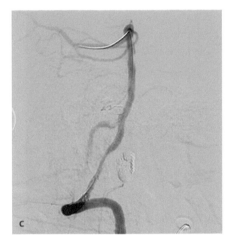

Response

This injection demonstrates a stent placed across the vertebral artery that has significant in-stent stenosis or thrombosis. There is significant risk of periprocedural stroke for this patient. In-stent angioplasty can be attempted for any stent-related complications causing stenosis, but if thrombosis is occurring, the endovascular team should immediately perform an intra-arterial injection of abciximab in an attempt to relieve the thrombosis.

Further Reading

Ashour R, Aziz-Sultan MA. Endovascular treatment of vertebrobasilar insufficiency. In: Spetzler R, Kalani M, Nakaji P, eds. Neurovascular Surgery. 2nd ed. New York, NY: Thieme; 2015:320–329

Potential Other Complications

Groin hematoma, vessel perforation, formation of emboli, brainstem stroke, Cushing response of vitals during endovascular management, dissection.

Case No. 9

A 72-year-old male farmer with a history of hypertension and coronary artery disease is referred to your clinic for a several month history of dizziness, vertigo, and nausea when he is working on the farm. When he stops to rest his symptoms go away. He is not sure what to make of it, but states that whenever he seems to be doing a strenuous activity with his left arm the symptoms again come. It seems worsened on the left compared to the right, but he can't be completely sure.

Response

The patient is reporting signs and symptoms of vertebrobasilar insufficiency, and the history may be suggestive of a flow reversal phenomenon, such as subclavian steal syndrome. The patient should have blood pressure testing in both arms as well as a complete neurological examination and vessel imaging to include the aortic arch, neck, and brain.

The patient's examination is normal in your clinic. Blood pressure testing demonstrates a pressure of 165/88 in the right arm, and 141/80 in the left arm. A CT angiogram is performed and the results are shown in the image.

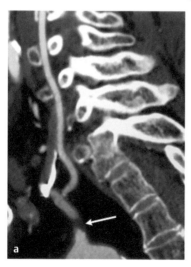 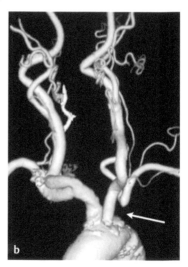

Response

The CT angiogram and 3D reconstruction demonstrate occlusion of the subclavian artery near its origin, and reconstitution of the distal subclavian flow via flow reversal in the vertebral artery. This is an example of subclavian steal syndrome. The >20 mm Hg difference in blood pressure between arms is consistent with the diagnosis, and the patient's symptoms also correlated with the findings on vascular imaging. The patient should be taken to the endovascular suite for an attempt at crossing the area of occlusion and performing an angioplasty and/or stenting procedure. (Examinee should explain the planned procedure step by step.)

Further Reading

Berlis A. Subclavian steal syndrome. In: Jansen O, Brückmann H, eds. Interventional Stroke Therapy. 1st ed. New York, NY: Thieme; 2013:17–182

The patient is taken to the endovascular suite and images from the successful angioplasty and stenting procedure are shown.

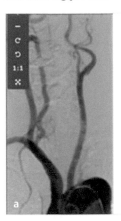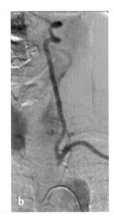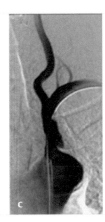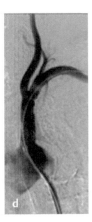

The final injection demonstrates an excellent result, with improved flow to the left arm, as well as symmetry in blood pressure readings between the two extremities. Your assistant notices that in the distal subclavian artery there appears to be contrast flowing into a false lumen in the vicinity of your guidewire.

Response

The distal subclavian artery may have an iatrogenic dissection, caused by aggressive manipulation of the guidewire in the vessel. The presence of the dissection puts the patient at risk for ischemic complications, and therefore he should continue on a heparin infusion or start antiplatelet agents to ensure no emboli form and cause peripheral ischemia. Stenting could be performed in the distal subclavian if required, but care must be taken to correctly identify the true lumen of the vessel, which will have active flow and no stasis.

Further Reading

Welch BG, Eddleman C. Endovascular management of extracranial carotid and vertebral artery aneurysms and dissections ⑨. Nader R, Gragnanielllo C, Berta S, et al., eds. Neurosurgery Tricks of the Trade. Cranial. 1st ed. New York, NY: Thieme; 2014:455–461

Potential Other Complications

Groin hematoma, vessel perforation, in-stent thrombosis, air emboli, renal failure, contrast allergy.

Case No. 10

You are called by the emergency department to evaluate a 48-year-old woman who is now being intubated for airway protection and a depressed neurologic examination. She reported to the emergency department that she had an extremely bad headache earlier in the day. Before she was intubated, she was very confused, drowsy, and demonstrating mild weakness of the left hemibody compared to the right.

Response

The patient's history is concerning for aneurysmal subarachnoid hemorrhage (aSAH), and intubation should be performed if deemed necessary by the emergency department team. The patient should proceed immediately to head CT and preparations should be made for possible external ventricular drain. If aSAH is confirmed, the patient was a Hunt and Hess grade III SAH prior to intubation, which portends a serious prognosis, with mortality at approximately 37%.

The patient is intubated and sedated. Her results for head CT are shown in the image.

Response

The head CT demonstrates evidence of subarachnoid hemorrhage that is likely aneurysmal. It can be difficult to determine the location of an aneurysm, but in this case there is significant clot burden in the interhemispheric fissure, as well as parenchymal hemorrhage into the gyrus rectus. This makes an anterior communicating artery aneurysm high on the differential. There is thick cisternal clot with hydrocephalus and also evidence of intraventricular hemorrhage in the fourth ventricle, making this a modified Fisher grade IV SAH, and at high risk for vasospasm. The dilation of the temporal horns is suggestive of hydrocephalus, and this patient should have an external ventricular drain

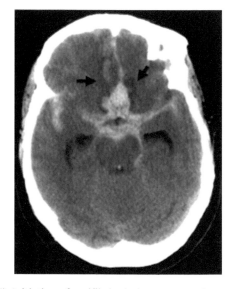

placed in the neuro intensive care unit (ICU). Initiation of antifibrinolytic agents, such as tranexamic acid, could be utilized until a potential aneurysm is secured, to decrease the risk of early re-bleeding. Nimodipine should be administered (60 mg PO Q4 or equivalent timing), and basic labs monitored daily. The patient should be scheduled for conventional angiogram as soon as feasible to both identify and potentially treat any identified aneurysm. Transcranial Dopplers should be scheduled to evaluate for vasospasm in the post-treatment phase.

Further Reading

Cohen M, Jethwa P, Prestigiacomo CJ, et al. Subarachnoid hemorrhage: workup and diagnosis. In: Harbaugh R, Shaffrey C, Couldwell W, et al., eds. Neurosurgery Knowledge Update. A Comprehensive Review. 1st ed. New York, NY: Thieme; 2015:39–43

The patient is stabilized, and an EVD is placed. She is taken to the endovascular suite where an angiogram demonstrates a large, irregular anterior communicating artery aneurysm. It has a favorable projection from the vessel, and it is successfully coiled by the endovascular team. She is returned to the neuro ICU. She is closely monitored, and her EVD remains at 10 mm Hg, and ICPs remain low. She is extubated and by post-bleed day 4 she is following commands reliably. On post-bleed day 8 she is drowsier and is clearly not moving the left arm as briskly as the day before. Transcranial dopplers (TCDs) are ordered and demonstrate increased velocities of the right MCA and anterior cerebral artery (ACA).

Response

The patient is likely experiencing vasospasm after a H+H grade III, modified Fisher grade 4 aneurysm. Her risk of vasospasm was approximately 40%. Initially she could be given fluids as well as permissive hypertension in an attempt to improve her perfusion, if this does not improve her condition she should be taken to the endovascular suite for evaluation and potential management. In the endovascular suite the areas of vasospasm could be identified and treated via angioplasty or intra-arterial injection of verapamil. TCDs should be continued as vasospasm could recur or develop in other vascular territories. (Examinee should explain the planned procedure step by step.)

Further Reading

Ringer AJ. Cerebral vasospasm. In: Harbaugh R, Shaffrey C, Couldwell W, et al., eds. Neurosurgery Knowledge Update. A Comprehensive Review. 1st ed. New York, NY: Thieme; 2015:49–53

Potential Other Complications

Aneurysmal re-bleed, cerebral salt wasting, syndrome of inappropriate antidiuretic hormone secretion (SIADH), coil migration, inability to coil the aneurysm, ischemic stroke.

Category 5: Tumor

Case No. 1

A 55-year-old man comes to your clinic with complaints of worsening vision. Specifically, he states that he is having difficulty seeing things in his peripheral vision, on both sides. It has been worsening over the past several months. He isn't sure if this is related, but also reports difficulty with impotence over that same time interval that has been worsening. He has never had either of these symptoms before.

Response

The patient should undergo a complete neurologic examination including visual field testing, imaging of the brain (preferably magnetic resonance imaging [MRI]), and likely an endocrine panel as his symptoms are concerning for a pituitary mass. If a mass is present, the endocrine panel will help identify if this is a functioning or nonfunctioning adenoma.

On examination the patient is neurologically intact, but has bitemporal hemianopsia that is fairly profound. He has an endocrine panel performed and growth hormone, adrenocorticotropic hormone (ACTH), luteinizing hormone, follicle-stimulating hormone, thyroid-stimulating hormone, thyroxine, cortisol, insulin-like growth factor 1, testosterone, and estradiol are within normal limits; however, prolactin is elevated at 98 µg/L. MRI was obtained and is shown in the image.

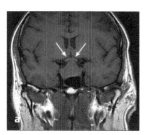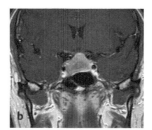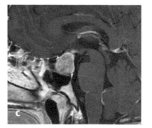

Response

The patient has a large, pituitary macroadenoma causing compression of the optic chiasm. The endocrine panel suggests a nonfunctioning adenoma as all labs are normal, with the exception of prolactin, which is elevated, but consistent with stalk effect rather than a functioning prolactinoma. Given the visual disturbances, this patient should proceed to the operating room (OR) for surgical resection. There are several techniques for this procedure, but given the location of the optic chiasm, a transsphenoidal approach (microscope or endoscope assisted) is likely the best. Postoperatively, the patient should be monitored and labs should be sent the next day, specifically cortisol and sodium in this case. (Examinee should explain the planned procedure step by step.)

Further Reading

Singer J, Selman W. Pituitary adenomas. In: Harbaugh R, Shaffrey C, Couldwell W, et al., eds. Neurosurgery Knowledge Update. A Comprehensive Review. 1st ed. New York, NY: Thieme; 2015:893–896

Khan OH, Zadeh G. Pituitary tumors. In: Bernstein M, Berger M, eds. Neuro-Oncology: The Essentials. 3rd ed. New York, NY: Thieme; 2015:410–417

The patient is taken to the OR for a microscope-assisted transsphenoidal resection of the pituitary adenoma. After the dura is opened, a significant portion of tumor is able to be expressed and is under mild pressure. Using ring curettes, the remainder of the tumor is resected and tissue is sent to pathology. When the anterosuperior region of the tumor is removed, the arachnoid is visualized, and a tear occurs. Cerebrospinal fluid (CSF) is seen leaking into the sella.

Response

Unfortunately a CSF leak has occurred and will need to be repaired. During a microscope-assisted procedure, subcutaneous fat can be taken from the abdomen and placed into the sella, then covered with a tissue sealant. Overpacking the sella with fat can lead to pituitary compression and hormonal failure. During endoscope-assisted surgery, fat is also used, and a nasoseptal flap may be required to treat the leak.

Potential Other Complications

Diabetes insipidus, hypocortisolemia, persistent CSF leak, carotid injury, early aggressive recurrence.

Case No. 2

You are consulted by the neurology service regarding a 69-year-old man with a 60-pack-year history of smoking and a known history of non-small cell lung cancer who was admitted to their service after having a complex partial seizure. Imaging was obtained and is shown in the image. On examination he has mild weakness of the right upper extremity but is otherwise full strength and neuro intact.

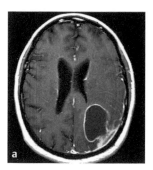 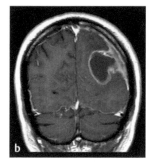

Response

This patient has a large, dural-based mass in the left parietal region. With a history of lung cancer, this mass is most likely to be a dural-based metastatic lesion. He should be started on an anti-epileptic drug (AED) as well as dexamethasone to decrease the peri-lesional edema and hopefully to improve his symptoms. Given the size of this lesion, stereotactic radiosurgery (SRS) is not likely a viable option owing to increased risk of complications and decreased efficacy when maximal diameter is >3 cm. The dural-based nature of the mass would also make targeting potentially difficult and local recurrence very likely. Surgical resection should be offered to this patient if he is medically able to tolerate such a procedure. This would include resection of the mass as well as the involved dura. The mass is close to the sensorimotor cortex, so monitoring could be considered, but most likely surgical resection remaining within the tumor margins will adequately decompress the surrounding brain and obtain adequate tissue for diagnosis. (Examinee should explain the planned procedure step by step.) Postoperative radiation will likely be necessary given the dural-based nature, and the type of radiation (whole brain vs. SRS) would likely depend on the presence of any other metastatic lesions, their number, and size. This is still a topic of active debate.

Further Reading

Patel AJ, Lang F, Sawaya R. Metastatic brain tumors. In: Bernstein M, Berger M, eds. Neuro-Oncology: The Essentials. 3rd ed. New York, NY: Thieme; 2015:451–461

Pabaney AH, Kalkanis SN. Management of brain metastases. In: Harbaugh R, Shaffrey C, Couldwell W, et al., eds. Neurosurgery Knowledge Update. A Comprehensive Review. 1st ed. New York, NY: Thieme; 2015:867–870

The patient is taken to the OR for open surgical resection. The mass and involved dura are readily identified and resected. In order to adequately resect the anterior margin, a fixed retractor is utilized for visualization. The patient recovers from surgery well, but has significantly worsened weakness in the right upper extremity. Postoperative imaging demonstrates no hematoma or diffusion restriction. There is continued edema around the resection cavity.

Response

The patient likely has temporarily worsened motor function in the right upper extremity due to retraction injury during surgery. The fixed retractor may have worsened the edema already present. The patient should be continued on dexamethasone and potentially even have the dose increased. Rehab services should be consulted and assist the patient in postoperative recovery. Long periods of fixed brain retraction should be avoided if possible.

Potential Other Complications

Intraoperative pathology demonstrates lymphoma, postop seizure, early local recurrence.

Case No. 3

A 32-year-old woman is sent to your clinic with a cerebellar mass that was discovered by her local primary care provider and neurologist. She has had persistent headaches and has developed right upper extremity intention tremor and ataxia. She has an otherwise normal neurologic examination. She has a history of retinal hemangioblastoma of the right eye discovered 5 years ago. MRI of the brain was performed and is shown in the image.

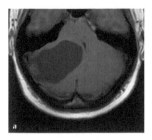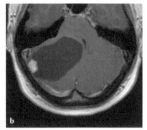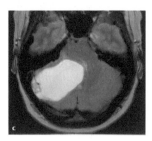

Response

The patient has a symptomatic posterior fossa mass with a large cystic component and enhancing mural nodule. This could represent a low-grade glioma, such as a pilocytic astrocytoma; however, with a history of retinal hemangioblastoma and the patient's age, this is most likely to be a cerebellar hemangioblastoma. It is also very likely that the patient has Von Hippel Lindau (VHL) syndrome. A genetics workup should be performed to evaluate for VHL, and further diagnostic imaging of the abdomen should be considered given the propensity for other mass abnormalities in these patients (clear cell renal tumors, pheochromocytomas, islet cell tumors of the pancreas). The posterior fossa mass will require treatment via resection, but approach should be planned carefully. There is a high likelihood that this patient will develop another hemangioblastoma of the cerebellum in the future, and may require reoperation. Approaches to the tumor should be tailored such that a return to the OR in the future is not hampered by the initial surgical resection. (Examinee should explain the planned procedure step by step.)

Further Reading

Naftel RP, Pollack IF. The phakomatoses > von Hippel-Lindau disease. In: Albright A, Pollack I, Adelson P, eds. Principles and Practice of Pediatric Neurosurgery. 3rd ed. New York, NY: Thieme; 2015:647–649

Snelling BM, Theodotou C, Komotar RJ. Posterior fossa tumors. In: Harbaugh R, Shaffrey C, Couldwell W, et al., eds. Neurosurgery Knowledge Update. A Comprehensive Review. 1st ed. New York, NY: Thieme; 2015:920–924

The patient is worked up by genetics and scanned for other masses, and VHL is confirmed, but no other masses are found. She is taken to the OR for tumor resection. When the dura is opened, the cerebellum immediately begins to herniate through the dural opening, and is under significant pressure.

Response

In this setting, the mass effect of the large cyst is causing increased posterior fossa pressure and causing the cerebellar cortex to herniate through the dural defect. Standard measures to decrease pressure, (i.e., hyperventilation, steroid administration, cerebrospinal fluid [CSF] drainage) will take time, and in the case of local CSF drainage, may be technically challenging and worsen the damage to the herniated cerebellar tissue. In this case the best maneuver would be to use a needle and syringe to puncture the cyst and aspirate cyst fluid contents. With enough aspiration, the posterior fossa pressure should substantially decrease and the herniated cerebellum will abate. Care should be taken to avoid puncturing the cyst through the mural nodule, which will likely be very vascular and could lead to significant hematoma formation.

Potential Other Complications

Severe hemorrhage from tumor during inspection, intraoperative pathology demonstrates pilocytic astrocytoma, CSF leak.

Case No. 4

A 28-year-old male is referred to your clinic after suffering a complex seizure with secondary generalization. He does not have a history of seizure disorder. The seizure started with speech arrest and was followed by a generalized tonic-clonic seizure that spontaneously aborted. He was taken to a local emergency department and was started on levetiracetam (Keppra) and had a computed tomography (CT) scan performed. Apparently it demonstrated an abnormality. He was discharged home and referred to you. He does not have the images with him at this appointment.

Response

It is concerning for this 28-year-old to have had a seizure and an abnormality on imaging. He should undergo a neurologic examination and further imaging, including an MRI. His outside CT scan should be uploaded and evaluated.

On examination the patient is neurologically intact. He has occasional difficulty with word finding and will substitute words when he gets stuck. The original CT scan is uploaded and results of the MRI are shown in the image. There is no evidence of contrast enhancement on contrasted scans.

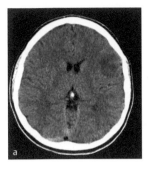 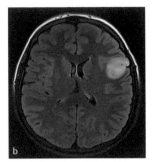 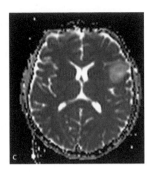

Response

The patient's CT scan demonstrates a hypodensity in the left frontal region. This is confirmed to be a mass lesion in the left frontal region based on the T2 FLAIR and apparent diffusion coefficient (ADC) scans. The report states no contrast enhancement. This is concerning for a glioma, likely low grade. Given the location of this lesion, language function may be at risk given the proximity to Broca's area in the left frontal operculum. Functional MRI (fMRI) could be performed to location of language. If an fMRI confirms left-sided location (roughly 80–90% of patients) considerations should be given to awake surgery with language mapping and monitoring. (Examinee should explain the planned procedure step by step.)

Further Reading

Ampie L, Sanai N. Low-grade gliomas. In: Harbaugh R, Shaffrey C, Couldwell W, et al., eds. Neurosurgery Knowledge Update. A Comprehensive Review. 1st ed. New York, NY: Thieme; 2015:876–881
Duffau H. Low-grade gliomas > The impact of surgical resection in low-grade glioma. In: Bernstein M, Berger M, eds. Neuro-Oncology: The Essentials. 3rd ed. New York, NY: Thieme; 2015:281–284
Bernstein M, Berger M. Neuro-oncology: the essentials. 3rd ed. New York, NY: Thieme; 2015

The patient would like to have surgery, and open surgical resection via awake craniotomy and language mapping is planned. Electroencephalographic (EEG) monitoring is employed during the procedure. Induction and craniotomy occurs without issue. During language mapping, the stimulator is applied to the exposed cortex. EEG reports sharp waves that are spreading. The patient begins slurring his words. EEG then states that seizure activity is occurring and spreading.

Response

The patient is having a stimulator-induced seizure. Iced saline should immediately be used to irrigate the cortex which can abort seizures. If they continue, anesthesia should begin administering benzodiazepine medications or possibly increase propofol;

however, care will need to be taken to ensure that the patient does not have significant enough respiratory depression to require intubation. Lastly, if the patient generalizes during the seizure, his Mayfield head holder should be disconnected from the operative table to avoid neck/spine injury during a generalized tonic-clonic seizure, or scalp injury from the patient ripping themselves out of the pinion head holder.

Potential Other Complications

Tumor region identified as Broca's area, postoperative MRI shows significant residual, oversedation leading to respiratory compromise.

Case No. 5

A 36-year-old woman has been experiencing mild right-sided hearing loss, tinnitus, and some gait imbalance over the past 3 months. It has been worsening and she was originally referred to a local ENT surgeon. After a significant workup, imaging (MRI) is performed and results are shown in the image. On examination, the mild hearing loss is confirmed and she is neurologically intact, including cranial nerves.

Response

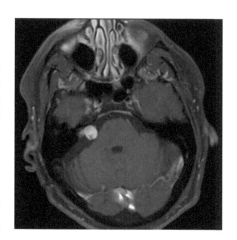

The patient has a mass in the right cerebellopontine angle (CP) that appears to emanate from the internal acoustic canal (IAC) and is contrast-enhancing. It has the appearance of a vestibular (acoustic) schwannoma. Her symptoms, including mild hearing loss, tinnitus, and gait imbalance, fit with the diagnosis of vestibular schwannoma (VS). It is approximately 1.5 cm in size at this time. The first step in management for this patient is likely observation. With one scan in time, it cannot be determined how quickly VS is growing. It could even stabilize. Initial observation with repeat imaging at 3 months is recommended.

Further Reading

Chen C-J, Ding D, Sheehan JP. Acoustic neuroma. In: Harbaugh R, Shaffrey C, Couldwell W, et al., eds. Neurosurgery Knowledge Update. A Comprehensive Review. 1st ed. New York, NY: Thieme; 2015:913–919

Rutkowski MJ, Oh T, Parsa AT. Vestibular schwannomas. In: Bernstein M, Berger M, eds. Neuro-Oncology: The Essentials. 3rd ed. New York, NY: Thieme; 2015:430–438

The patient returns at 3 months as instructed, and a repeat MRI is performed which demonstrates growth of the tumor by 2.5 mm, it is now approximately 1.8 cm. She continues to have her previous symptoms, and hearing testing demonstrates further worsening of her hearing.

Response

The patient now has a rapidly expanding VS with associated symptoms, and should undergo treatment. Given the size of the tumor, several options are available, including microsurgical resection (Examinee should explain the planned procedure step by step.) or stereotactic radiosurgery (SRS) (Examinee should explain the planned procedure step by step.) There are risks and benefits to either approach.

The patient is concerned about SRS, and feels more comfortable with open surgical resection. She is taken to the OR for resection via retrosigmoid craniotomy. When the IAC is being drilled out, it becomes apparent that the semicircular canals have been breached by the drill.

Response

With breach of the semicircular canals, it is very likely that this patient will suffer complete ipsilateral hearing loss. The canal cannot be left open to intracranial contents, and will need to be closed with bone wax or other substance that can cause a water-tight seal. Otherwise the risk of CSF leak is significantly elevated.

Further Reading

Di Ieva A, Lee J, Cusimano M. Posterior skull base surgery > Vestibular schwannoma. In: Handbook of Skull Base Surgery. 1st ed. New York, NY: Thieme; 2016:552–565

Potential Other Complications

Intraoperative stimulation discovers facial nerve schwannoma, swollen cerebellum, entirety of tumor capsule stimulates as CN VII.

Case No. 6

A 20-year-old man is referred to your clinic after having persistent headaches that have worsened over the past month. They are present when he is lying down, but seem to slightly improve when standing. He was initially referred to a local neurologist who discovered papilledema but an otherwise intact neuro examination and obtained an MRI, which is shown in the image.

Response

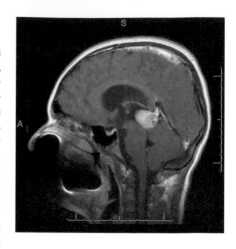

The patient has signs of hydrocephalus on history and physical examination, and imaging demonstrates triventricular hydrocephalus. There is also a contrast-enhancing mass in the pineal region causing compression of the aqueduct, likely leading to obstructive hydrocephalus. This mass could represent many different pathologies. Initial evaluation could include serum markers for alpha fetoprotein, beta human chorionic gonadotropin (b-HCG), and placental alkaline phosphatase (PLAP); however, CSF values of these markers would be more sensitive to detect a germ cell tumor. CSF can be sampled while simultaneously treating the hydrocephalus via endoscopic third ventriculostomy (ETV) with CSF sampling. An attempt could be made to obtain tumor tissue for histopathological diagnosis during the ETV; however, there is a risk of bleeding and forniceal injury when attempting to reach the mass. (Examinee should explain the planned procedure step by step.) If both are performed, the ETV should be performed first, as the mass biopsy could lead to bleeding which would make the ETV very difficult.

Further Reading

Weinberg JS. Pineal region tumors. In: Harbaugh R, Shaffrey C, Couldwell W, et al., eds. Neurosurgery Knowledge Update. A Comprehensive Review. 1st ed. New York, NY: Thieme; 2015:907–912

Tomita T. Pineal region tumors. In: Albright A, Pollack I, Adelson P, eds. Principles and Practice of Pediatric Neurosurgery. 3rd ed. New York, NY: Thieme; 2015:509–525

The patient is taken to the OR for ETV, CSF sampling, and biopsy of the mass. The ETV is performed successfully, CSF markers and serum markers are negative, and a biopsy specimen is obtained. The final pathology is found to be pineoblastoma.

Response

The patient does not have a tumor that can be treated solely with radiation and chemotherapy (such as some germ cell tumors); therefore surgical resection should be performed. There are several approaches to this region, including interhemispheric transcallosal, as well as supracerebellar, infratentorial. Depending on the location of the internal cerebral veins and the vein of Galen, each approach has risks and benefits. (Examinee should explain the planned procedure step by step.) Surgery will obtain further tissue to guide radiation and chemotherapy as well as cytoreduction and aqueductal decompression.

Further Reading

Weinberg JS. Pineal region tumors. In: Harbaugh R, Shaffrey C, Couldwell W, et al., eds. Neurosurgery Knowledge Update. A Comprehensive Review. 1st ed. New York, NY: Thieme; 2015:907–912

The patient is taken to the OR for mass resection via supracerebellar, infratentorial approach. The mass is completely resected. Postoperatively, the patient recovers well, but you notice on postoperative day 1 that the patient is not able to elevate either eye. All other eye movements are intact, but upgaze is absent.

Response

The patient is likely to have developed Parinaud syndrome, or upgaze palsy, from edema or damage to the tectal plate. Imaging should be obtained to rule out any compressive hematoma or other injuries, and if absent, dexamethasone should be administered to decrease cerebral edema. The patient should be observed for spontaneous improvement/resolution of the upgaze palsy.

Further Reading

Elhadi AM, Zaidi HA, Nakaji P. Neuroendoscopic approaches to the pineal region. In: Torres-Corzo J, Rangel-Castilla L, Nakaji P, eds. Neuroendoscopic Surgery. 1st ed. New York, NY: Thieme; 2016:160–170

Potential Other Complications

Bleeding during tumor biopsy, vein of Galen injury, postoperative cerebellar subdural hematoma.

Case No. 7

A 21-year-old man presents to your clinic with complaints of headache for the past month, and increasing episodes of vomiting over the past 2 weeks. He does not feel as though he has been recently ill. He also says he feels that his voice is getting hoarse, and has been coughing quite a bit when he is trying to drink liquids.

Response

The patient's constellation of symptoms is concerning. He should have a complete neurologic examination and an MRI of the brain.

On examination, the patient is full strength in all four extremities and is alert and orient-ed. His CNs are intact with the exception of mild palatal deviation and mild dysarthria. Papilledema is present. MRI is performed and is shown in the image.

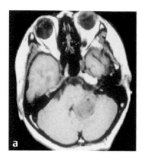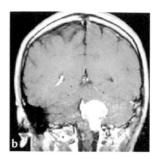

Response

On MRI the patient has an enhancing, fourth ventricular mass that is extending laterally through the foramen of Luschka. There may be associated ventriculomegaly; however, that is not readily apparent on the selected MRI scans. Vomiting is common in cases of ependymoma with involvement of the floor of the fourth ventricle, making that diag-nosis likely. Dysarthria and mild dysphagia can also be explained by invasion of the floor of the fourth ventricle. The patient should have MRI of the entire spine to deter-mine if any CSF dissemination has occurred. Surgery should be planned for histologic diagnosis, likely via a midline, fourth ventricular approach, or potentially a more lateral exposure via a far-lateral approach. (Examinee should explain the planned procedure step by step.)

Further Reading

Wait SD, Taylor M, Boop FA. Ependymomas. In: Albright A, Pollack I, Adelson P, eds. Principles and Practice of Pediatric Neurosurgery. 3rd ed. New York, NY: Thieme; 2015:535–552
Parsa AT, Arnaout O. Ventricular tumors (colloid cyst, ependymoma, central neurocytoma, miscellaneous ventricular tumors). In: Harbaugh R, Shaffrey C, Couldwell W, et al., eds. Neurosurgery Knowledge Update. A Comprehensive Review. 1st ed. New York, NY: Thieme; 2015:903–906

The patient is taken to the OR for tumor resection via a midline suboccipital approach. After the craniotomy is completed, bone is being removed near the transverse sinus, and the anesthesiologist notifies you that the oxygen saturation is decreasing. The end-tidal CO$_2$ has dropped significantly. The transesophageal echocardiogram is demonstrating evidence of air.

Response

The patient is experiencing a venous air embolism, potentially via emissary veins in the bone. The operative field should be heavily irrigated and bone surfaces should be cov-ered in bone wax. The head of the bed can be lowered, and anesthesia should provide supportive care. Discussions should be had about any potential need for rapid closure and removal from Mayfield pinions for further resuscitation if necessary.

Further Reading

Flexman AM, Talke PO. Neuroanesthesia > Anesthesia considerations for operations in the posterior fossa. In: Spetzler R, Kalani M, Nakaji P, eds. Neurovascular Surgery. 2nd ed. New York, NY: Thieme; 2015:147

Potential Other Complications

Posterior inferior cerebellar artery (PICA) injury, tumor invasion of the floor of the fourth ventricle, drop metastases.

Case No. 8

A 53-year-old woman is referred to your clinic by her neurologist with worsening visual acuity in the left eye as well as mild temporal visual field loss in her right eye. She also has headaches and has occasionally been found to have mild word finding difficulties. She is otherwise neurologically intact on examination. All of these findings prompted an MRI of the brain and the results are shown in the image.

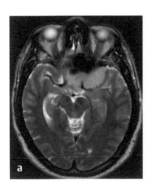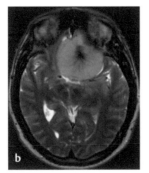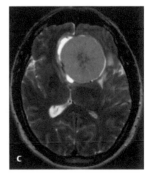

Response

This patient has a very large, medial sphenoid wing mass that appears to be consistent with a meningioma, although contrasted scans are not present in this series. The middle MR image demonstrates a likely dural origin along the middle sphenoid wing. There appears to be a CSF plane around the mass in the far right image, but also flow voids around and through the mass which likely represent displaced arteries that may or may not be feeding the tumor. Given this patient's worsening symptoms and mass effect, a surgical resection should be attempted. It may be prudent to first obtain an angiogram and potential embolization of the meningioma; however, this tumor is likely to be fed by branches of the middle meningeal artery (which is easy to obliterate during surgery) as well as dural branches from the cavernous ICA (which are difficult to embolize without risk to upper cranial nerves). Further, if a mass of this size is embolized preoperatively, either close observation or immediate surgery should occur as the mass could swell and cause further mass effect and deficits. Resection of this tumor will likely require drilling of the sphenoid wing and anterior clinoid process as well as decompression of the optic canal. (Examinee should explain the planned procedure step by step.)

Further Reading

DeMonte F, McDermott M, Al-Mefty O. Al-Mefty's meningiomas. 2nd ed. New York, NY: Thieme; 2011

Ali F. Krisht. Clinoidal meningiomas. In: DeMonte F, McDermott M, Al-Mefty O, eds. Al-Mefty's Meningiomas. 2nd ed. New York, NY: Thieme; 2011:228–236

Di Ieva A, Lee J, Cusimano M. Middle skull base surgery > Meningiomas involving the sphenoid bone. In: Handbook of Skull Base Surgery. 1st ed. New York, NY: Thieme; 2016:489–498

The patient is taken to surgery for resection of the mass. Embolization of the middle meningeal artery is performed preoperatively, but branches from the cavernous ICA could not be safely embolized. The mass is completely resected with significant difficulty and moderate blood loss. The anterior clinoid is removed and the optic canal is decompressed. Inspection of the operative cavity after tumor resection is performed demonstrates a completely intact optic chiasm and optic nerves bilaterally. When the patient recovers from surgery, she endorses complete visual loss in the left eye.

Response

Unfortunately the optic nerve was damaged during the surgical resection, either via tumor manipulation, stretch, or heat transfer from the drill bit when the sphenoid wing is drilled. Care should be taken to avoid significant manipulation of the optic nerve during resection if possible, and irrigation should be used during bony drilling around the optic nerve to avoid heat damage. With an intact optic nerve and visual loss, dexamethasone and observation should be utilized in hopes of return of function.

Potential Other Complications

Carotid injury, cavernous sinus bleeding, breach into ethmoid air cells during clinoidectomy, brain invasion by meningioma, ACA injury.

Case No. 9

A 35-year-old man presents to your clinic with progressively worsening hearing loss on the right, and his family members have noticed that when he smiles the right side of his face doesn't move as well. He also reports being slightly unsteady on his feet and has had a headache over the same time interval.

Response

The patient is describing cranial nerve palsies and should undergo a complete neurologic examination as well as imaging of the brain with MRI.

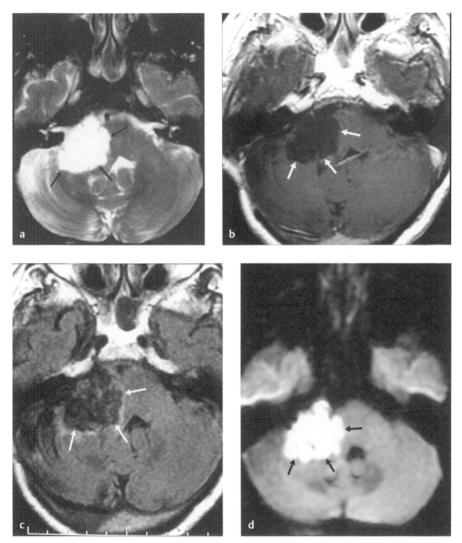

On examination, the patient is alert and oriented with full strength in all four extremities. He has a right-sided lateral gaze palsy (cannot bury the eye), a House-Brackmann grade II right facial palsy, right hearing loss, and palatal elevation to the left side. MRI is performed and shown in the image.

Response

The patient has a CP angle mass that does not enhance and is restricts diffusion on DWI. This is a classic appearance for an epidermoid tumor of the CP angle. The mass effect from the tumor contents are likely causing is cranial neuropathies, and resection should be attempted. It is important to counsel the patient that the risk of recurrence of this tumor is very high, as it can be unacceptably morbid to attempt to resect the entirety of the tumor capsule which may be invested with the brainstem or other critical structures. Unfortunately, unless the entirety of the capsule is resected, the tumor is likely to recur. There are several approaches to resect this tumor. (Examinee should explain the planned procedure step by step.)

Further Reading

Almefty KK, Erkmen K, Al-Mefty O. Skull base meningiomas and other tumors > Epidermoid and dermoid tumors. In: Bernstein M, Berger M, eds. Neuro-Oncology: The Essentials. 3rd ed. New York, NY: Thieme; 2015:405–407

The patient is taken to the OR for resection of the tumor. During exposure and bone removal over the transverse sinus, a segment of bone is removed and the operative field is suddenly filled with dark blood.

Response

It is likely that a sinus injury has occurred. Anesthesia should be notified of the potential for significant blood loss. If there is an obvious tear that is easily accessible, an attempt at suture repair could be considered, but this is almost never possible. A piece of Gelfoam should be placed over the laceration followed by a cottonoid patty and suction to provide counter pressure and contain the bleeding. Tack holes should be drilled into the bone and dural tack-up sutures placed to fold the dura over the point of laceration. When the tack-up sutures are tightened, the Gelfoam should seal the laceration. The tack sutures should be left in place permanently.

Further Reading

Davidson L, Armonda RA. Management of venous sinus injuries. In: Ullman J, Raksin P, eds. Atlas of Emergency Neurosurgery. 1st ed. New York, NY: Thieme; 2015:153–168

Potential Other Complications

CSF leak/pseudomeningocele, AICA injury, tumor extending anteriorly into suprasellar region.

Case No. 10

You are consulted by neurology regarding a 59-year-old man who was admitted to their service with persistent headache and has the MRI shown in the image. His examination is otherwise neurologically intact.

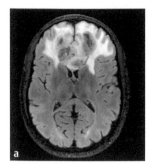 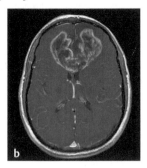

Response

The patient has a butterfly appearing mass crossing the corpus callosum with rim-enhancement on MRI. This is almost certainly a glioblastoma in this 59-year-old man. Unfortunately, with the location of this tumor, surgical resection is not an option. Tissue should be obtained for diagnostic purposes and could be achieved via a stereotactic needle biopsy of the lesion. (Examinee should explain the planned procedure step by step.)

Further Reading

Lüppert A, Rähn T. Frame-based stereotactic brain biopsy Ⓐ. In: Nader R, Gragnanielllo C, Berta S, et al., eds. Neurosurgery Tricks of the Trade. Cranial. 1st ed. New York, NY: Thieme; 2014:550–553

McDermott MW, Garcia RM, Bernstein M. Imaged-guided surgery: frame and frameless > Stereotactic brain lesion biopsy. In: Bernstein M, Berger M, eds. Neuro-Oncology: The Essentials. 3rd ed. New York, NY: Thieme; 2015:114–121

The patient is taken to the OR for stereotactic needle biopsy of the lesion. The first sample is taken without issue and appears abnormal. During aspiration of the second sample, blood is present in the syringe. When the inner portion of the biopsy needle is removed, blood is found to be coming out of the biopsy instrument.

Response

The outer biopsy instrument with open side port should be left in place to allow a tract for blood to escape. Gentle irrigation down the needle can be performed to provide back pressure, attempting to stop the bleeding. This should be applied continuously until bleeding is no longer encountered. The patient should be taken to the CT scanner for immediate imaging.

Further Reading

McDermott MW, Garcia RM, Bernstein M. Imaged-guided surgery: frame and frameless > Stereotactic brain lesion biopsy. In: Bernstein M, Berger M, eds. Neuro-Oncology: The Essentials. 3rd ed. New York, NY: Thieme; 2015:114–121

Potential Other Complications

Negative biopsy, intraventricular puncture.

Category 6: Pediatrics

Case No. 1

A 16-year-old teenager with a history of L1 myelomeningocele repair at birth, developmental delay, and shunted hydrocephalus comes to the emergency department with his mother, who states that over the past 3 days he has been more irritable, and seems to be complaining of a headache. His last shunt replacement was performed 5 years ago.

Response

The patient should be evaluated for a possible shunt malfunction. This includes a physical examination, basic labs including infectious markers, shunt series, and head computed tomography (CT).

On examination, the patient is wheelchair-bound, not moving either lower extremity. He moves both upper extremities purposefully, but holds them to his head. He responds to basic questioning and has his eyes open, but appears irritable. Basic labs are normal, including erythrocyte sedimentation rate/C-reactive protein (ESR/CRP) and he is afebrile. Shunt series does not demonstrate any disconnection. Head CT is shown in the image (previous head CT demonstrates normal ventricular size).

Response

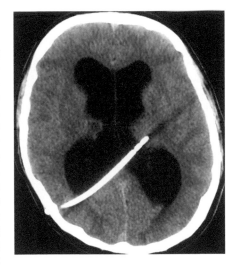

The patient's examination and imaging are suggestive of a shunt malfunction. The head CT demonstrates ventriculomegaly, and the shunt catheter appears to have backed out of its previous location. The patient should be scheduled for the operating room as soon as possible for shunt evaluation and revision. During the procedure the catheter can be redirected to a more advantageous position. In the operating room, the patient should be prepped and draped as if the entire shunt system will need to be replaced. During the procedure, cerebrospinal fluid (CSF) should be sent for culture to rule out infection. (Examinee should explain the planned procedure step by step.)

Further Reading

Kalra RS, Kestle J. Treatment of hydrocephalus with shunts > Shunt failure. In: Albright A, Pollack I, Adelson P, eds. Principles and Practice of Pediatric Neurosurgery. 3rd ed. New York, NY: Thieme; 2015:111–114

The patient is taken to the operating room and the cranial incision is opened. The distal catheter is disconnected from the valve, and spontaneous flow from the valve and proximal catheter are observed. A pressure manometer is filled up with saline and connected to the distal catheter, and no flow is observed distally.

Response

It appears to be a distal shunt obstruction; however, the proximal catheter is not in an ideal position. The entire shunt should be replaced. If it were simply a proximal catheter or valve problem, those elements could be removed and connected to the distal catheter.

Further Reading

Sivakumar W, Riva-Cambrin J, Ravindra VM, Kestle J. Ventricular shunting for hydrocephalus. In: Cohen A, ed. Pediatric Neurosurgery: Tricks of the Trade. 1st ed. New York, NY: Thieme; 2016:316–320

Case No. 2

A 12-year-old girl is brought to your office by her mother who states that she has been having daily left-sided headaches for the past 3 months. The patient points to a region just above and behind her left eye as the origin point of her symptoms. She has been evaluated by a multidisciplinary team who obtained imaging that demonstrated some type of cystic abnormality; however, the CT scans are not available for your review. She has been put on several medications with no improvement in her symptoms. She was referred to you by her local neurologist who is helping to manage her care.

Response

Unfortunately the images are not available for review, so an imaging study will need to be repeated, preferably a magnetic resonance imaging (MRI) of the brain. She should also undergo a complete neurologic examination.

Her neurologic examination is completely normal, and an MRI of the brain is obtained and shown in the image.

Response

The MRI is suggestive of a left-sided arachnoid cyst in the region of the middle fossa. This is a developmental abnormality, but they are rarely symptomatic, with only approximately 7% being thought to have associated symptoms. In many cases of incidental discovery they can simply be monitored. In this patient's case, she is clearly symptomatic, and demonstrates a headache origin directly over the cyst

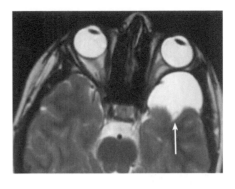

region. A case could still be made for observation in this patient, but the option of surgical exploration and fenestration via multiple techniques should be considered. For a cyst in this region, successful surgery is approximately 75% or less. (Examinee should explain the planned procedure step by step.)

Further Reading

Garton HJL. The Dandy–Walker complex and arachnoid cysts > Arachnoid cysts. In: Albright A, Pollack I, Adelson P, eds. Principles and Practice of Pediatric Neurosurgery. 3rd ed. New York, NY: Thieme; 2015:149–157
Sgouros S, Tsitouras V. Congenital intracranial cysts. In: Cohen A, ed. Pediatric Neurosurgery: Tricks of the Trade. 1st ed. New York, NY: Thieme; 2016:325–329

The patient and family members decide that medical management has not been working and they would like to proceed with surgery. The patient is taken to the operating room for an endoscopic cyst fenestration into the basal cisterns. The procedure is completed as planned, and a large fenestration into the basal cisterns is created. She recovers well initially from the procedure, but the evening of surgery, you are called by nursing who state that she has a significant headache and has vomited several times. The overnight resident obtained a head CT which was negative for any acute intracranial abnormality, and demonstrates the fenestration is open. The size of the cyst even appears to have decreased somewhat.

Response

While postoperative hemorrhage would immediately need to be considered, the head CT was negative for hemorrhage, and the fenestration appears to remain open. When a cyst has successfully been fenestrated, the intracranial contents can take time to re-equilibrate. This can cause headaches and vomiting in the postoperative period. The normal head CT is reassuring, and the patient should be treated for nausea and observed, as the symptoms will likely improve.

Potential Other Complications

Cyst recurrence, cyst hemorrhage.

Case No. 3

You are consulted by the pediatric neurology team regarding a 6-year-old boy who was admitted to their service with persistent headaches, occasional vomiting, and some difficulty swallowing. On examination he is awake, but has a headache, will respond to basic questions, and demonstrates spontaneous, full strength movements of all four extremities. His cranial nerves are intact with the exception of slight deviation of the uvula to the left side. They obtained an MRI which is shown in the image.

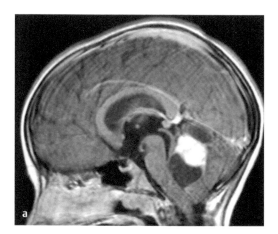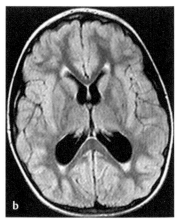

Response

The patient has symptoms consistent with hydrocephalus, and on examination he has deviation of the uvula suggesting some brainstem and/or cranial nerve dysfunction. The MRI demonstrates a cystic mass with an enhancing nodule causing mass effect, some evidence of brainstem compression. There is also evidence of hydrocephalus with an expanded aqueduct and trans-ependymal flow in the supratentorial compartment. The mass is consistent with a likely WHO grade I pilocytic astrocytoma. The patient could be started on appropriate doses of dexamethasone to decrease edema and potentially symptoms, but the patient should be schedule for surgery during this hospitalization. External ventricular drainage preoperatively could be considered, but the patient could also be observed until surgical resection can be performed. (Examinee should explain the planned procedure step by step.)

Further Reading

Da Silva SL, Krieger MD. Cerebellar astrocytoma. In: Cohen A, ed. Pediatric Neurosurgery: Tricks of the Trade. 1st ed. New York, NY: Thieme; 2016:481–487

Peruzzi P, Boué DR, Raffel C. Cerebellar astrocytomas > Treatment. In: Albright A, Pollack I, Adelson P, eds. Principles and Practice of Pediatric Neurosurgery. 3rd ed. New York, NY: Thieme; 2015:568–570

The patient is taken to the operating room for a suboccipital craniotomy and tumor resection. The tumor is exposed and all enhancing portions are completely resected. There appears to be good CSF flow through the fourth ventricle and resection cavity. The patient recovers from the surgery well and the headaches/cranial nerve dysfunction improve substantially. Pathology demonstrates WHO grade I pilocytic astrocytoma. Postoperative MRI demonstrated complete resection. During a 6 week postoperative visit, the patient's incision is well-healed, but his mother reports that his headaches have returned. A repeat MRI is obtained and is shown in the image.

Response

The patient has slightly enlarged ventricles and continued trans-ependymal flow. It is likely that he has developed post-resection hydrocephalus, most likely in a communicating fashion. This could be due to blood products or proteinaceous material during resection obstructing the arachnoid villi. This patient will likely require a ventriculo-peritoneal (VP) shunt unless an obvious area of obstruction is demonstrated.

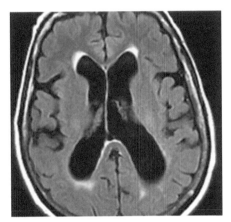

Potential Other Complications

Cerebellar mutism, postoperative hemorrhage.

Case No. 4

You are consulted by the pediatric neurology service regarding a newborn male with an enlarging head circumference. At birth, his head circumference was 37 cm, and now 1 week later, his head circumference is 39 cm. There are no apparent abnormalities on physical examination. The primary team obtained an MRI scan which is shown in the image.

Response

The patient has a large head circumference at birth, and is enlarging at a fast rate. The MRI demonstrates substantial triventricular hydrocephalus. There is aqueductal stenosis present, leading to the triventricular nature of the hydrocephalus. Given that this patient's fontanelles are open, the risk of acute intracranial pressure (ICP) is lessened. However, this patient should receive treatment for the hydrocephalus. Given that the patient is a newborn, a VP shunt may not be feasible. Also, considering the hydrocephalus and enlarged ventricular system, an endoscopic third ventriculostomy (ETV) could be performed. The family members should be counseled that this procedure has an 80 to 90% success rate at avoiding a VP shunt, and the rate of patency of the fenestration is approximately 75% at 1 year postprocedure. (Examinee should explain the planned procedure step by step.)

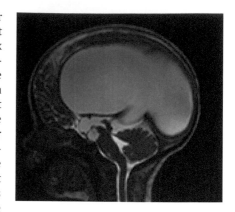

Further Reading

Cohen A, Vogel TW. Neuroendoscopy > Endoscopic procedures. In: Albright A, Pollack I, Adelson P, eds. Principles and Practice of Pediatric Neurosurgery. 3rd ed. New York, NY: Thieme; 2015:122–131

The patient is taken to the operating room for an ETV. It is performed successfully and there is clear flow through the fenestration at the end of the case. The patient tolerates the procedure well, and head circumference remains stable/within the normal range. At 6 months, the patient returns with continued increased head circumference above normal. Gradient-echo MRI appears to demonstrate closure of the fenestration and recurrent hydrocephalus.

Response

Unfortunately the patient likely has a failed ETV. Based on the ETV success score, this patient had several factors going against success, mostly related to young age. At this point, he is likely big enough to tolerate a VP shunt procedure, and a shunt should be placed to treat the hydrocephalus.

Further Reading

Hardesty D, Little AS. Endoscopic third ventriculostomy. In: Torres-Corzo J, Rangel-Castilla L, Nakaji P, ed. Neuroendoscopic Surgery. 1st ed. New York, NY: Thieme; 2016:225–232

Potential Other Complications

CSF leak, hemorrhage during ETV.

Case No. 5

You are consulted by the pediatric service regarding a newborn female with little to no prenatal care who was born with the abnormality shown in the image. They are unsure how to manage this situation.

Response

The patient has a myelomeningocele, or open neural tube defect. Several things should occur initially. The newborn should be placed in the prone position, with a warmer, and the defect should be evaluated for any evidence of rupture, or CSF leak. The defect should be covered with sterile gauze and direct pressure on the defect should be avoided. Depressing the fontanelle can help identify any evidence of CSF leak. If a leak is present, the patient should be started on antibiotics to avoid the development of ventriculitis, which can negatively affect outcome. Physical examination should be attempted, however, it may need to occur based mostly on observation of spontaneous movement.

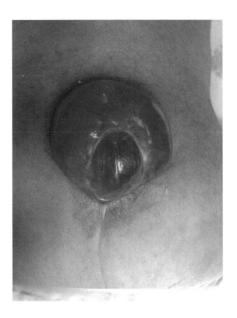

Further Reading

Foster KA, Boop FA. The perinatal management of a child born with a myelomeningocele. In: Loftus C, ed. Neurosurgical Emergencies. 3rd ed. New York, NY: Thieme; 2018:337–346

The patient is placed in the prone position and the defect is covered with sterile dressing. There is no evidence of CSF leak.

Response

Antibiotics can currently be avoided, as the defect appears to be intact, but continued observation of the defect for any signs of leak should occur. Repairing the myelomeningocele should occur urgently, but does not need to happen emergently in this case. The patient should be stabilized and prepared for a semi-elective case by the primary team. (Examinee should explain the planned procedure step by step.)

Further Reading

Warf BC. Myelomeningocele. In: Cohen A, ed. Pediatric Neurosurgery: Tricks of the Trade. 1st ed. New York, NY: Thieme; 2016:269–273

The patient is stabilized by the pediatric team; however, later in the evening you are notified that the defect has started to leak CSF.

Response

Now the patient should be started on antibiotics. Choice of antibiotics may differ based on institution, but ampicillin and gentamicin would be adequate starting choices. Most infections are caused by *Escherichia coli*, group b streptococcus, or staphylococcus bacterium. Broad-spectrum antibiotics should be initiated, and the closure of the defect should be scheduled for the next day if possible.

Potential Other Complications

Skin cannot cover defect.

Case No. 6

A 7-year-old girl comes to your office complaining of headaches and irritability over the past month. Her mother reports that the headaches are daily, and getting worse. They seem to be worsened when she lies down, and improved slightly when she is sits upright. Otherwise on examination she is neurologically intact.

Response

The patient has symptoms of increased ICP leading to headaches, specifically with positional worsening of her symptoms. The remainder of the neurologic examination is reassuring, but positional headaches in a 7-year-old are concerning for a mass causing obstructive hydrocephalus. The patient should have an imaging study, preferably an MRI of the brain.

The patient undergoes an MRI of the brain and results are shown in the image.

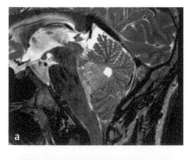
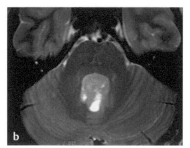
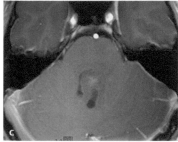

Response

The MRI scan demonstrates a fourth ventricular mass obstructing CSF flow with patchy enhancement. It is located in the midline, and this makes a medulloblastoma a distinct possibility. Given the patient's symptoms, she should be scheduled for surgical resection in the near future. Resection would achieve decompression of CSF pathways as well as tissue diagnosis for any potential further treatment. Consideration should be given to prepping in a Frasier burr hole if necessary for emergent CSF diversion. (Examinee should explain the planned procedure step by step.)

Further Reading

Ostling L, Raffel C. Medulloblastoma. In: Cohen A, ed. Pediatric Neurosurgery: Tricks of the Trade. 1st ed. New York, NY: Thieme; 2016:488–495

The patient goes to the operating room and undergoes a suboccipital craniotomy and tumor resection via a midline cerebellar approach. The final pathology was consistent with a WNT subtype.

Response

There are several major groups of medulloblastoma, WNT, SHH, and Group 3/4. Of these, the WNT subtype has the best prognosis, with approximately 95% 5-year survival. Currently, the recommendations for postoperative adjuvant radiation and chemotherapy are actively being studied and altered, with the idea of reducing potential radiation doses in patients who have an excellent prognosis with complete tumor resection. Consultation with pediatric neuro-oncology and radiation therapy should be performed to get the most up-to-date recommendations on adjuvant therapy for this patient. A full spine MRI should be considered to look for drop metastases.

Further Reading

Merchant TE, Murphy ES. Radiotherapy of pediatric brain tumors > Medulloblastoma. In: Albright A, Pollack I, Adelson P, eds. Principles and Practice of Pediatric Neurosurgery. 3rd ed. New York, NY: Thieme; 2015:676–677

On postoperative day #1, you are rounding on the patient and she is not verbal. She is also very irritable and family/nursing state that since approximately midnight she has been very upset and emotionally labile. It does not appear to be due to pain. She also has some mild nystagmus and ataxia on examination.

Response

The patient underwent a midline cerebellar approach to her tumor, and it appears that she has developed cerebellar mutism, also known as posterior fossa syndrome. It is characterized by decreased speech production, ataxia, and severe irritability/emotional swings. It can occur in up to 20% of these cases. Imaging should be performed to ensure no postoperative complications have occurred in the operative cavity; however if none are identified, observation will be recommended for this patient. Recovery can take significant time, up to 8 weeks in many cases.

Further Reading

Ramaswamy V, Taylor M. Medulloblastomas > Complication: posterior fossa syndrome. In: Albright A, Pollack I, Adelson P, eds. Principles and Practice of Pediatric Neurosurgery. 3rd ed. New York, NY: Thieme; 2015:533

Potential Other Complications

Hydrocephalus, cerebellar herniation upon opening dura.

Case No. 7

A 3-month-old baby is brought to your clinic by his parents because he has an oddly shaped head. He appears to have a pointed forehead and a broadened posterior skull. He is neurologically normal and meeting all milestones.

Response

The patient may have a form of craniosynostosis. With the description, it could be metopic craniosynostosis causing trigonocephaly. The patient should undergo dedicated CT scan of the head to evaluate the sutures to identify the involved suture.

He undergoes a CT scan with 3D reconstruction and results are shown in the image.

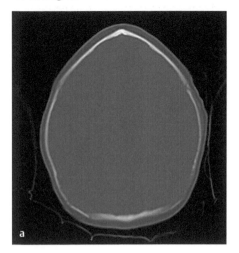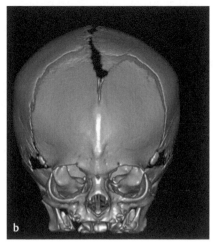

Response

The CT scan demonstrates fusion of the metopic suture causing trigonocephaly. The other sutures remain open. The patient should undergo a reconstruction of the metopic suture, either via open or endoscopic techniques. This procedure can be followed by helmet use to help reshape the skull cosmetically. (Examinee should explain the planned procedure step by step.)

Further Reading

Baird I C, Proctor MR. Craniosynostosis > Surgical treatment. In: Albright A, Pollack I, Adelson P, eds. Principles and Practice of Pediatric Neurosurgery. 3rd ed. New York, NY: Thieme; 2015:239–244

Krieger MD, Ritter AM, Brzezicki G, Conley A. Positional plagiocephaly, craniosynostosis, syndromic craniosynostosis. In: Harbaugh R, Shaffrey C, Couldwell W, et al., eds. Neurosurgery Knowledge Update. A Comprehensive Review. 1st ed. New York, NY: Thieme; 2015:381–389

The patient is taken to the operating room with the assistance of plastic surgery for reconstruction of the metopic suture via a mini-open approach. The suture is successfully reconstructed, but at the end of the procedure, it is noticed that there is a durotomy off midline, likely from retraction of the dura during drilling of the suture. There does not appear to be any underlying brain injury.

Response

A durotomy occurred during the suture reconstruction, and should be repaired during this procedure. Using the durotomy, the underlying brain could be inspected to ensure no vascular injury occurred. If the dura is not repaired, a CSF leak, pseudomeningocele, or growing skull fracture could occur. These can be avoided via direct repair at time of injury.

Potential Other Complications

Sinus injury, incomplete resection of suture.

Case No. 8

You are consulted by the pediatric service regarding an 11-month-old boy (22 lbs) who was admitted to their service for lethargy, decreased oral intake, and irritability. On further examination he is found to move the left side less than the right side, although spontaneous, purposeful movements are still noted to be present. The primary team obtained an MRI scan of the brain requiring intubation, results are shown in the image.

Response

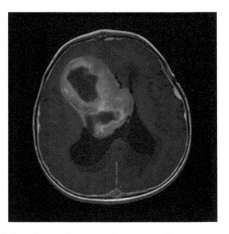

This 11-month-old child has a large, contrast-enhancing mass in the supratentorial space that is most likely a supratentorial primitive neuroectodermal tumor. The mass extends into the ventricle, or possibly arises from the ventricle, so a choroid plexus papilloma/carcinoma could also be considered; however, it lacks the frond-like appearance for these tumors. Regardless, this patient will need surgical excision of the mass for tissue diagnosis as well as decompression of the intracranial contents. At 11 months of age, the anterior fontanelle is likely still open, and may be bulging due to increased pressure, but emergent CSF diversion is not likely required in this case. Prompt surgical resection should be considered. (Examinee should explain the planned procedure step by step.)

Further Reading

Bhat S, Ann Ahern V, Kellie SJ. Supratentorial primitive neuroectodermal tumors. In: Keating R, Goodrich J, Packer R, eds. Tumors of the Pediatric Central Nervous System. 2nd ed. New York, NY: Thieme; 2013:216–229

Wait SD, Boop FA, Klimo P Jr. Supratentorial nonglial hemispheric neoplasms > Supratentorial primitive neuroectodermal tumors. In: Albright A, Pollack I, Adelson P, eds. Principles and Practice of Pediatric Neurosurgery. 3rd ed. New York, NY: Thieme; 2015:460–461

The patient is taken to the operating room for surgical resection of the mass. Upon exposure of the tumor, it is found to be very vascular. Resection will likely be bloody. Anesthesiologist asks if they should be concerned about operative blood loss.

Response

The patient is 11 months old, and likely has approximately 80 mL/kg blood volume. At 22 lbs, he is approximately 10 kg, and therefore has only 800 cc of total blood volume. Anesthesiologist should be made aware of the potential for significant blood loss during a resection of a tumor of this size in a young patient. Blood should be in the room cross-matched and ready for transfusion if necessary. Extreme care will need to be taken during exposure and resection to ensure minimal blood loss. Despite these maneuvers, transfusion is very likely to be required.

Potential Other Complications

Postoperative hydrocephalus, postoperative seizures.

Case No. 9

You are consulted by maternal-fetal medicine regarding a woman who is 30 weeks pregnant and prenatal ultrasound detected an abnormality of the brain. An MRI was obtained and is shown in the image.

Response

The patient has a small occipital encephalocele on MRI. It does not appear to have any brain tissue herniating through the defect currently. The pregnancy should continue, and at this time there is no indication for fetal surgery. Delivery should occur, however, the maternal-fetal medicine team feels is appropriate, and the encephalocele can be addressed after birth likely via an elective repair unless there is evidence of CSF leak.

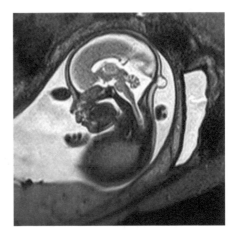

Further Reading

Jimenez DF, Barone CM. Encephaloceles, meningoceles, and dermal sinuses > Encephaloceles. In: Albright A, Pollack I, Adelson P, eds. Principles and Practice of Pediatric Neurosurgery. 3rd ed. New York, NY: Thieme; 2015:205–223

The patient is delivered via vaginal delivery with no complications. The patient is monitored by the pediatrician, and you are notified that the encephalocele appears to be increasing in size. Repeat MRI is performed at 1 month and is shown below.

Response

Unfortunately the encephalocele has increased in size, and now there is evidence of brain herniation through the defect. This encephalocele should be repaired as soon as feasible to stop the progression of brain herniation and close the defect. (Examinee should explain the planned procedure step by step.)

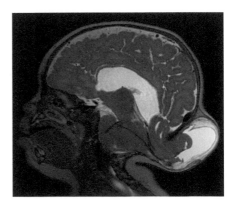

Further Reading

Balogun JA, Drake JM. Occipital encephalocele. In: Cohen A, ed. Pediatric Neurosurgery: Tricks of the Trade. 1st ed. New York, NY: Thieme; 2016:197–202

The patient is taken to the operating room and a circumferential excision of the encephalocele is performed. The herniated brain does not appear pulsatile or viable, and is removed. The dura is repaired and the skin is closed over the defect. On postoperative day #3, nursing notices clear fluid draining from the wound and a neurologic change, the patient is more lethargic. Immediate imaging demonstrates pneumocephalus.

Response

The CSF leak may be due to incomplete repair of the defect in the postoperative setting, but also due to the risk of the patient developing hydrocephalus, which can occur in up to 30% of these patients. There are several options, including returning to the operating room for wound evaluation and attempted re-closure or CSF diversion without direct revision of the wound. It is likely that the patient will need some combination of wound revision and CSF diversion either for the short-term or long-term.

Potential Other Complications

Cranial nerve deficits, CSF leak preoperatively.

Case No. 10

An 8-year-old girl is referred to your clinic after being found to have multiple lower cranial neuropathies, including a left hypoglossal nerve palsy, mild right facial palsy, and difficulty swallowing. The pediatric neurologist obtained an MRI scan and results are shown in the images.

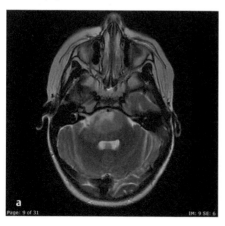
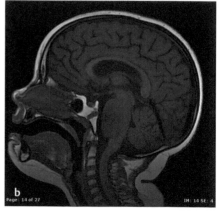

Response

Imaging in this patient demonstrates diffuse expansion of the pons and minimal/patchy enhancement. These findings, along with cranial neuropathies are concerning for a brainstem glioma, specifically diffuse intrinsic pontine glioma (DIPG). Unfortunately, the prognosis for this patient with a DIPG is grim, with a median survival of 10 months. There has been considerable discussion regarding whether or not open surgical biopsy is required, or if the diagnosis can be made on imaging alone. It has been demonstrated that radiographic diagnosis can be made with approximately 90% sensitivity, and approximately 50% specificity, with an overall positive predictive value of ~96%. Imaging alone cannot provide information on prognosis without histopathological confirmation and grading. If no surgical biopsy is performed, the patient will likely undergo conventional radiation; however, this is deemed palliative radiation in many cases.

Further Reading

Saratsis AM, Nazarian J, Magge SN. Brainstem gliomas. In: Keating R, Goodrich J, Packer R, eds. Tumors of the Pediatric Central Nervous System. 2nd ed. New York, NY: Thieme; 2013: 347–353

McCrea HJ, Souweidane MM. Brainstem gliomas. In: Albright A, Pollack I, Adelson P, eds. Principles and Practice of Pediatric Neurosurgery. 3rd ed. New York, NY: Thieme; 2015:553–562

The family understands regarding the likely diagnosis and prognosis. Despite your counseling, they are very insistent on obtaining a confirmation via tissue diagnosis. You heavily counsel them regarding the risks of the procedure, and they continue to ask for tissue confirmation. You realize that it is within your rights to deny surgery, but you elect to take the patient to the operating room in an attempt to obtain tissue for diagnosis via a small, retrosigmoid craniotomy for direct visualization. You encounter an enlarged pons with some abnormal appearing tissue. You are able to obtain a very small piece of tissue from the surface, but after you grasp the specimen and remove it, the anesthesiologist informs you that the patient's blood pressure has significantly increased, and the patient is also bradycardic.

Response

The patient has likely experienced a Cushing response to brainstem displacement during removal of the tissue specimen. At this point, it is likely not safe to continue with the procedure, and whatever tissue has already been obtained will have to suffice for diagnosis. Further samples could cause an intraoperative death or severe morbidity.

Potential Other Complications

CSF leak from biopsy delaying radiation, worsened cranial neuropathies postop.

Category 7: Functional

Case No. 1

A 63-year-old man is referred to your clinic for consideration of deep brain stimulation (DBS) for his Parkinsonism. He is currently managed by a movement disorder neurologist, and has been on carbidopa-levodopa for around 5 years. He is having decreased effect from the medications and is having increasing side effects, including dyskinesias.

Response

The patient has signs/symptoms of advanced Parkinsonism, and meets criteria for consideration of DBS. Multiple targets could be considered for Parkinsonism, but specific targeting depends on symptoms, as different targets may work better for specific Parkinsonian features. These targets include ventral intermedius nucleus (VIM) (mainly for tremor), internal globus pallidus (GPI) (if there is concern for emotional lability, dystonia, or medication reduction is not required), and subthalamic nucleus (STN) (greatest chance of reducing medication use). This patient should be scheduled for preoperative evaluation as well as for bilateral STN DBS. (Examinee should explain the planned procedure step by step.)

Further Reading

De La Cruz P, Plakas C, Ramirez Zamora A, Pilitsis JG. Deep brain stimulation for Parkinson disease. In: Harbaugh R, Shaffrey C, Couldwell W, et al., eds. Neurosurgery Knowledge Update. A Comprehensive Review. 1st ed. New York, NY: Thieme; 2015:279–283

Awan NR, Al Otaibi FA, Soualmi L, Sabbagh AJ. Deep brain stimulation for movement disorders (A). In: Nader R, Gragnaniello C, Berta S et al. eds. Neurosurgery Tricks of the Trade. Cranial. 1st ed. New York, NY: Thieme; 2014:598–603

The patient is taken to the operating room (OR) for bilateral STN DBS. The left lead is placed first, and intraoperative stimulation demonstrates improvement in rigidity. When the right lead is placed and stimulated, the patient reports diplopia. On examination, the patient has medial deviation of the right eye, with no deviation of the left eye.

Response

The right-sided lead is likely placed too medial from STN and is causing excitation of the fibers of the III nerve. This is leading to the medial deviation of the eye and diplopia. The lead should be removed from that tract and moved laterally.

Potential Other Complications

Hemorrhage, lead back out, lead too lateral, too anterior, too posterior.

Case No. 2

A 14-year-old girl is sent to your clinic by a neurologist. She has medically refractory epilepsy, currently on levetiracetam (Keppra) and lacosamide (Vimpat). She previously took lamotrigine (Lamictal) with little effect, and significant side effects. She underwent an stereoelectroencephalography (SEEG) procedure that was suggestive of left-sided origin; however, no specific region could be localized. There is no evidence of mesial temporal sclerosis on imaging, and the patient/family is not interested in a large craniotomy for grid placement. Currently, she is experiencing approximately 10 seizures per month.

Response

The patient has ongoing, medically refractory epilepsy from what is currently thought to be a diffuse, but possibly left-sided, source. While craniotomy for grid placement could be considered, this patient does not want this procedure. Addition of further antiepileptic agents would likely not have any efficacy, and may increase the risk of side effects. The only surgical option for this patient currently would be placement of a vagal nerve stimulator (VNS).

Further Reading

Lew SM. Pediatric epilepsy: surgical management. In: Harbaugh R, Shaffrey C, Couldwell W, et al., eds. Neurosurgery Knowledge Update. A Comprehensive Review. 1st ed. New York, NY: Thieme; 2015:407–412

The patient and family are interested in pursuing implantation of a VNS, but they have read opinions on the Internet that are positive and negative regarding VNS. They are wondering what they can expect in regards to improvement in seizures?

Response

VNS is a well-tolerated procedure, but only 1 to 2% of patients will become seizure-free after implantation. Approximately 40 to 50% of patients will achieve an approximately 50% reduction of seizure frequency by 3 years after stimulation. It is a treatment that can help reduce seizure frequency and potentially decrease medication doses/side effects. (Examinee should explain the planned procedure step by step.)

Further Reading

Limbrick D Jr, Smyth MD. Neuromodulation procedures: vagus nerve stimulation. In: Cataltepe O, Jallo G, eds. Pediatric Epilepsy Surgery. Preoperative Assessment and Surgical Treatment. 1st ed. New York, NY: Thieme; 2010:279–289

The patient is taken to the OR for left-sided VNS implantation. The procedure occurs without difficulty. After recovery, it is discovered that the patient has a hoarse voice.

Response

There are several reasons the patient could have a hoarse voice. The endotracheal (ET) tube can cause irritation, but also, hoarseness is the most likely complication of the procedure. Initially the hoarseness should be observed. If persistent, ear, nose, and throat (ENT) specialist can be consulted to perform a vocal cord check for paralysis. If this is not present, the hoarseness should improve over time.

Potential Other Complications

Infection, tethered wires, internal jugular vein injury.

Case No. 3

A 44-year-old woman is sent to your clinic by neurology with medically refractory epilepsy. She has generalized tonic-clonic seizures, approximately three times per month. These episodes are precipitated by nausea and a déjà vu experience. Electroencephalogram (EEG) suggested right temporal lobe origin. She is currently on levetiracetam (Keppra) and lamotrigine (Lamictal), previously was on phenytoin (Dilantin), but had to stop due to side effects. Imaging was obtained and the MRI is shown in the image.

Response

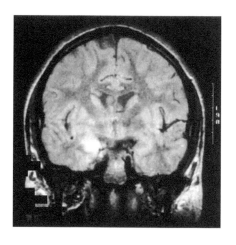

On magnetic resonance imaging (MRI), the patient has evidence of mesial temporal sclerosis. Clinically, she has evidence of temporal lobe origin of her seizures. Given her medically refractory status, surgical resection should be considered. Based on current research, approximately 50 to 75% of patients who undergo resection for temporal lobe epilepsy will be seizure-free 10 years after resection. Intraoperative EEG with depth electrodes and surface grid electrodes over the right temporal lobe should be utilized. If the anterior temporal neocortex demonstrates sharp waves or other evidence of epileptogenic activity, a complete anterior temporal lobectomy should be performed rather than a selective amygdalohippocampectomy. (Examinee should explain the planned procedure step by step.)

Further Reading

Mistry AM. Neimat J. Epilepsy surgery. In: Harbaugh R, Shaffrey C, Couldwell W, et al., eds. Neurosurgery Knowledge Update. A Comprehensive Review. 1st ed. New York, NY: Thieme; 2015:269–275

The patient is taken to surgery and a complete anterior temporal lobectomy is performed successfully. When she is taken to the post anesthesia care unit, she is noted to not be moving her left side, and appears to have a homonymous hemianopia.

Response

The patient has an examination that is consistent with an anterior choroidal artery injury. The anterior choroidal artery is at risk during the medial dissection of the amyg-dalohippocampal complex. Attempts should be made to preserve the arachnoid plane between the basal cisterns and the temporal lobe. Regardless, straying too medial can risk the anterior choroidal artery. Injury to this vessel can cause contralateral hemiparesis and visual abnormalities. Imaging should be obtained to rule out a hemorrhage or mass lesion initially, and if negative, rehab should be consulted for this patient.

Further Reading

Grand W, Hopkins L, Siddiqui A, et al. Posterior communicating artery and anterior choroidal artery > Anterior choroidal artery. In: Vasculature of the Brain and Cranial Base. Variations in Clinical Anatomy. 2nd ed. New York, NY: Thieme; 2016:85–101

Potential Other Complications

Third nerve injury, persistent seizures, superior quadrantanopsia.

Case No. 4

A 52-year-old concert violinist is sent to your clinic by his neurologist with difficult to treat essential tremor. The tremor occurs in both hands, and it is negatively affecting his career as a violinist. He reports that if he plays after having a glass of wine, his tremor is much improved. He was initially managed by his neurologist using propranolol and primidone, however, the tremor has persisted. It occurs when his arms are outstretched, and is approximately 4–12hz. If his tremor can't be treated, he is considering retirement.

Response

This patient appears to have essential tremor, and it is clearly affecting his ability to play the violin. He has had adequate trials of medications which have not provided any significant relief. Only about 40% of patients will respond completely to medical therapy. This patient could be considered for DBS for his essential tremor, targeting the ventral intermediate (VIM) nucleus of the thalamus bilaterally.

Further Reading

Videnovic A. Movement disorders > Essential tremor. In: Borsody M, ed. Comprehensive Board Review in Neurology. 2nd ed. New York, NY: Thieme; 2013:215–216

The patient is interested in pursuing DBS, but is wondering the efficacy and the risk of the procedure.

Response

Most patients tolerate the procedure quite well, and between 60 and 90% of patients will experience a significant reduction in tremor after surgery. (Examinee should explain the planned procedure step by step.) The biggest risk of the procedure is infection leading to reoperation and potential removal of the hardware.

Further Reading

Phookan S, Plakas C, Ramirez Zamora A, Pilitsis JG. Deep brain stimulation for essential tremor. In: Harbaugh R, Shaffrey C, Couldwell W, et al., eds. Neurosurgery Knowledge Update. A Comprehensive Review. 1st ed. New York, NY: Thieme; 2015:284–290

The patient is taken to the OR for bilateral VIM DBS with microelectrode recording. Intra-operative stimulation demonstrated excellent tremor control in the right hand. When the right-sided lead is tested, the patient demonstrates tetanic motor contractions of the left arm, as well as facial pulling.

Response

It is likely that the right-sided lead has been placed too lateral, and is causing stimulation of the internal capsule. The lead should be moved medially to minimize activation of the internal capsule.

Potential Other Complications

Hemorrhage around lead, lead back out, infection.

Case No. 5

A 58-year-old woman comes to your clinic with a 3-month history of severe, lancinating pain into the jaw. It shoots into the inferior aspect of her jaw on the left. It is intermittent, and feels like an electric shock. It is severe enough that she has been having difficulty eating, and has lost 15 lbs over that time frame. The pain is triggered by brushing her teeth, or sometimes even by wind hitting her face. She is asking for any sort of relief available.

Response

The patient has symptoms concerning for classic, type I trigeminal neuralgia (TN) in a V3 distribution on the left. More information should be gathered, however, since up to 5% of patients with these symptoms can harbor cerebellopontine angle tumors, and a subset of patients may have neuroinflammatory conditions, such as multiple sclerosis that can cause symptoms. The patient should have a physical examination and undergo an MRI scan of the brain with gradient-echo, or other specialized MRI to evaluate for a compressing vessel.

On physical examination, the patient is neurologically intact with no cranial nerve abnormalities. Sensation to V1–2 is intact on the left, but the patient refuses to allow you to test V3 distribution out of concern for pain. MRI scan is obtained and is shown in the image.

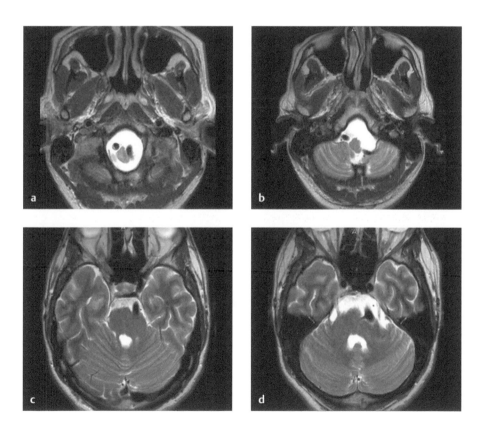

Response

The patient has evidence of an ectatic left vertebral artery that is causing compression of the trigeminal nerve entry zone into the brainstem. On examination she has findings consistent with left TN. This patient should initially be started on carbamazepine (Tegretol). There can be side effects, but these are often diminished by starting the medication slowly. The patient could take 100 mg twice daily, increasing by 100 mg twice daily up to a total dose of 1200 mg daily. This medication can be very effective for TN but side effects can limit its use. Gabapentin (Neurontin) has fewer efficacies, but a better side-effect profile. Medication should be the initial management choice.

Further Reading

Jannetta PJ. Trigeminal and glossopharyngeal neuralgia > Medical treatment of trigeminal neuralgia. In: Spetzler R, Kalani M, Nakaji P, eds. Neurovascular Surgery. 2nd ed. New York, NY: Thieme; 2015:1000–1001

The patient tries carbamazepine and initially experiences some relief, however, the pain returns approximately 2 months later. Further increases in the medications have led to side effects.

Response

With the failure of medications, the patient should be considered for left-sided microvascular decompression (MVD) via a retrosigmoidal approach. Given the large, compressive vessel on imaging and classic symptoms, this patient should expect a high rate of improvement in symptoms with effective microvascular decompression. (Examinee should explain the planned procedure step by step.) The MVD would be considered a nondestructive treatment, compared to destructive treatments, including glycerol rhizotomy, balloon compression, radiofrequency ablation, or stereotactic radiosurgery. The potential benefit of nondestructive treatment is preservation of normal sensation in the distribution of the trigeminal nerve.

Further Reading

Fukushima T, Watanabe K. Microvascular decompression for trigeminal neuralgia: operative results in 2,488 cases. In: Spetzler R, Kalani M, Nakaji P, eds. Neurovascular Surgery. 2nd ed. New York, NY: Thieme; 2015:1007–1015

The patient is taken to the OR for a left-sided MVD. The dura is opened, and as a cottonoid patty is placed over the cerebellar hemisphere to retract and remove cerebrospinal fluid (CSF), sudden, brisk bleeding is encountered.

Response

It is likely that retraction of the cerebellar hemisphere has caused avulsion of the petrosal vein at the junction of the tentorium and the petrous bone. A large suction should be used to control the bleeding and identify the likely source. A piece of Gelfoam can be placed over the area of bleeding and gentle pressure can be applied to the avulsed segment of the petrosal vein. If a segment can be identified, it can be coagulated, however, if it is avulsed from its entry, the Gelfoam should be left in place to control the bleeding.

Potential Other Complications

No intraoperative vessel, CSF leak, loss of brainstem auditory evoked responses (BAERs).

Case No. 6

A 62-year-old man is sent to your clinic by a pain specialist with persistent, medically refractory face pain that he has experienced since suffering a left middle cerebral artery (MCA) stroke approximately 2 years ago. It is the only symptom that persists from the stroke. It is present constantly, and covers the top of his head down to the bottom of his right jaw. It is throbbing and burning in nature. He has tried multiple medications via a comprehensive pain management team, as well as cognitive behavioral therapy as well as physical therapy over the past 3 months. All of these have failed. There is no evidence of any new lesions or abnormalities on recent MRI.

Response

The patient has an intractable pain syndrome likely from deafferentation from his prior stroke. It seems to cover the entirety of his right face, crossing all trigeminal distributions, and further, there is no evidence of TN on imaging. The patient does not have many options for treating his persistent face pain; however, placement of a motor cortex stimulator is possible. He should undergo a further 3 months of attempted multidisciplinary treatment prior to consideration for motor cortex stimulation, for 6 months of conservative management before surgical intervention.

Further Reading

Kalia SK, Hamani C, Rezai A, Lozano AM. Deep brain stimulation for chronic pain. In: Burchiel K, ed. Surgical Management of Pain. 2nd ed. New York, NY: Thieme; 2015:380–390

The patient undergoes another 3 months of attempted therapy, and fails. He returns to your office desperate for relief, and is interested in having a motor cortex stimulator placed.

Response

The patient should be considered for motor cortex stimulator on the left side; however, the patient should be informed that the results of this procedure for pain are that approximately 50% of patients will experience 50% improvement in their pain. This is weighed against the risk of hardware implantation and infection. (Examinee should explain the planned procedure step by step.)

Further Reading

Sindou M, Maarrawi J, Mertens P. Motor cortex stimulation. In: Burchiel K, ed. Surgical
    Management of Pain. 2nd ed. New York, NY: Thieme; 2015:366–379

The patient is taken to the OR for placement of a left-sided motor cortex stimulator. The procedure is tolerated well and 1 month after implantation the patient is experiencing some relief of his face pain. On 3-month follow-up, the patient is doing well, but upon examination of the cranial wound, there is evidence of a motor cortex stimulator wire that has eroded through the scalp and is intermixed with the patient's hair. There is evidence of pus, and a culture taken in the office is positive for Staphylococcus aureus.

Response

The patient has exposed hardware and evidence of an infection. If the infection were contained within the battery pocket only, consideration could be given to removing the battery, washing out the wound and putting the patient on antibiotics to clear the infection before battery replacement, without total hardware removal. In this case, however, the cranial wires are exposed and infected, and all of the hardware should be removed due to significant risk of the infection spreading intradurally. When the infection is cleared, the stimulator could be replaced if the patient is interested in undergoing further surgery.

Potential Other Complications

Seizures, worsened facial pain, tethered wires.

Case No. 7

A 34-year-old man comes to your office 2 years after a complete brachial plexus avulsion from a motorcycle accident. He has evidence of pseudomeningoceles from C5 to T1 on the right side and has a flail arm. He underwent attempted nerve transfers to regain some shoulder/elbow function; however, these procedures were not successful. He is complaining of severe burning pain in the right upper extremity that is excruciating. He has seen pain specialists and analgesics are not having any significant effect. His current pain specialists do not suspect complex regional pain syndrome at this time. He comes to your clinic asking if there are any other options.

Response

The patient likely is experiencing deafferentation pain of the right upper extremity. This may occur in up to 90% of patients with preganglionic injuries to the brachial plexus. This patient may be suitable for dorsal root entry zone (DREZ) lesioning in an attempt to decrease the pain.

Further Reading

Sindou M. Dorsal root entry zone lesions. In: Burchiel K, ed. Surgical Management of Pain. 2nd ed. New York, NY: Thieme; 2015:576–592

The patient is interested in this procedure, but would like to know the chance of success, as well as the risks.

Response

The DREZ lesion procedure is well-tolerated, with the primary risks being infection, CSF leak, and a small risk of lower extremity weakness due to propagation of the lesion into the corticospinal tract. (Examinee should explain the planned procedure step by step.) Outcomes of this procedure are excellent, with 75 to 85% of patients having pain relief allowing the withdrawal of opioids by 8 years. Up to 75% of patients may have a complete cure, with no further medication requirement.

The patient is taken to the OR and a right-sided DREZ lesion is performed from C5-T1, along the avulsed roots. In recovery, the patient demonstrates some leg weakness in the right leg.

Response

It is likely that there was some propagation of the lesion toward the ipsilateral corticospinal tract. It is not initially certain if the tract itself was lesioned or if there is local edema and tract dysfunction. The patient should be started on a short taper of steroids, and physical therapy should be consulted. If the injury is due to edema, it should resolve over time with steroids and physical therapy.

Case No. 8

A 38-year-old woman has a long history of refractory epilepsy. It starts with rhythmic contractions of the left hand, travels up the arm before generalizing into a tonic-clonic seizure. She has dealt with 10 to 15 seizures per month and is currently on phenytoin (Dilantin) and levetiracetam (Keppra). She has had minimal, if any improvement in her seizure frequency on these medications. Video EEG monitoring has captured a seizure and is suggestive of right hemisphere onset. Single photon emission computed tomography (SPECT) and positron emission tomography (PET) studies have failed to further delineate a region of onset.

Response

The patient has medically refractory epilepsy that appears to be of extratemporal origin. Multiple imaging and EEG studies have failed to further identify a region of onset. The patient has two options. The first is to try another antiepileptic; however, the chance of improvement in her epilepsy with the addition of a third antiepileptic drug (AED) is only approximately 5%. The second option is for the patient to undergo a craniotomy and cortical grid placement for further monitoring to better identify a region of onset. (Examinee should explain the planned procedure step by step.) The patient should be counseled that this procedure introduces a risk of infection or brain injury, but also that the monitoring could identify seizures originating from eloquent cortex, which would mean resection is not possible.

Further Reading

Mistry AM. Neimat J. Epilepsy surgery. In: Harbaugh R, Shaffrey C, Couldwell W, et al., eds. Neurosurgery Knowledge Update. A Comprehensive Review. 1st ed. New York, NY: Thieme; 2015:269–275

The patient elects to undergo a craniotomy for grid placement. She is taken to the OR and several grids are successfully placed. Postoperative X-ray is shown in the image. The patient is taken to the neuro intensive care unit (ICU) for monitoring. On postoperative day #3, she has two seizures and the neurology team achieves enough data to suggest that the region of onset is located in the premotor cortex, in a region representing the hand knob.

Response

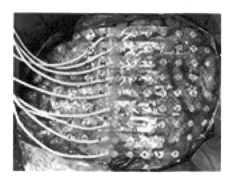

Unfortunately the patient has a seizure onset region that is located in eloquent cortex, specifically the motor strip. It would be unacceptably morbid for the patient to undergo resection of the motor cortex to stop her seizures. She should be taken back to the OR for grid removal with no attempted resection. Further AEDs and/or placement of a vagal nerves stimulator should be considered.

Potential Other Complications

Infection, hemorrhage under grid, grid movement, sinus injury during craniotomy.

Case No. 9

A 14-year-old boy is sent to your clinic with a history of refractory epilepsy. His seizure semiology consists of episodes of inappropriate laughter. He has been trialed on several medications with no effect. Imaging was obtained by his neurologist and is shown in the image. On examination he is neurologically intact.

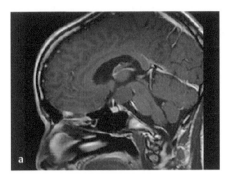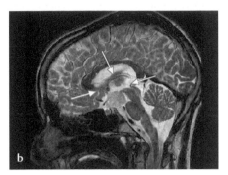

Response

The patient has a suprasellar mass making the differential for this lesion large. The symptoms, including gelastic seizures, however, make a hypothalamic or tuber cinereum hamartoma most likely. Imaging demonstrates no contrast enhancement which further suggests hamartoma in this case. The patient should still undergo CSF sampling (for germ cell markers) prior to treatment decision-making to help ensure the diagnosis.

The patient has a lumbar puncture for CSF sampling, and alpha-fetoprotein, beta human chorionic gonadotropin (b-HCG), and alkaline phosphatase are all within normal limits. There are not enough cells on flow cytometry to make any diagnosis. The remainder of the CSF labs are within normal limits.

Response

Assuming this mass is a hypothalamic hamartoma causing gelastic seizures, there are several treatment options. They include open surgical resection via multiple approaches, stereotactic radiosurgery (however, this hamartoma is likely on the larger side for SRS), and potentially even MR-guided laser ablation if a safe approach can be utilized. (Examinee should explain the planned procedure step by step.) There is a risk to hypothalamic structures in any approach, and the patient should be counseled about these risks, specifically about hypothalamic obesity syndrome.

Further Reading

Shetter AG, McBride HL, Kerrigan JF. Stereotactic radiosurgery for hypothalamic hamartomas. In: Lunsford L, Sheehan J, eds. Intracranial Stereotactic Radiosurgery. 2nd ed. New York, NY: Thieme; 2016:182–192

Mittal S, Montes JL, Farmer J-P, Sabbagh AJ. Hypothalamic hamartomas. In: Baltuch G, Villemure J, eds. Operative Techniques in Epilepsy Surgery. 1st ed. New York, NY: Thieme; 2009:8–98

The patient is taken to the OR for open resection of the hamartoma. It is readily identified and is distinct from the infundibulum. It is successfully resected and the hypothalamus appears to be intact. He tolerates the procedure very well. The evening of surgery, his nurse calls and states that he has been to the bathroom four times overnight, and in each instance, his urine appears as clear as water.

Response

It is likely that the patient is developing central diabetes insipidus, either from irritation of the hypothalamus or displacement of the infundibulum. The patient should have basic labs obtained, specifically sodium, as well as monitoring of urine output. A urine specific gravity should be sent the next time the patient voids. If it is less than 1.005, the patient should be considered for desmopressin (DDAVP) administration (0.1 mg PO BID if conscious). For the conscious patient who can drink to thirst, the patient should be instructed to drink water and keep up with losses. Simultaneously, sodium should be checked every 6 hours initially to make sure the hypernatremia isn't getting out of control. Consideration should be given to the triphasic response as well, so that during the second phase, the patient isn't over treated into hyponatremia.

Further Reading

Greenberg M. Sodium homeostasis and osmolality > Hypernatremia > Diabetes insipidus. In: Handbook of Neurosurgery. 8th ed. New York, NY: Thieme; 2016:120–125

Potential Other Complications

Total pituitary failure, hypothalamic obesity, continued seizures (remnant left), Addisonian crisis.

Case No. 10

A 78-year-old woman presents to your clinic with severe, lancinating pain into the lower right jaw that has been persistent for the past year. It occurs when she brushes her teeth or eats. It is severe, but intermittent. She has been treated by a local neurologist and pain specialist, including the use of carbamazepine. She had some relief of her pain on this medication, but it had to be decreased due to side effects. Imaging does not demonstrate any evidence of vascular compression or brainstem abnormalities.

Response

The patient has symptoms consistent with classic TN on the right side. Unfortunately, imaging does not demonstrate a point of vascular compression, although this does not mean a vascular compression is not present. The patient likely needs another form of treatment, either open surgery, or needle-based procedures to help treat her pain.

Further Reading

Burchiel K, McCartney S. Trigeminal neuralgia. In: Burchiel K, ed. Surgical Management of Pain. 2nd ed. New York, NY: Thieme; 2015:175–179

The patient is interested in another form of treatment, but would not like to undergo craniotomy as she feels it is too invasive and she is worried about her perioperative risk. She wonders if there are any other procedures available for her.

Response

This patient could be considered for a percutaneous needle-based procedure, either radiofrequency ablation, glycerol rhizotomy, or balloon compression, all of which are destructive lesions, and numbness in the nerve distribution should be discussed with the patient. (Examinee should explain the planned procedure step by step.)

Further Reading

Brown JA, Stetson ND, Cheyuo C. Percutaneous balloon compression for trigeminal neuralgia > Technique and results. In: Burchiel K, ed. Surgical Management of Pain. 2nd ed. New York, NY: Thieme; 2015:476–487

The patient undergoes a percutaneous balloon compression of the right trigeminal nerve. Intraoperative image is shown. Initially after the procedure she reports improvement in her face pain and even some numbness in V1–2 on the right. At 1 month after the procedure, she comes to your office with complaints of severe, burning pain in the V1 distribution on the right side of her face. Her right eye is irritated and injected. There is no evidence of infectious cause.

Response

Unfortunately this patient has symptoms consistent with anesthesia dolorosa (AD), likely caused by deafferentation of V1 on the right during the balloon compression. This complication is more common in radiofrequency ablation (1.6% compared to 0.1% for balloon compression). AD is a difficult complication to treat, and her pain may be permanent. Care will need to be taken to ensure that she does not damage her eye, sense it will likely be insensate. She will need to be managed by a pain specialist as there are no surgical options to treat this complication. Management will likely include an AED such as gabapentin, as well as pain-modulating antidepressants, among other medications.

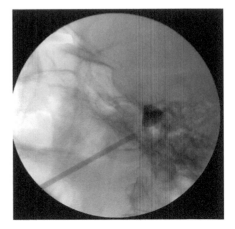

Further Reading

Levine DA, Argoff CE, Pilitsis J. Trigeminal neuropathic pain and anesthesia dolorosa > Anesthesia dolorosa. In: Burchiel K, ed. Surgical Management of Pain. 2nd ed. New York, NY: Thieme; 2015:184–187

Potential Other Complications

Intracranial bleeding, recurrent trigeminal pain, intraoral breach by needle during procedure, temporal lobe injury.

Category 8: Peripheral Nerve

Case No. 1

You are covering peripheral nerve cell and are consulted by the emergency department (ED) for a 25- year-old man who presents with trauma to the right leg and a right foot drop. He was intoxicated and attempted to kick through a plate glass window, shattering it, and sustaining a deep laceration to the lateral aspect of the proximal leg. His friends brought him to the ED.

Response

A laceration to the lateral knee with associated foot drop is concerning for a sharp injury to the peroneal nerve. The patient should be examined as thoroughly as possible, and given the deep nature of the injury with peripheral nerve deficit, othopedics and vascular surgery should be made aware of the patient in case of injury/contamination of local bony structures or the potential for vascular injury.

The patient is examined and demonstrates intact sensation across the toes, the dorsum of the foot, and anterolateral aspect of the leg. On motor examination foot eversion is 5/5 strength, while ankle dorsiflexion is 0/5 strength. Orthopaedics and vascular surgery are consulted. Vascular surgery finds no evidence of vessel injury. Orthopaedics would like to take the patient for a wound debridement and closure.

Response

The patient has sustained an injury to the peroneal nerve, most likely caused by the glass window. With foot eversion intact, either it is an incomplete injury, or the injury is distal to the branch point of the common peroneal nerve and the deep branch is selectively involved. That being stated, the sensation in the first web space is preserved, suggesting some potential continuity of the deep branch, or aberrant anatomy. Given the relative clean laceration, the patient should be explored and an early nerve repair (within 72 hours) could be performed if feasible. (Examinee should explain the planned procedure step by step.) Electromyography/nerve conduction study (EMG/NCS) would not suffice at early stage. Imaging is not needed. Ultrasound (if available) is being used at some centers to help define the injury.

Further Reading

Addas BMJ. Nerve injuries: anatomy, pathophysiology, and classification > Laceration injury. In: Socolovsky M, Rasulic L, Midha R, et al., eds. Manual of Peripheral Nerve Surgery. From the Basics to Complex Procedures. 1st ed. Stuttgart: Thieme; 2018:20

Russell S. Sciatic nerve > Motor innervation and testing. In: Examination of Peripheral Nerve Injuries: An Anatomical Approach. 2nd ed. New York, NY: Thieme; 2015:146–160

The patient is taken to the operating room the next morning for exploration, washout, and closure. The common peroneal nerve is exposed and the intraoperative photograph is shown in the image. What is the next best step in management?

Response

The intraoperative photo demonstrates an incomplete laceration of the common peroneal nerve. This explains the examination findings. Repair can still be performed, but care should be taken not to disrupt the intact fascicles. Intrafascicular dissection should be performed, and the proximal and distal ends should be mobilized (dissected 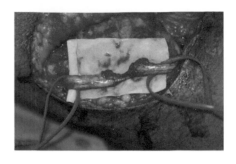 free from surrounding tissue in order to increase available length) and provide a tension-free repair if possible. Despite these maneuvers, suture repair of the common peroneal nerve may only lead to 36% of patients achieving M3 or greater strength in the tibialis anterior musculature. An ankle/foot orthotic could be prescribed for short-term during recovery or long-term if no muscle improvement is demonstrated; it will also keep the heel cord supple. Sensory recovery is useful for extremity protection, and may have a higher rate of recovery than motor function. Tendon transfer can be considered by an orthopaedist or a plastic surgeon if there is no recovery following nerve reconstruction; typically the posterior tibialis tendon (tibial innervated) is utilized.

Further Reading

Rasulic L, Samardzic M. Outcomes in the repair of nerve injuries. In: Socolovsky M, Rasulic L, Midha R, et al., eds. Manual of Peripheral Nerve Surgery. From the Basics to Complex Procedures. 1st ed. Stuttgart: Thieme; 2018:90–97

Other Potential Complications

Vascular injury, bony injury, edematous nerve, neuroma in continuity, stump retraction.

Case No. 2

A 38-year-old man presents to your clinic with a 3-month history of deep aching pain in his left wrist. He also states that his pinky finger feels numb and when he tries to wave to someone with his left hand, it looks odd, because his "ring and pinky finger seem stuck in the bent position."

Response

The patient has symptoms referable to an ulnar nerve lesion, and further examination should be performed to help localize the lesion. A full motor examination should be performed, but sensation can give clues to the location of the lesion. What is the pattern of abnormal sensation? Is sensation preserved over the dorsum of the hand and/or hypothenar eminence? An EMG could be performed as well to confirm findings on physical examination. Imaging of the wrist via magnetic resonance imaging (MRI) or ultrasound could be considered.

On examination, the patient has intact sensation to the dorsum of the hand and the hypothenar eminence, but has diminished sensation to the fifth digit and medial half of the fourth digit, including the nail beds. Froment and Wartenberg signs are positive, and images of the patient attempting to extend both hands are shown in the image.

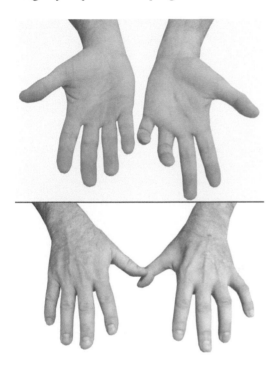

Response

The patient has examination findings consistent with an ulnar neuropathy at the wrist. Preservation of sensation over the hypothenar eminence and dorsum of the hand suggest wrist pathology, and weakness of hand intrinsics as well as positive Froment sign (flexion of the thumb to compensate for weakness of adductor pollicis) and Wartenberg sign (unopposed action by extensor digiti minimi causing abduction of fifth digit). EMG could be performed to confirm, and imaging via MRI or ultrasound could help guide therapy. Regardless, this patient would likely benefit from decompression of Guyon canal. (Examinee should explain the planned procedure step by step.)

Further Reading

Costales JR, Domitrovic L, Costales DR, Fernández Fernández J, Ibáñez Plágaro J. Clinical aspects of peripheral nerve lesions in the upper limb > Ulnar nerve. In: Socolovsky M,

Rasulic L, Midha R, et al., eds. Manual of Peripheral Nerve Surgery. From the Basics to Complex Procedures. 1st ed. Stuttgart: Thieme; 2018:31–36

Russell S. Ulnar nerve > Clinical findings and syndromes. In: Examination of Peripheral Nerve Injuries: An Anatomical Approach. 2nd ed. New York, NY: Thieme; 2015:50–58

The patient undergoes ultrasound of the wrist and a cystic mass is demonstrated underneath the ulnar nerve, suspicious for a compressive ganglion cyst in Guyon canal. The patient is set up for surgery and a decompression of Guyon canal is performed. A ganglion cyst is resected at the level of the wrist joint. When the decompression is completed, the nerve stimulator is used on the ulnar nerve before it branches. Motor response was seen in the hand intrinsics, but the abductor pollicis brevis also fires any time the ulnar nerve is stimulated.

Response

This patient must have an ulnar-to-median nerve anastomosis in the hand, commonly known as the Riche-Cannieu anastomosis. It is often a connection between the deep motor branch of the ulnar nerve and the recurrent motor branch of the median nerve, and it may be fairly common in the population.

Further Reading

Davidge KM, Boyd KU. Ulnar nerve entrapment and injury. In: Mackinnon S, ed. Nerve Surgery. 1st ed. New York, NY: Thieme; 2015:251–288

Potential Other Complications

Intraoperative nerve injury, elbow pathology, martin-gruber anastomosis, medial cord lesion, vascular injury.

Case No. 3

A 42-year-old drummer in a jazz band presents to your clinic with pain in her right hand that wakes her up at night. Initially she thought it was due to soreness from playing a long set at the jazz club, but now she notices that the pain in her hand has persisted despite her taking a break from drumming. She reports that when it wakes her up, she shakes her hand a few times and that seems to help relieve the pain.

Response

The patient is reporting symptoms that could be consistent with carpal tunnel syndrome, but further examination and studies should be performed to ensure that. A complete median nerve motor examination should be performed with special attention placed on the median nerve at the wrist. Sensory examination is helpful as well, specifically the palmar cutaneous branch. Provocative maneuvers should be done. EMG would be useful to confirm findings on examination. Imaging is not typically needed.

The patient's examination demonstrates thenar atrophy and moderate weakness of thumb abduction. A photograph of attempted right thumb abduction in the plane of the palm is shown. Sensory examination demonstrates diminished two-point discrimination in the first three digits and radial half of the fourth digit. Sensation is preserved over the thenar eminence. Phalen test leads to symptom recurrence after 70 seconds. Tinel sign is positive over the carpal tunnel. EMG demonstrates prolonged sensory latency of the median nerve at the wrist.

Response

The patient has classic carpal tunnel syndrome, confirmed by examination, EMG, and provocative testing. The patient should have a trial of conservative management, including wrist splinting, nonsteroidal anti-inflammatory drugs (NSAIDs), and activity modification; however, the presence of atrophy may lead to surgical intervention more acutely.

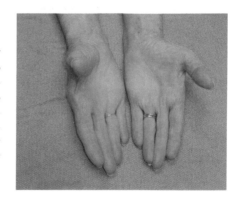

Further Reading

Russell S. Median nerve. In: Examination of Peripheral Nerve Injuries: An Anatomical Approach. 2nd ed. New York, NY: Thieme; 2015:1–22

Davidge KM, Sammer DM. Median nerve entrapment and injury > Carpal tunnel syndrome. In: Mackinnon S, ed. Nerve Surgery. 1st ed. New York, NY: Thieme; 2015:212–235

The patient trials NSAIDs, wrist splinting, and has taken a break from jazz drumming. Three months later she returns to your clinic with persistent symptoms. She also states that she would like to get back to drumming, as not being able to perform is causing financial stress.

Response

The patient should undergo carpal tunnel release. There are several techniques available, open or endoscopic, each with pros and cons. Multiple studies have been performed comparing the two approaches, with no clear difference in outcomes or complications. Regardless of approach, care must be taken to plan the incision so that the palmar cutaneous branch is protected superficially, and the thenar motor branch is avoided during division of the transverse carpal ligament. (Examinee should explain the planned procedure step by step.)

The patient undergoes endoscopic carpal tunnel release and tolerates the procedure well. The patient is discharged home the same day. Three days later she calls the office and states that she is having incisional pain, but also that her nocturnal symptoms have persisted, even on the night of surgery. The aching pain continues as she is nervous to shake it away. It feels just like it did before surgery, except now she has incisional pain as well.

Response

It is possible that this patient has an incompletely divided transverse carpal ligament, as the symptoms never improved after surgery. Initial management should be conservative to watch for improvement. However, if symptoms persist, repeat EMG/NCS can be considered to compare values and imaging could be performed to evaluate for an incompletely divided TCL. If this is the case, the patient should undergo reoperation, likely via open approach, to complete the division of the transverse carpal ligament.

Potential Other Complications

Entrance into Guyon canal, median nerve injury, proximal lesion, Martin-Gruber anastomosis.

Case No. 4

You are evaluating a 55-year-old man in your clinic who had lost control of his motorcycle on loose gravel and crashed. He was wearing protective gear and a helmet, but landed hard on his right shoulder. He was stabilized in the ED, but was noted to have a "weak arm." His hand works just fine but his upper arm is weak. CT of the brain and spine, and radiographs of the shoulder in the ED were negative, and after a short hospital stay he was discharged and outpatient consultation in your clinic was arranged. The injury was a week ago.

Response

The patient has symptoms concerning for a potential right brachial plexus injury that occurred a week ago. A detailed brachial plexus examination should be performed. Given that the injury occurred a week ago, it is too early for an initial EMG, which should be arranged for approximately 1 month post-injury, to allow for any Wallerian degeneration to occur. He should be scheduled for an EMG and office visit at that time.

On examination 1 week after injury, the patient's arm is adducted, extended, and internally rotated. There is 0/5 strength in external rotation of the arm, shoulder abduction, and elbow flexion. There is 5/5 strength for extension of the arm, and all functions of the hand are full strength with the exception of some weakness of wrist and finger extension. Sensory examination demonstrates paresthesias over the deltoid and thumb/index finger. An image is demonstrated.

EMG at 1 month demonstrates evidence of denervation of paraspinals, rhomboids, supra/infraspinatus, deltoid, and biceps muscles. Sensory nerve action potentials are preserved. MRI has evidence of pseudomeningoceles at C5 and 6.

Response

The patient has evidence of a multilevel preganglionic injury that is suggestive of brachial plexus avulsion. Based on current literature, up to 40% of closed C5–6 injuries may recover to some degree by 3 to 4 months and should initially be monitored. If there is no improvement on clinical examination or EMG, the patient should be taken for surgical exploration and repair depending on intraoperative results. Repair could entail nerve grafting or nerve transfers. (Examinee should explain the planned procedure step by step.)

Further Reading

Siqueira MG, Martins RS. Traumatic brachial plexus lesions: clinical aspects, assessment, and timing of surgical repair. In: Socolovsky M, Rasulic L, Midha R, et al., eds. Manual of Peripheral Nerve Surgery. From the Basics to Complex Procedures. 1st ed. Stuttgart: Thieme; 2018:135–140

Tung T, Moore AM. Brachial plexus injuries. In: Mackinnon S, ed. Nerve Surgery. 1st ed. New York, NY: Thieme; 2015:391–467

Garozzo D. Traumatic brachial plexus injuries: surgical techniques and strategies. In: Socolovsky M, Rasulic L, Midha R, et al., eds. Manual of Peripheral Nerve Surgery. From the Basics to Complex Procedures. 1st ed. Stuttgart: Thieme; 2018:141–148

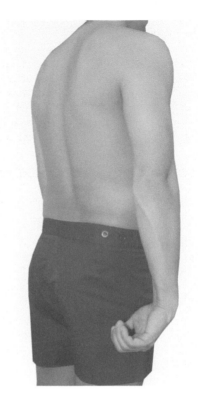

The patient is monitored, and repeat EMG at 3 months demonstrates no evidence of re-innervation potentials. Clinical examination remains unchanged. The patient is taken for exploration of the plexus and complete avulsion of C5–6 is confirmed intraoperatively with intraoperative testing. A spinal accessory to suprascapular nerve transfer is performed along with a triceps branch nerve transfer to the axillary nerve for shoulder abduction/external rotation, as well as an Oberlin transfer for elbow flexion (ulnar fascicular branch transfer to the biceps motor branch). The patient tolerates the procedure well and is admitted to the hospital overnight for monitoring. You are called by the nurse who states that the patient is having desaturations and is coughing quite a bit. She has started oxygen by nasal cannula.

Response

The patient is having respiratory difficulties which could arise for several different reasons. A chest X-ray (CXR) should be performed to evaluate the lungs.

A CXR is performed and the result is shown in the image.

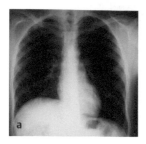 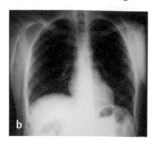

Response

The patient has no evidence of pneumonia or pneumothorax. There is elevation of the right hemidiaphragm which suggests possible phrenic nerve injury during the surgical exploration. Alternatively, the phrenic nerve could be involved from the original trauma and C5/6 avulsion injury (although the elevated hemidiaphragm was not seen on initial imaging). Initial management should include respiratory support and observation for spontaneous improvement.

Potential Other Complications

Vascular injury, neuroma-in-continuity, positive action potentials across neuroma, pneumothorax.

Case No. 5

You are asked to evaluate a 41-year-old woman who has had the onset of right foot drop over the past week. She has shooting pain going down the anterolateral aspect of her lower leg into the top of the foot. There was no precipitating injury to the leg that she can recall.

Response

The patient has findings that are referable to nerve pathology, either in the lumbar spine or in the common peroneal nerve. A full physical examination should be performed to help determine the location of the lesion. Evaluation of foot inversion and hip abduction can differentiate between common peroneal and L5 nerve involvement. An EMG can help localize pain as well.

On examination, the patient has 3/5 strength of foot eversion, 1/5 strength of ankle dorsiflexion, and toe extension. Inversion in plantarflexion is normal (posterior tibialis testing).

Sensation is diminished and dysesthetic over the anterolateral leg and top of the foot. Foot inversion was 5/5 strength. Tinel sign is positive at the fibular neck. Straight leg raise is negative. EMG is suggestive of a lesion at the common peroneal nerve.

Response

The patient's physical examination and EMG findings suggest a lesion of the common peroneal nerve. With no history of recent trauma, MRI could be obtained to determine any focal lesions of the nerve or to potentially identify any areas of compression.

An MRI of the lower extremity is shown in the image.

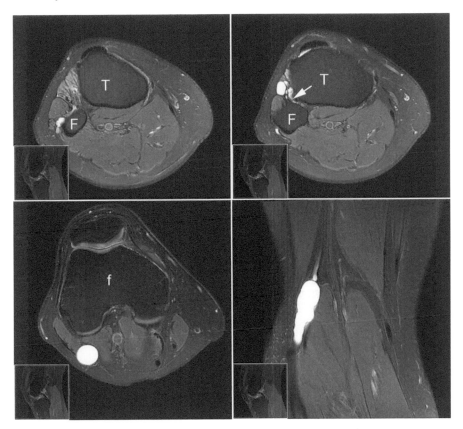

Response

The MRI scan of the leg demonstrates an intraneural ganglion cyst of the common peroneal nerve. It has been suggested that these lesions arise from an abnormal connection to the superior tibiofibular joint (STFJ) by cystic dilation of the articular branch of the nerve. In the past, extensive intraneural dissection was performed, but it is now believed that simple disconnection of the articular connection should lead to resolution of the cyst. Direct cyst decompression is not thought to be necessary. The patient should be scheduled for surgery. (Examinee should explain the planned procedure step by step.)

Further Reading

Spinner RJ. Peroneal intraneural ganglia. In: Harbaugh R, Shaffrey C, Couldwell W, et al., eds. Neurosurgery Knowledge Update. A Comprehensive Review. 1st ed. New York, NY: Thieme; 2015:728–732

Barbour JR, Boyd KU. Tumors of the peripheral nervous system > Neoplasms of nonneural origin. In: Mackinnon S, ed. Nerve Surgery. 1st ed. New York, NY: Thieme; 2015:557–569

The patient is taken to the operating room for exposure of the common peroneal nerve at the fibular neck. A large, dilated nerve is found, and unfortunately, the cyst is breached during dissection and mucous material is removed from the nerve. The patient tolerates the procedure well and has some improvement in symptoms in the initial postoperative phase. Post 3 months the patient returns with recurrent, worsening symptoms that are the same as before the operation. Another MRI is performed and there is evidence of cyst recurrence. A dilation of the articular branch is re-demonstrated on this subsequent MRI.

Response

The unfortunate recurrence of symptoms and cyst contents on MRI are suggestive of a failure to remove the articular connection in the initial procedure. The patient should be taken back the operating room and further dissection should be performed to properly identify the articular connection, and disconnect it. Orthopaedics should be involved to obliterate the STFJ to substantially decrease the rate of recurrence of this lesion.

Potential Other Complications

Intraoperative nerve injury.

Case No. 6

You are asked to evaluate a 29-year-old woman with right leg pain in a sciatic distribution and an asymmetrically larger right thigh compared to the left. She feels like there is a bump just above her knee that has been getting larger over the past month. The pain has limited her from walking distances that she is used to, but she isn't sure that she has any weakness of the leg.

Response

A painful, growing mass of the thigh with nerve pain could be suggestive of a peripheral nerve lesion. A full physical examination should be performed and further history should be obtained. Does the patient have any familial syndromes, specifically neurofibromatosis (NF)?

The patient carries a diagnosis of neurofibromatosis type I. On examination, there is a clear distal thigh mass that seems to be immobile. Palpation of the mass is associated with shooting pain in a sciatic distribution. There is 4/5 strength of right ankle plantarflexion, but hamstring strength is preserved. Sensation is diminished over the posterior calf.

Response

In a patient with NF type I, an enlarging mass with peripheral nerve symptoms is concerning either for a compressive lesion caused by a benign neurofibroma, or an aggressive lesion such as a malignant peripheral nerve sheath tumor (MPNST). The patient should undergo imaging, specifically a lower extremity MRI.

MRI of the right leg is shown in the image.

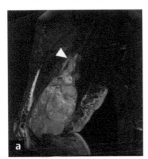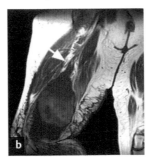

Response

The MRI scan demonstrates a large, heterogenous mass associated with the sciatic nerve, causing enlargement of the thigh. In this patient a mass of this size is likely consistent with a MPNST. Histopathologic confirmation should be obtained via biopsy to confirm pathology and help with treatment decisions. It will be important for the biopsy team to mark the biopsy tract and use a trajectory that would likely be used during a potential surgical resection, so the entire biopsy tract can be excised if necessary.

The patient undergoes a needle biopsy with identification of the biopsy tract. Histopathological evaluation confirms MPNST.

Response

Staging studies are necessary to ensure that distant metastases are not present. Usually these consist of CT chest/abdomen/pelvis and/or a positron emission tomography (PET) scans. The case is best managed by a multidisciplinary approach. For an MPNST without metastases, the patient will need a wide local excision of the mass, with attempts at negative margins. This is a very aggressive tumor with high rates of local recurrence and distant metastases. Neoadjuvant radiation to the tumor can be considered prior to surgery in cases where postoperative radiation might be harmful (in cases where a free flap or complicated closure will be required). An en-bloc resection of the tumor with negative nerve margins should be performed, as well as excision of the biopsy tract. Other surgical disciplines, such as orthopaedics and plastic surgery may be helpful to have involved in this case. The patient should be counseled regarding loss of distal function. Nerve grafting could be considered, but is not often performed due to the need for adjuvant radiation/chemotherapy which can make any meaningful functional recovery challenging. Nerve transfers or tendon transfers could be considered in select cases. (Examinee should explain the planned procedure step by step.)

Further Reading

Barbour JR, Boyd KU. Tumors of the peripheral nervous system > Neoplasms of nerve sheath origin. In: Mackinnon S, ed. Nerve Surgery. 1st ed. New York, NY: Thieme; 2015:530–557
Hong J, Pisapia J, Niziolek PJ, et al. Malignant peripheral nerve sheath tumors. In: Socolovsky M, Rasulic L, Midha R, et al., eds. Manual of Peripheral Nerve Surgery. From the Basics to Complex Procedures. 1st ed. Stuttgart: Thieme; 2018:196–209

The patient has a wide local excision, and adjuvant external beam radiation/chemotherapy with doxorubicin and ifosfamide. Initial postoperative scan at 3 months demonstrates no evidence of recurrence. At 6 months, an interval MRI demonstrates local tumor recurrence. Further imaging does not demonstrate any evidence of distant metastases.

Response

Unfortunately the patient has a local recurrence, which is seen in up to two-thirds of patients despite adequate treatment. If there is no current evidence of distant metastases, proximal amputation of the lower extremity should be considered as a means of attempted local control. Distant metastases are still possible (likely) after amputation, but this surgery is a logical next step.

Potential Other Complications

MPNST on pathology while resecting a presumed benign tumor, intradural extension of MPNST, distant metastases from MPNST at presentation.

Case No. 7

You are evaluating a 32-year-old man with severe pain of the right hand. He does not report any weakness, just severe pain on the dorsal aspect of the hand near his thumb. The pain started approximately 2 months ago when he was arrested and handcuffs were placed very tightly around his wrists. He initially had numbness in this region, but it has subsequently developed into severe, burning pain.

Response

The patient should undergo a detailed neurologic examination with a focus on sensory evaluation of the distal radial sensory nerve and lateral antebrachial cutaneous nerve. Tinel sign should be present over the location of the lesion. A nerve block could be used to help differentiate between the lateral antebrachial cutaneous (LABC) and the superficial radial sensory nerve. Ultrasound imaging could be performed to look for a neuroma.

The patient's motor examination is normal. Sensory examination demonstrates extreme dysesthesia of the right dorsal aspect of the hand and thumb. The patient cannot tolerate a more extensive evaluation due to pain. Tinel sign is positive 1 cm proximal to the anatomical snuffbox, and the patient refuses to let you try another Tinel sign. Ultrasound is difficult due to pain, but appears to demonstrate enlargement of the nerve in the region of Tinel sign. Nerve block of the LABC has no effect on the pain.

Response

The tests performed are suggestive of a neuroma of the superficial radial sensory nerve. The patient should be counseled regarding nonoperative management. If symptoms do not respond to these attempts, neuroma excision should be considered. Surgery should be targeted to the area of positive Tinel sign with a plan for excision of the neuroma with burial of the proximal stump in muscle, deep and away from a joint. The patient should be counseled in the preoperative stage regarding persistent numbness in the painful region. (Examinee should explain the planned procedure step by step.)

Further Reading

Colbert SH. Painful sequelae of peripheral nerve injuries. In: Mackinnon S, ed. Nerve Surgery. 1st ed. New York, NY: Thieme; 2015:591–619

The patient is not interested in conservative management, as the pain is ruining his life. He would like surgery and accepts the possibility of persistent numbness in the distal territory. Surgery is performed and an incision is made over the area of maximum Tinel sign. The nerve is readily identified and enlargement is demonstrated. The neuroma extends to the edges of the incision, and appears to continue proximal to the current incision, approximately 6 cm.

Response

The patient has evidence of a large neuroma intraoperatively. The incision should be extended until normal radial sensory nerve is encountered. The neuroma resection should continue to the point of normal nerve. If the gap is substantial, nerve grafting is likely not an option. Attempts should be made to reduce the risk of repeat neuroma formation. This can be performed by burying the cut end of the nerve in a local muscle, pulling the nerve and cutting proximally, allowing for retraction into uninvolved tissue. The mainstay of the procedure should be focused on adequate neuroma resection and maneuvers/strategies to prevent the development of a recurrent painful neuroma.

Potential Other Complications

Neuroma recurrence, complex regional pain syndrome.

Case No. 8

You are consulted in the ED regarding a 27-year-old man who was hunting and had an accidental discharge of his firearm, resulting in gunshot wound to his right arm just above the elbow. He is awake and his pain is well controlled on IV medications. There is no significant arterial bleeding.

Response

The patient likely has a severe soft tissue injury to the right distal arm. The injury location could involve branches of the radial, median, or ulnar nerves, or any number of combinations of each. A detailed examination should be performed to identify any nerve injuries. Orthopaedics, plastic surgery, and potentially vascular surgery should be consulted, as this patient will need operative intervention. (Examinee should explain the planned procedure step by step.)

On examination, the patient has adequate function of the flexor digitorum profundus in digits 2–5. Sensation to the volar palm is intact. The patient has complete wrist and finger drop. Forearm fractures and potential vascular injury are identified. Orthopaedics surgery, plastic surgery, and vascular surgery are consulted, and plan to take the patient to the operating room for exploration, wound debridement, and initial closure. Then ask if you will perform a nerve repair for this patient?

Response

The patient has evidence of neurologic injury, likely the radial nerve. Given that a gunshot wound injury to the peripheral nerve can lead to more damage than just the transected region (via concussive shock to local soft tissue), definitive repair should not occur during initial exposure. Exposure of the neurologic injury should be performed if the patient is going to the operating room with other surgical disciplines, but the injured nerve ends should be tagged and sutured to surrounding tissue to avoid retraction and allow for healing of the initial injury. When the patient has recovered from initial stabilization procedures, an EMG could be performed to determine the degree of nerve involvement, and definitive repair could be planned for 3 to 4 weeks after surgery. At the subsequent surgery, the nerve ends are identified, and damaged nerve tissue is trimmed back until normal fascicles are seen. A graft repair could be performed at that time if deemed possible.

Further Reading

Samardzic M, Rasulic L. Gunshot and other missile wounds to the peripheral nerves. In: Socolovsky M, Rasulic L, Midha R, et al., eds. Manual of Peripheral Nerve Surgery. From the Basics to Complex Procedures. 1st ed. Stuttgart: Thieme; 2018:98–104

Initial exploration, debridement and closure are performed, and the transected ends of the radial nerve are identified and tagged. No other others appear involved in the injury. The patient undergoes a subsequent operation for tissue coverage. Three weeks post-injury the radial nerve deficit continues, and an EMG confirms absence of function in the distal radial nerve. The patient is taken to the operating room for exploration and nerve repair. Both nerve ends are inspected and trimmed to normal fascicles, and a 7-cm gap is created.

Response

Given the gap length, a graft repair could be considered using a sural nerve graft from the patient. Several cable grafts are needed to fill the diameter of the radial nerve. Typically 35 cm of sural nerve can be harvested from one leg. Despite the length of the graft and the scarring from previous operations in the region, radial nerve recovers relatively well. Maximal recovery may take several years.

The patient has a sural nerve graft performed and a tension-free repair is achieved. He tolerated the procedure well and recovers well. He is followed for the 18 months, and over that time he demonstrates no evidence of re-innervation on clinical examination. There is no advancement of a Tinel sign. There is no recovery on EMG.

Response

The nerve repair has unfortunately failed. The patient should be evaluated for potential tendon transfers that could help restore metacarpophalangeal (MCP) finger extension and wrist extension. He could also use a radial nerve brace that provides wrist dorsiflexion and finger extension, and keeps hand supple.

Further Reading

Patterson JM, Boyer MI, Goldfarb CA, Sammer DM. Tendon transfers for functional reconstruction > Principles of tendon transfer. In: Mackinnon S, ed. Nerve Surgery. 1st ed. New York, NY: Thieme; 2015:504-529

Case No. 9

A 52-year-old smoker is brought to your office due to an onset of right arm weakness. She tells you that she had a bad upper respiratory tract infection about 1 month ago which resolved spontaneously. Then, about 2 weeks ago, she woke up in the middle of the night with severe right shoulder pain that was excruciating. It moved down her arm to the elbow, and lasted for a couple of days before resolving. Now, starting 3 days ago, she has had difficulty brushing her hair with her right arm. She is having difficulty grasping the hairbrush, and also can't seem to get the brush to the top of her head.

Response

The patient has symptoms concerning for idiopathic brachial plexitis, or Parsonage-Turner syndrome. She had the onset of a viral illness, followed by severe shoulder pain and late weakness. She should undergo a detailed physical examination, MRI likely of the brachial plexus, and EMG if possible.

On examination, the patient has 3/5 strength of the right deltoid, 4-/5 strength in the supra/infraspinatus, and 3/5 finger flexion in the second and third digit. MRI of the right brachial plexus is shown in the image. EMG is suggestive of involvement of multiple nerve territories.

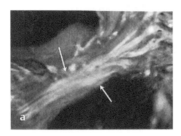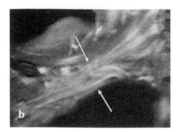

Response

The examination and EMG suggest involvement of multiple nerves, and the MRI confirms this. There is thickening and enlargement of the upper and lower trunks, as well as some contrast enhancement in those regions. All of the evidence helps confirm the evidence of idiopathic brachial plexitis in this case. The patient should have physical therapy and be monitored, given that maximal recovery may take up to 2 or 3 years. Surgical intervention is very unlikely to be necessary in this patient. The majority of patients with Parsonage-Turner syndrome make good recovery without surgical intervention.

Further Reading

Tung T, Moore AM. Brachial plexus injuries > Epidemiology and classification > Neuralgic amyotrophy (Parsonage-Turner syndrome). In: Mackinnon S, ed. Nerve Surgery. 1st ed. New York, NY: Thieme; 2015:403–404

The patient is monitored and undergoes physical therapy as well as pain management. She demonstrates some improvement in her right upper extremity function over the next 3 months. When she returns to visit with you, she has developed severe pain in the median nerve distribution, with edema and erythema. She has significant allodynia and cannot complete a full examination due to pain.

Response

Unfortunately it seems as though the patient has developed complex regional pain syndrome (CRPS) of the right upper extremity. CRPS can be difficult to treat, and likely will require multimodality treatment. Medications have had some efficacy, including pregabalin and courses of steroids. The patient should be evaluated by the anesthesia-pain specialists to help with treatment strategies. If medications don't work, a sympathetic blockade or even varying stimulation devices could be considered. (Examinee should explain the planned procedure step by step.)

Further Reading

Colbert SH. Painful sequelae of peripheral nerve injuries > Abnormal pain response > Pathophysiology of complex regional pain syndrome. In: Mackinnon S, ed. Nerve Surgery. 1st ed. New York, NY: Thieme; 2015:608–611
Colbert SH. Painful sequelae of peripheral nerve injuries > Abnormal pain response > Treatment of complex regional pain syndrome. In: Mackinnon S, ed. Nerve Surgery. 1st ed. New York, NY: Thieme; 2015:614–616

Case No. 10

A 41-year-old man comes to your office with a 2-month history of right hand pain and a proximal forearm mass. He says that he feels like the mass has been increasing in size, and when he moves it around, he gets an electric-like sensation shooting into the dorsum of his right hand.

Response

The patient should have a dedicated neurologic examination performed and he should be asked about any familial genetic syndromes, such as neurofibromatosis. He should also undergo an MRI of the right forearm to better identify any mass lesions.

On examination, the patient has a palpable mass in the dorsomedial aspect of the right forearm that is mildly mobile. It has a Tinel sign that causes sensory abnormalities in a superficial radial nerve distribution of the right hand. There is no associated motor weakness in a radial nerve distribution. An MRI is performed and the results are shown in the image.

Response

The patient's examination is suggestive of a mass involving the superficial radial sensory nerve, distal to the takeoff of the posterior interosseous nerve (PIN), as there appears to be no associated motor deficit. The MRI demonstrates a homogeneously enhancing mass of the radial sensory nerve, but also demonstrates the deep branch (PIN) displaced adjacent to the tumor. The tumor has an imaging appearance of a benign schwannoma, but

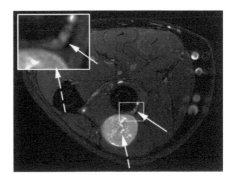

full diagnosis cannot be confirmed until tissue is obtained. Given its appearance, a needle biopsy is likely not required, and open surgical resection should be performed. The patient should be counseled about the possibility of persistent numbness in the superficial radial sensory nerve distribution and the potential for injury to local nerves during the tumor dissection. (Examinee should explain the planned procedure step by step.)

Further Reading

Barbour JR, Boyd KU. Tumors of the peripheral nervous system. In: Mackinnon S, ed. Nerve Surgery. 1st ed. New York, NY: Thieme; 2015:530–571

The patient is taken to the operating room and exposure of the tumor (and normal nerves proximal and distal to the tumor) is performed. There is evidence of displaced fascicles around the edge of the tumor. Prior to tumor excision, local nerves were identified, and the posterior interosseous nerve is identified deep to the tumor. The tumor is isolated from surrounding fascicles and completely excised including the entering and exiting fascicle from which the tumor arose. After the tumor is removed, inspection is performed, and it is discovered that manipulation of the nerve during tumor resection caused a transection of the posterior interosseous nerve. Readily identifiable ends are observed.

Response

Unfortunately, an iatrogenic nerve injury has occurred. In this case, a nerve repair should be performed as the transection is readily apparent; cut ends are both identified, and the injury has occurred in a controlled environment. The nerve ends should be mobilized and coapted, with special attempts made to correctly line up the fascicular anatomy during repair. A tension-free repair should be performed. The patient will unfortunately have a postoperative motor deficit that will hopefully recover over time.

Further Reading

Ramachandran S, Midha R. Surgical repair of nerve lesions: neurolysis and neurorrhaphy with grafts or tubes. In: Socolovsky M, Rasulic L, Midha R, et al., eds. Manual of Peripheral Nerve Surgery. From the Basics to Complex Procedures. 1st ed. Stuttgart: Thieme; 2018:74–83

Image Credits: Cases 1–8

Category 1: General Cases

- Case No. 1: Case 142. A 35-year-old who fell from a height of 14 feet. In: Riascos R, Bonfante E, Calle S, ed. RadCases Plus Q&A: Neuro Imaging. 2nd Edition. Thieme; 2018. Figure 2.
- Case No. 2: Extra-axial hematomas. In: Loftus C, ed. Neurosurgical Emergencies. 3rd Edition. Thieme; 2017. Figure 7.5.
- Case No. 3: Supratentorial astrocytomas. In: Keating R, Goodrich J, Packer R, ed. Tumors of the Pediatric Central Nervous System. 2nd Edition. Thieme; 2013. Figure 16.2.
- Case No. 4: Fetal Brain MRI. In: Meyers S, ed. Differential Diagnosis in Neuroimaging: Brain and Meninges. 1st Edition. Thieme; 2016. Figure 1.229.
- Case No. 5: Imaging. In: Forsting M, Jansen O, ed. MR Neuroimaging: Brain, Spine, Peripheral Nerves. 1st Edition. Thieme; 2016. Figure 10.24.
- Case No. 5: Dural and intradural extramedullary lesions. In: Meyers S, ed. Differential Diagnosis in Neuroimaging: Spine. 1st Edition. Thieme; 2016. Figure 1.165
- Case No. 6: Pathophysiology of spinal pain and pain pathways. In: Kim D, Abdi S, Schütze G, ed. Epiduroscopy: Atlas of Procedures. 1st Edition. Thieme; 2017. Figure 3.4.
- Case No. 6: Pathophysiology of spinal pain and pain pathways. In: Kim D, Abdi S, Schütze G, ed. Epiduroscopy: Atlas of Procedures. 1st Edition. Thieme; 2017. Figure 3.5.
- Case No. 7: Surgical therapies for middle cerebral artery aneurysms. In: Spetzler R, Kalani M, Nakaji P, ed. Neurovascular Surgery. 2nd Edition. Thieme; 2015. Figures 48.2 a–c.
- Case No. 8: Case 168. A 75-year-old woman presenting with transient left hemiparesis. In: Riascos R, Bonfante E, Calle S, ed. RadCases Plus Q&A: Neuro Imaging. 2nd Edition. Thieme; 2018. Figure 7.
- Case No. 9: Diffusion weighted and diffusion tensor imaging in infectious diseases. In: Leite C, Castillo M, ed. Diffusion Weighted and Diffusion Tensor Imaging. A Clinical Guide. 1st Edition. Figure 8.11.
- Case No. 10: Introduction and background. In: Cohen A, ed. Pediatric Neurosurgery: Tricks of the Trade. 1st Edition. Thieme; 2015. Figure 24.1.

Category 2: Neurology Mimics

- Case No. 1: Conventional morphological imaging: MRI remains the workhorse. In: Jain R, Essig M, ed. Brain Tumor Imaging. 1st Edition. Thieme; 2015. Figure 1.13.
- Case No. 1: Introduction. In: Meyers S, ed. Differential Diagnosis in Neuroimaging: Brain and Meninges. 1st Edition. Thieme; 2016. Figure 4.9.
- Case No. 2: Glossopharyngeal nerve: pathologic images. In: Binder D, Sonne D, Fischbein N, ed. Cranial Nerves: Anatomy, Pathology, Imaging. 1st Edition. Thieme; 2010. Figure 9.20.
- Case No. 5: Intramedullary space. In: Forsting M, Jansen O, ed. MR Neuroimaging: Brain, Spine, Peripheral Nerves. 1st Edition. Thieme; 2016. Figure 16.4.
- Case No. 7: Osseous tumors. In: Choudhri A, ed. Pediatric Neuroradiology. Clinical Practice Essentials. 1st Edition. Thieme; 2016. Figure 27.10.
- Case No. 9: Prion disease. In: Kanekar S, ed. Imaging of Neurodegenerative Disorders. 1st Edition. Thieme; 2015. Figure 27.2.
- Case No. 10: Skull base and cranial nerves. In: Choudhri A, ed. Pediatric Neuroradiology. Clinical Practice Essentials. 1st Edition. Thieme; 2016.Figure 16.14.

Category 3: Spine

- Case No. 1: Intramedullary space. In: Forsting M, Jansen O, ed. MR Neuroimaging: Brain, Spine, Peripheral Nerves. 1st Edition. Thieme; 2016. Figure 14.27.
- Case No. 2: Extradural space. In: Forsting M, Jansen O, ed. MR Neuroimaging: Brain, Spine, Peripheral Nerves. 1st Edition. Thieme; 2016. Figure 16.12.

- Case No. 3: Cervical fracture/dislocation Ⓟ. In: Nader R, Berta S, Gragnanielllo C et al., ed. Neurosurgery Tricks of the Trade. Spine and Peripheral Nerves. 1st Edition. Thieme; 2014. Figure 47.1.
- Case No. 4: Intramedullary spinal tumors. In: Dickman C, Fehlings M, Gokaslan Z, ed. Spinal Cord and Spinal Column Tumors. 1st Edition. Thieme; 2006. Figure 5.15.
- Case No. 5: Degenerative. In: Shaya M, Gragnanielllo C, Nader R, ed. Neurosurgery Rounds: Questions and Answers. 2nd Edition. Thieme; 2017. Figure 6.14.
- Case No. 5: Decision making in adult deformity surgery: decompression versus short or long fusion. In: Vialle L, ed. AOSpine Masters Series, Volume 4: Adult Spinal Deformities. 1st Edition. Thieme; 2015. Figure 2.5.
- Case No. 6: Tumors of the craniovertebral junction. In: Goel A, Cacciola F, ed. The Craniovertebral Junction. Diagnosis–Pathology–Surgical Techniques. 1st Edition. Thieme; 2011. Figure 38.5.
- Case No. 6: Meninges. In: Meyers S, ed. Differential Diagnosis in Neuroimaging: Brain and Meninges. 1st Edition. Thieme; 2016. Figure 4.17.
- Case No. 7: Degenerative spinal and foraminal stenoses. In: Forsting M, Jansen O, ed. MR Neuroimaging: Brain, Spine, Peripheral Nerves. 1st Edition. Thieme; 2016. Figure 12.33.
- Case No. 8: Multilevel cervical spondylosis: anterior approach. In: Albert T, Lee J, Lim M, ed. Cervical Spine Surgery Challenges. Diagnosis and Management. 1st Edition. Thieme; 2008. Figure 3.3.
- Case No. 8: Surgical management of cervical ossification of posterior longitudinal ligament Ⓟ. In: Nader R, Berta S, Gragnanielllo C et al., ed. Neurosurgery Tricks of the Trade. Spine and Peripheral Nerves. 1st Edition. Thieme; 2014. Figure 84.2.
- Case No. 9: Thoracic disc. In: Abdulhak M, Marzouk S, ed. Challenging Cases in Spine Surgery. 1st Edition. Thieme; 2005. Figure 34.1.
- Case No. 9: Koktekir E, Tatarli N, Ceylan D et al. Symptomatic Pneumorrhachis. Journal of Neurological Surgery Part A Central European Neurosurgery 2014; 75(02): 140–145. Figure 3.
- Case No. 10: Spinal imaging. In: Baaj A, Mummaneni P, Uribe J et al., ed. Handbook of Spine Surgery. 2nd Edition. Thieme; 2016. Figure 8.1.
- Case No. 10: Junctional issues following adult deformity surgery. In: Vialle L, ed. AOSpine Masters Series, Volume 4: Adult Spinal Deformities. 1st Edition. Thieme; 2015. Figure 9.1 a,b.

Category 4: Vascular

- Case No. 1: Skull-base trauma. In: Anzai Y, Tozer-Fink K, ed. Imaging of Traumatic Brain Injury. 1st Edition. Thieme; 2015. Figure 9.26.
- Case No. 2: Bonadio L, Mello L, Boer V et al. Pericallosal Aneurysms: Effectiveness of Endovascular Management. Arquivos Brasileiros de Neurocirurgia: Brazilian Neurosurgery 2017; 36(01): 07–13. Figure 2.
- Case No. 3: Distal anterior circulation and posterior circulation aneurysms. In: Park M, Taussky P, Albuquerque F et al., ed. Flow Diversion of Cerebral Aneurysms. 1st Edition. Thieme; 2017. Figure 6.8.
- Case No. 3: III CNS locations for infection. In: Hall W, Kim P, ed. Neurosurgical Infectious Disease. Surgical and Nonsurgical Management. 1st Edition. Thieme; 2013. Figure 11.5.
- Case No. 4: Computed tomography (CT). In: Runge V, ed. Imaging of Cerebrovascular Disease. 1st Edition. Thieme; 2016. Figure 1.22.
- Case No. 4: Angioplasty and stenting for management of intracranial arterial stenosis. In: Bendok B, Naidech A, Walker M et al., ed. Hemorrhagic and Ischemic Stroke. Medical, Imaging, Surgical and Interventional Approaches. 1st Edition. Thieme; 2011. Figure 31.6.
- Case No. 5: Aydin S, Abuzayed B, Kiziltan G et al. Unilateral Thalamic Vim and GPi Stimulation for the Treatment of Holmes' Tremor Caused by Midbrain Cavernoma: Case Report and Review of the Literature. Journal of Neurological Surgery Part A Central European Neurosurgery 2013; 74(04): 271–276. Figure 1.
- Case No. 6: Radiosurgery of arteriovenous malformations without embolization. In: Sheehan J, Gerszten P, ed. Controversies in Stereotactic Radiosurgery. Best Evidence Recommendations. 1st Edition. Thieme; 2014. Figure 13.1.
- Case No. 6: Liquid embolization of vascular lesions Ⓐ. In: Nader R, Gragnanielllo C, Berta S et al., ed. Neurosurgery Tricks of the Trade. Cranial. 1st Edition. Thieme; 2013. Figure 101.1.
- Case No. 6: Classification of brain arteriovenous malformations and fistulas. In: Dumont

A, Lanzino G, Sheehan J, ed. Brain Arteriovenous Malformations and Arteriovenous Fistulas. 1st Edition. Thieme; 2017. Figure 12.3.
- Case No. 7: 6.3 Results. In: Dumont A, Lanzino G, Sheehan J, ed. Brain Arteriovenous Malformations and Arteriovenous Fistulas. 1st Edition. Thieme; 2017. Figure 6.3.
- Case No. 8: Management of vertebral artery dissections and vascular insufficiency. In: Bambakidis N, Dickman C, Spetzler R et al., ed. Surgery of the Craniovertebral Junction. 2nd Edition. Thieme; 2012. Figure 14.4.
- Case No. 8: Extracranial vertebral artery angioplasty and stenting. In: Nussbaum E, Mocco J, ed. Cerebral Revascularization: Microsurgical and Endovascular Techniques. 1st Edition. Thieme; 2011. Figure 13.3.
- Case No. 9: Vascular abnormalities. In: Meyers S, ed. Differential Diagnosis in Neuroimaging: Brain and Meninges. 1st Edition. Thieme; 2016. Figure 5.51.
- Case No. 9: Proximal stenosis of supra-aortic vessels. In: Jansen O, Brückmann H, ed. Interventional Stroke Therapy. 1st Edition. Thieme; 2012. Figure 15.2.
- Case No. 10: Case 057. A young woman who has fallen from a height after "the worst headache of her life." In: Riascos R, Bonfante E, ed. RadCases: Neuro Imaging. 1st Edition. Thieme; 2010.

Category 5: Tumor

- Case No. 1: Tumors of the sellar region. In: Forsting M, Jansen O, ed. MR Neuroimaging: Brain, Spine, Peripheral Nerves. 1st Edition. Thieme; 2016. Figure 3.44.
- Case No. 2: Case 8. In: Tsiouris A, Sanelli P, Comunale J, ed. Case-Based Brain Imaging. 2nd Edition. Thieme; 2013. Figure 8.2.
- Case No. 3: Miscellaneous tumors. In: Forsting M, Jansen O, Hrsg. MR Neuroimaging: Brain, Spine, Peripheral Nerves. 1st Edition. Thieme; 2016. Figure 3.67.
- Case No. 4: Other tumors (mainly supratentorial). In: Choudhri A, Hrsg. Pediatric Neuroradiology. Clinical Practice Essentials. 1st Edition. Thieme; 2016. Figure 8.13.
- Case No. 5: Microsurgery for acoustic neuromas. In: Sheehan J, Gerszten P, ed. Controversies in Stereotactic Radiosurgery. Best Evidence Recommendations. 1st Edition. Thieme; 2014. Figure 8.1.
- Case No. 6: Pineal region tumors. In: Harbaugh R, Shaffrey C, Couldwell W et al., ed. Neurosurgery Knowledge Update. A Comprehensive Review. 1st Edition. Thieme; 2015. Figure 154.1.
- Case No. 7: X. Oncology. In: Citow J, Macdonald R, Refai D, ed. Comprehensive Neurosurgery Board Review. 2nd Edition. Thieme; 2009. Figure 3.72.
- Case No. 8: 21.7 Case examples. In: Sekhar L, Fessler R, ed. Atlas of Neurosurgical Techniques: Brain, Volume 2. 2nd Edition. Thieme; 2015. Figure 21.26.
- Case No. 9: Section IV: Inner ear and petrous bone. Chapter 45: Epidermoid. In: Hoeffner E, Mukherji S, ed. Temporal Bone Imaging. 1st Edition. Thieme; 2008. Figure 45.1.
- Case No. 10: Tumors of the neuroepithelial tissue. In: Jain R, Essig M, ed. Brain Tumor Imaging. 1st Edition. Thieme; 2015. Figure 1.5.

Category 6: Pediatrics

- Case No. 1: Introduction. In: Meyers S, ed. Differential Diagnosis in Neuroimaging: Brain and Meninges. 1st Edition. Thieme; 2016. Figure 2.42.
- Case No. 2: Table 2.3 Extraocular lesions involving the orbit. In: Meyers S, ed. Differential Diagnosis in Neuroimaging: Head and Neck. 1st Edition. Thieme; 2016. Figure 2.87.
- Case No. 3: Hydrocephalus and intracranial hypotension. In: Forsting M, Jansen O, ed. MR Neuroimaging: Brain, Spine, Peripheral Nerves. 1st Edition. Thieme; 2016. Figure 10.17.
- Case No. 3: Normal pressure hydrocephalus. In: Kanekar S, ed. Imaging of Neurodegenerative Disorders. 1st Edition. Thieme; 2015. Figure 29.4.
- Case No. 4: Ventricular anatomy and neuroendoscopy. In: Harbaugh R, Shaffrey C, Couldwell W et al., ed. Neurosurgery Knowledge Update. A Comprehensive Review. 1st Edition. Thieme; 2015. Figure 52.1.

- Case No. 5: Congenital abnormalities of the thoracic and thoracolumbar spine. In: Fessler R, Sekhar L, ed. Atlas of Neurosurgical Techniques. Spine and Peripheral Nerves. 2nd Edition. Thieme; 2016. Figure 47.7.
- Case No. 6: Embryonal tumors. In: Forsting M, Jansen O, ed. MR Neuroimaging: Brain, Spine, Peripheral Nerves. 1st Edition. Thieme; 2016. Figure 3.25.
- Case No. 7: Skull and scalp. In: Choudhri A, ed. Pediatric Neuroradiology. Clinical Practice Essentials. 1st Edition. Thieme; 2016. Figure 15.5.
- Case No. 8: 55.1 Background. In: Cohen A, ed. Pediatric Neurosurgery: Tricks of the Trade. 1st Edition. Thieme; 2015. Figure 55.3.
- Case No. 9: Occipital encephalocele. In: Cohen A, ed. Pediatric Neurosurgery: Tricks of the Trade. 1st Edition. Thieme; 2015. Figure 22.3.
- Case No. 9: Case No. 9: Fetal imaging. In: Choudhri A, ed. Pediatric Neuroradiology. Clinical Practice Essentials. 1st Edition. Thieme; 2016. Figure 5.7.
- Case No. 10: Radiographic findings. In: Keating R, Goodrich J, Packer R, Hrsg. Tumors of the Pediatric Central Nervous System. 2nd Edition. Thieme; 2013. Figure 33.1.

Category 7: Functional

- Case No. 3: VII. Seizures. In: Citow J, Macdonald R, Refai D, ed. Comprehensive Neurosurgery Board Review. 2nd Edition. Thieme; 2009. Figure 4.6.
- Case No. 5: Case examples. In: Spetzler R, Kalani M, Nakaji P et al., ed. Color Atlas of Brainstem Surgery. 1st Edition. Thieme; 2017. Figure 5.40.
- Case No. 8: 84.7 Operative detail and preparation. In: Cohen A, ed. Pediatric Neurosurgery: Tricks of the Trade. 1st Edition. Thieme; 2015. Figure 84.4.
- Case No. 9: Neuroepithelial tumors. In: Forsting M, Jansen O, ed. MR Neuroimaging: Brain, Spine, Peripheral Nerves. 1st Edition. Thieme; 2016. Figure 3.24.
- Case No. 10: 50.3 Surgical technique. In: Sekhar L, Fessler R, ed. Atlas of Neurosurgical Techniques: Brain, Volume 2. 2nd Edition. Thieme; 2015. Figure 50.3.

Category 8: Peripheral Nerve

- Case No. 1: Laceration injury. In: Socolovsky M, Rasulic L, Midha R et al., ed. Manual of Peripheral Nerve Surgery. From the Basics to Complex Procedures. 1st Edition. Thieme; 2017. Figure 3.4.
- Case No. 2: Ulnar nerve. In: Russell S, ed. Examination of Peripheral Nerve Injuries: An Anatomical Approach. 2nd Edition. Thieme; 2015. Figure 2.22.
- Case No. 3: Carpal tunnel syndrome. In: Mackinnon S, ed. Nerve Surgery. 1st Edition. Thieme; 2015. Figure 9.8.
- Case No. 4: 5.1 Proximal brachial plexus palsies. In: Russell S, ed. Examination of Peripheral Nerve Injuries: An Anatomical Approach. 2nd Edition. Thieme; 2015. Figure 5.4.
- Case No. 4: Traumatic brachial plexus lesions: Clinical Aspects, Assessment, and Timing of Surgical Repair. In: Socolovsky M, Rasulic L, Midha R et al., ed. Manual of Peripheral Nerve Surgery. From the Basics to Complex Procedures. 1st Edition. Thieme; 2017. Figure 16.1.
- Case No. 5: Peroneal intraneural ganglia. In: Harbaugh R, Shaffrey C, Couldwell W et al., ed. Neurosurgery Knowledge Update. A Comprehensive Review. 1st Edition. Thieme; 2015. Figure 120.1.
- Case No. 6: Malignant peripheral nerve sheath tumors. In: Socolovsky M, Rasulic L, Midha R et al., ed. Manual of Peripheral Nerve Surgery. From the Basics to Complex Procedures. 1st Edition. Thieme; 2017. Figure 23.3.
- Case No. 9: Table 7.1 Brachial plexus abnormalities. In: Meyers S, ed. Differential Diagnosis in Neuroimaging: Head and Neck. 1st Edition. Thieme; 2016. Figure 7.13.
- Case No. 10: Diseases of the peripheral nervous system. In: Forsting M, Jansen O, ed. MR Neuroimaging: Brain, Spine, Peripheral Nerves. 1st Edition. Thieme; 2016. Figure 18.7.

Quick Reference Guide

General

GCS

Glasgow coma[a] scale1 (recommended for age ≥ 4 yrs)

Points[b]	Best eye opening	Best verbal	Best motor
6	–	–	obeys
5	–	oriented	localizes pain
4	spontaneous	confused	withdraws to pain
3	to speech	inappropriate	flexion (decorticate)
2	to pain[c]	incomprehensible	extensor (decerebrate)
1	none	none	none[d]

[a]technically, this is a scale of impaired consciousness, whereas "coma" implies unresponsiveness
[b]range of total points: 3 (worst) to 15 (normal)
[c]when testing eye opening to pain, use peripheral stimulus (the grimace associated with central pain may cause eye closure)
[d]if no motor response, important to exclude spinal cord transection
Source: Greenberg MS. Coma. In: Handbook of Neurosurgery, 8th ed. New York, NY: Thieme; 2016:296. Table 18.1

Children's coma scale[a] (for age < 4 yrs)

Points[b]	Best eye	Best verbal	Best motor	Points[b]
6	–	–	obeys	6
5	–	smiles, oriented to sound, follows objects, interacts		localizes pain
		Crying	**Interaction**	
4	spontaneous	consolable	inappropriate	withdraws to pain
3	to speech	inconsistently consolable	moaning	flexion (decorticate)
2	to pain	inconsolable	restless	extensor (decerebrate)
1	none	none	none	none

[a]same as adult Glasgow coma scale except for verbal response[3]
[b]range of total points: 3 (worst) to 15 (normal)
Source: Greenberg MS. Coma. In: Handbook of Neurosurgery, 8th ed. New York, NY: Thieme; 2016:296. Table 18.2

Muscle Grading

Muscle grading (modified Medical Research Council system)

Grade	Strength		
0	no contraction (total paralysis)		
1	flicker or trace contraction (palpable or visible)		
2	active movement with gravity eliminated		
3	active movement through full ROM against gravity		
4	active movement against resistance; subdivisions →	4– Slight resistance	
		4 Moderate resistance	
		4+ Slight resistance	
5	normal strength (against full resistance)		
NT	not testable		

Source: Greenberg MS. Peripheral nerves. In: Handbook of Neurosurgery, 8th ed. New York, NY: Thieme; 2016:505. Table 29.2

Acute ICP Elevation

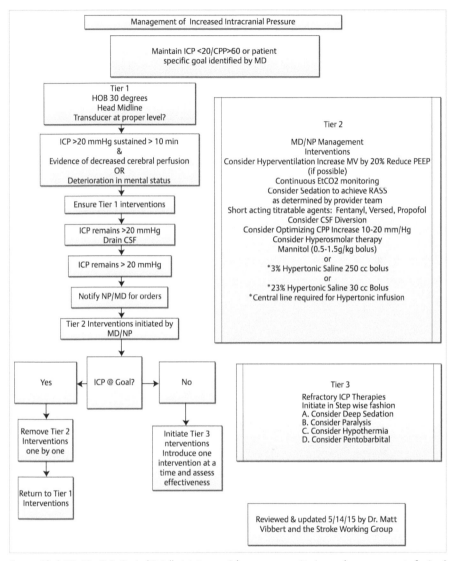

Management of Increased Intracranial Pressure

Maintain ICP <20/CPP>60 or patient specific goal identified by MD

Tier 1
HOB 30 degrees
Head Midline
Transducer at proper level?

ICP >20 mmHg sustained > 10 min
&
Evidence of decreased cerebral perfusion
OR
Deterioration in mental status

Ensure Tier 1 interventions

ICP remains >20 mmHg
Drain CSF

ICP remains > 20 mmHg

Notify NP/MD for orders

Tier 2 Interventions initiated by MD/NP

ICP @ Goal? — Yes / No

Yes → Remove Tier 2 Interventions one by one → Return to Tier 1 Interventions

No → Initiate Tier 3 nterventions Introduce one intervention at a time and assess effectiveness

Tier 2
MD/NP Management
Interventions
Consider Hyperventilation Increase MV by 20% Reduce PEEP (if possible)
Continuous EtCO2 monitoring
Consider Sedation to achieve RASS as determined by provider team
Short acting titratable agents: Fentanyl, Versed, Propofol
Consider CSF Diversion
Consider Optimizing CPP Increase 10-20 mm/Hg
Consider Hyperosmolar therapy
Mannitol (0.5-1.5g/kg bolus)
or
*3% Hypertonic Saline 250 cc bolus
or
*23% Hypertonic Saline 30 cc Bolus
*Central line required for Hypertonic infusion

Tier 3
Refractory ICP Therapies
Initiate in Step wise fashion
A. Consider Deep Sedation
B. Consider Paralysis
C. Consider Hypothermia
D. Consider Pentobarbital

Reviewed & updated 5/14/15 by Dr. Matt Vibbert and the Stroke Working Group

Source: Shah SO, Kim B-S, Govind B, Jallo J. Intracranial pressure monitoring and management of raised intracranial pressure. In: Loftus C, ed. Neurosurgical Emergencies. 3rd ed. New York, NY: Thieme; 2017:13. Figure 2.5

Status Epilepticus Management

Summary of initial steps for status epilepticus (adults and children > 13 kg; see text for details)

ABC's. Start O_2. Turn patient on their side. Check VS. Do a neuro exam.

Monitor/labs: Pulse oximetry. EKG/telemetry. ✓ Fingerstick glucose.
Blood tests (do not wait for results to begin ℞): ✓ electrolytes, ✓ CBC, ✓ ABG, ✓ AED levels,
   ✓ LFTs, ✓ Mg^{++}, ✓ Ca^{++}, ✓ head CT

Large bore IV X 2. Start IV fluids:

   thiamine 100 mg IV and/or 50 ml of 50% dextrose (if needed based on fingerstick glucose)

First-line AED:

lorazepam (Ativan®) 4 mg IV for adults, 2 mg IV for children > 13 kg @ < 2 mg/min

OR

midazolam (Versed®) 10 mg IM for adults, 5 mg IM for children > 13 kg OR (if no IV access or
   midazolam injections not available)

diazepam can be given rectally in Diastat® gel formulation (0.2–0.5mg/kg)

Repeat loading dose of benzodiazepine if necessary.

Second-line AED: given with failure of (or simultaneously with administration of) repeat dose of
   benzodiazepine

fosphenytoin: 15–20mg PE/kg IV @ < 150mg PE/min (preferred drug: faster infusion rate, less
   irritation)

OR

phenytoin: 15–20mg/kg IV @ < 50mg/min (less expensive) If no response to loading dose, an
   additional 10mg/kg IV may be given after 20min.

NB: following infusion rate guidelines is imperative. Significant cardiovascular risk is associated
   with rapid infusion of phenytoin/fosphenytoin.

✓ phenytoin level ≈ 10 min after PHT loading dose; repeat 10 min later additional dose if required

Alternative second-line AEDs:

sodium valproate: 20–30 mg/kg IV bolus (max rate: 100 mg/min) – has been shown to be equal or
   superior to phenytoin in a few small studies

OR

phenobarbital: 20 mg/kg IV (start infusing @ 50–100 mg/min) – commonly used 2nd or 3rd line
   AED. A repeat dose of 25–30mg/kg can be given 10min after first dose.

OR

Levetiracetam (Keppra®): 20mg/kg IV bolus of over 15 minutes – evidence for Keppra as a first or
   second line drug is less clear

If seizures continue > 30 mins and are refractory to 1st and 2nd line AEDs: intubate in ICU and
   begin continuous infusion therapy (CIT) of:

Midazolam: 0.2mg/kg IV loading dose followed by 0.2–0.6 mg/kg/hr

OR

Propofol: 2mg/kg IV loading dose followed by 2–5mg/kg/hr

If Sz persist, ensure that correctable conditions have been ruled-out and/or treated

novel therapeutic options (not systematically studied): shock therapy...

Source: Greenberg MS. Special types of seizures. In: Handbook of Neurosurgery, 8th ed. New York, NY:
Thieme; 2016:469. Table 27.5

Drug Induced Coma

Clinical features of coma from drug overdoses

Syndrome	Sympathomimetic	Sympatholytic	Anticholinergic	Cholinergic
Causative drugs	Cocaine, amphetamine, ephedrine	Opiates, benzodiazepines, alcohol	Antihistamines, neuroleptics, TCAs	Insecticides (organophosphates)
Heart rate	↑ ↑	Normal or ↓	↑	Either: ↑ ↓
BP	↑ ↑	↓	↑	Either: ↑ ↓
Pupils	Large	Pinpoint	Very large to fixed	Small
Diaphoresis[a]	↑	Normal	↓ ↓	↑ ↑
GI/GU motility[a]	↑	Normal or ↓	↓	↑ ↑
Other features			TCAs: wide QRS on EKG	Fasciculations, lacrimation, salivation

Abbreviations: BP, blood pressure; EKG, electrocardiogram; CI, gastrointestinal; GU, genitourinary; TCA, tricyclic antidepressant.
Data from Gerace RW. Drugs part A: poisoning. In: Young GB, Ropper AH, Bolton CF, eds. Coma and Impaired Consciousness. New York, NY: McGraw-Hill; 1998: 457–469.
[a]Reduced diaphoresis leads to hot, dry, flushed skin. Increased GI/GU motility includes nausea and vomiting, cramps, and diarrhea. Decreased GI/GU motility includes ileus and bladder atony. Seizures and cardiac arrhythmias may occur with any syndrome.
Source: Merchut MP, Biller J. Assessment of acute loss of consciousness. In: Loftus C, ed. Neurosurgical Emergencies. 3rd ed. New York, NY: Thieme; 2017:6. Table 1.1

Trauma

Cranial Surgical Indications

Surgical lesion	Guidelines
Acute epidural hematoma	Serial head CT and clinical examination: EDH < 30 cm³, clot thickness < 15 mm, midline shift < 5 mm, GCS score > 8, and without focal neurologic deficit Emergent surgical evacuation: All EDH > 30 cm³, GCS score < 9 with anisocoria
Acute subdural hematoma	ICP monitoring: GCS score < 9 Emergent surgical evacuation: SDH of > 10 mm thickness, or with > 5 mm MLS GCS score < 9, and a SDH of < 10 mm thickness and < 5 mm MLS, if GCS score decreased by > 2, if ICP > 20 mm Hg, or if anisocoric
Traumatic parenchymal lesions	Close observation: Neurologically stable without midline shift, mass effect, elevated ICP Emergent surgical intervention: Neurologic deficit/decline, mass effect, or intractable ICP GCS score 6–8 with frontal or temporal IPH > 20 cm³ and either > 5 mm MLS or cistern compression on head CT IPH > 50 cm³
Posterior fossa mass lesion	Observation: Patients without mass effect or neurologic deficit Emergent operative intervention: Patients with mass effect or neurologic deficit
Depressed skull fractures	Observation: < 1 cm depression, no dural tear, large hematoma, frontal sinus involvement, pneumocephalus, or wound infection/contamination Operative intervention: Open fractures displaced greater than the thickness of the skull should undergo surgery

Abbreviations: CT, computed tomography; GCS, Glasgow Coma Scale; ICP, intracranial pressure; IPH, intraparenchymal hemorrhage; MLS, midline shift; SDH, acute subdural hematoma.
Source: Pendleton C, Jallo J. Summary and synopsis of the brain trauma foundation head injury guidelines. In: Loftus C, ed. Neurosurgical Emergencies. 3rd ed. New York, NY: Thieme; 2017:192. Table 19.2

Spine Injury Scales

ASIA impairment scale

Class	Description
A	Complete: no motor or sensory function preserved
B	Incomplete: sensory but no motor function preserved below the neurologic level (includes sacral segments S4–5)
C	Incomplete: motor function preserved below the neurologic level (more than half of key muscles below the neurologic level have a muscle strength grade < 3)
D	Incomplete: motor function preserved below the neurologic level (more than half of key muscles below the neurologic level have a muscle strength grade ≥ 3)
E	Normal: Sensory & motor function normal

Source: Greenberg MS. General information, neurologic assessment, whiplash and sports-related injuries, pediatric spine injuries. In: Handbook of Neurosurgery, 8th ed. New York, NY: Thieme; 2016:944. Table 62.13

Thoracolumbar injury classification & severity score (TLICS)

Category	Finding	Points
Radiographic findings	compression fx	1
	burst component or lateral angulation > 15°	1
	distraction injury	2
	translational/rotational injury	3
Neurologic status	intact	0
	root injury	2
	complete SCI	2
	incomplete SCI	3
	cauda equina syndrome	3
Integrity of posterior ligamantous complex	intact	0
	undetermined	2
	definite injury	3
TLICS = Total Points →		

Source: Greenberg MS. Thoracic, lumbar and sacral spine fractures. In: Handbook of Neurosurgery, 8th ed. New York, NY: Thieme; 2016:1007. Table 66.3

Subaxial injury classification (SLIC)

Injury (rate *the most severe injury* at that level)	Points
Morphology	
No abnormality	0
Simple compression (compression fx, endplate disruption, sagittal or coronal plane VB fx.)	1
Burst fracture	2
Distraction (perched facet, posterior element fx.)	3
Rotation/translation (facet dislocation, teardrop fx., advanced compression injury, bilateral pedicle fx., floating lateral mass. Guidelines: relative axial rotation ≥ 11°[4] or any translation not related to degenerative causes	4
Discoligamentous complex (DLC)	
Intact	0
Indeterminate (isolated interspinous widening with < 11° relative angulation & no abnormal facet alignment, ↑ signal on T2WI MRI in ligaments...)	1
Disrupted (perched or dislocated facet, < 50% articular apposition, facet diastasis > 2 mm, widened anterior disc space, ↑ signal on T2WI MRI through entire disc...)	2
Neurologic status	
Intact	0
Root injury	1
Complete spinal cord injury	2
Incomplete spinal cord injury	3
Continuous cord compression with neuro deficit	+1

Source: Greenberg MS. Subaxial (C3 through C7) injuries/fractures. In: Handbook of Neurosurgery, 8th ed. New York, NY: Thieme; 2016:986. Table 65.1

Management based on TLICS

TLICS	Management
≤ 3	nonoperative candidates
4	"grey zone" may be considered for operative or nonoperative management
≥ 5	surgical candidates

Source: Greenberg MS. Thoracic, lumbar and sacral spine fractures. In: Handbook of Neurosurgery, 8th ed. New York, NY: Thieme; 2016:1007. Table 66.4

Ventricular Access

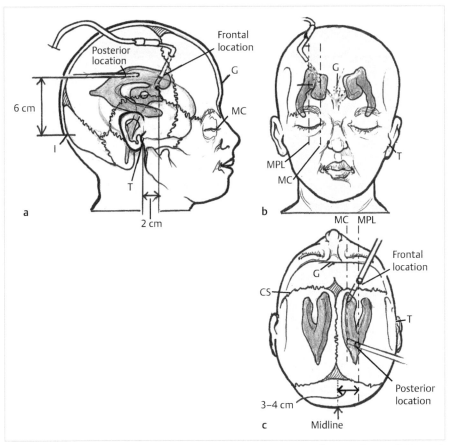

Source: Sciubba D. External ventricular drain (ventriculostomy). In: Connolly E, McKhann II G, Huang J, et al., eds. Fundamentals of Operative Techniques in Neurosurgery. 2nd ed. Thieme; 2010:372. Figure 83.1)

Spine

Cervical Disc Syndromes

Cervical disc syndromes

Syndrome	Cervical disc syndromes			
	C4–5	C5–6	C6–7	C7-T1w
% of cervical discs	2%	19%	69%	10%
compressed root	C5	C6	C7	C8
reflex diminished	deltoid & pectoralis	biceps & brachioradialis	triceps	finger-jerk[a]
motor weakness	deltoid	forearm flexion	forearm ext (wrist drop)	hand intrinsics
paresthesia & hypesthesia	shoulder	upper arm, thumb, radial forearm	fingers 2 & 3, all fingertips	fingers 4 & 5

[a]not everyone has a finger flexor reflex. Description: gently lift the fingertips of the patient's pronated hand and tap the underside of the fingers with a reflex hammer. When present, fingers flex in response
Source: Greenberg MS. Cervical disc herniation. In: Handbook of Neurosurgery, 8th ed. New York, NY: Thieme; 2016:1069. Table 70.1

Lumbar Disc Syndromes

Lumbar disc syndromes

Syndrome	Level of herniated lumbar disc		
	L3–4	L4–5	L5-S1
root usually compressed	L4	L5	S1
% of lumbar discs	3–10% (5% average)	40–45%	45–50%
reflex diminished	knee jerk[a] (Westphal's sign)	medial hamstring[b]	Achilles[a] (ankle jerk)
motor weakness	quadriceps femoris (knee extension)	tibialis anterior (foot drop) & EHL	gastrocnemius (plantarflexion), ± EHL
decreased sensation[c]	medial malleolus & medial foot	large toe web & dorsum of foot	lateral malleolus & lateral foot
pain distribution	anterior thigh	posterior LE	posterior LE, often to ankle

[a] Jendrassik maneuver may reinforce
[b]medial hamstring reflex is unreliable (not always pure L5), may also stimulate adductors when eliciting
[c]sensory impairment is most common in the distal extremes of the dermatome
Source: Greenberg MS. Lumbar and thoracic intervertebral disk herniation/radiculopathy. In: Handbook of Neurosurgery. 8th ed. New York, NY: Thieme; 2016:1050. Table 69.3

Deformity Measurements

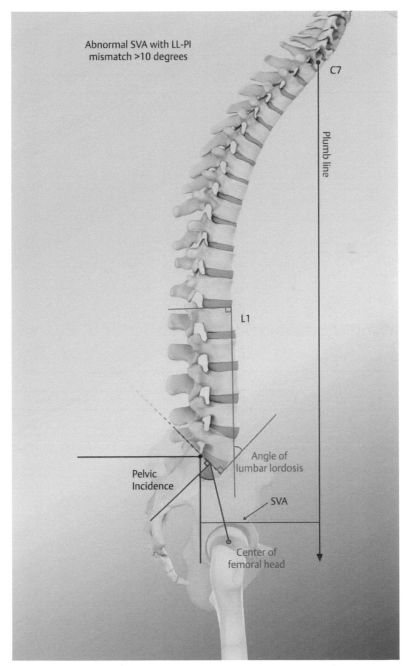

Abnormal SVA with LL-PI
mismatch >10 degrees

C7

Plumb line

L1

Angle of
lumbar lordosis

Pelvic
Incidence

SVA

Center of
femoral head

Source: Lau D, Kuntz C IV, Shaffrey C, Mummaneni PV. Sagittal spinopelvic parameters and measurements. In: Harbaugh R, Shaffrey C, Couldwell W et al., eds. Neurosurgery Knowledge Update. A Comprehensive Review. 1st ed. New York, NY:Thieme; 2015:546. Figure 87.2

Deformity Surgery Decision Making

Anteroposterior Radiography Features in Spinal Trauma

Radiological Features
Fractures of the transverse process, isolated lamina
Loss of vertebral body height (compare with the adjacent normal vertebra)
Widening of interpedicular distance
Vertebral translation
Loss of alignment of spinous processes
Increased interspinous distance
Horizontal split in the body

Source: Rajasekaran S, Kanna RM, Maheswaran A, Shetty AP. Radiographic assessment of thoracolumbar fractures. In: Vialle L, ed. AOSpine Masters Series, Volume 6: Thoracolumbar Spine Trauma. 1st ed. New York, NY: Thieme; 2015:10. Table 2.1

Vascular

Acute Ischemic Stroke Treatment Timeline

Differentiating aggressive from benign DAVF

"Aggressive" symptoms	"Benign" symptoms
Cortical venous reflux (CVR): the hallmark of an aggressive DAVF	Pulsatile bruit
Intracerebral hemorrhage	Orbital congestion (without increased intraocular pressure)
Focal neurological deficit	Cranial nerve palsy
Dementia	Chronic headaches
Papilledema	
Increased intraocular pressure	

Source: Greenberg MS. Endovascular neurosurgery. In: Handbook of Neurosurgery, 8th ed. New York, NY: Thieme; 2016:1590. Table 102.3

Carotid Stenosis Trials

Summary of Major Trials Comparing CEA and Medical Therapy for Carotid Stenosis

	Purpose	Eligibility	Results	Criticism
Asymptomatic Carotid Atherosclerosis Study (ACAS)11	Randomized prospective 5-year multicenter study comparing medical management to CEA for asymptomatic patients with carotid stenosis (via ultrasound and arteriogram) in 1662 patients.	Patients had at least 60% asymptomatic carotid stenosis and were randomized to aspirin only (325 mg daily) or aspirin plus CEA. Barred further participation of some surgeons who had adverse outcomes during the trial.	For the CEA group, the risk of death, any perioperative stroke or ipsilateral stroke over 5 years was half that of the aspirin-only group (5.1% in the surgery group versus 11% in the non-surgical group). There was no significant benefit of CEA in women.	(1) Absolute risk reduction with CEA was only .1% per year. (2) The low operative risk may not be matched in "real world" practice. (3) Non-significant absolute risk reduction of disabling or fatal stroke with surgery (2.7%). (4) The trial had insufficient power for subgroup analysis compared with ACST.
Asymptomatic Carotid Surgery Trial (ACST)12	A 5-year prospective, randomized trial that included 126 hospitals and randomized 3120 asymptomatic patients with carotid stenosis (by ultrasound) to either receive immediate CEA or deferral of CEA until treatment was indicated.	At least 60% unilateral or bilateral carotid stenosis without any TIA or stroke within 6 months prior to the study. Very few exclusion criteria.	Similar results to ACAS. Absolute reduction in 5 year stroke risk was 6.4% in the CEA group versus 11.8% in the deferral group. Unlike ACAS, there was a significant absolute reduction with CEA in risk of disabling or fatal stroke. Because of larger enrollment, the study had sufficient power for subgroup analysis.	(1) Medical management in the deferral group was variable. (2) The study excluded patients who had neurological symptoms or stroke for up to 6 months prior to the study; however, around 300 patients were admitted into the study who had neurological symptoms more than 6 months prior to the study onset.

(Continued)

(*Continued*) Summary of Major Trials Comparing CEA and Medical Therapy for Carotid Stenosis

	Purpose	Eligibility	Results	Criticism
North American Symptomatic Carotid Endarterectomy Trial (NASCET)4	One of the original multicenter, randomized, controlled prospective trials designed to compare CEA to medical therapy for secondary stroke prevention in patients with symptomatic carotid stenosis. The trial studied 2885 patients at 106 centers. Primary outcome was fatal or nonfatal stroke ipsilateral to the stenosis for which patient was treated. Secondary outcome was all strokes and deaths.	Hemispheric or retinal TIA or nondisabling stroke within 120 days prior to enrollment. Patients were divided into two categories based on severity of carotid stenosis: 30–69% and 70–99%. 659 patients were randomized in the high-grade category, and 858 patients were in the 50–69% category. The remainder were in the <50% stenosis group.	The 2-year ipsilateral stroke risk was significantly lower in the CEA group compared with medical group (9% in the surgery group versus 26% in the medical group, p < 0.001). The moderate stenosis group achieved a statistically significant 5-year stroke risk reduction with CEA (15.7% versus 22.2% in medical group). CEA was clearly beneficial for symptomatic high-grade (≥70%) stenosis. CEA was beneficial in carefully selected patients with symptomatic moderate stenosis. There was no benefit with CEA for stenosis <50%.	(1) There were no standardized guidelines for the medical management group. (2) Patients ≥80 years and medical comorbidities were excluded; study population not reflective of entire population at risk of stroke from carotid stenosis. (3) The low surgical complication rates in the trial are not reflective of "real world" practice. (4) Medical management has improved since this trial and the results in the medical arm may no longer be applicable.

(*Continued*)

(*Continued*) Summary of Major Trials Comparing CEA and Medical Therapy for Carotid Stenosis

	Purpose	Eligibility	Results	Criticism
European Carotid Surgery Trial (ECST)5	ECST was a randomized, multicenter, prospective trial that compared CEA to medical management in 3024 patients with symptomatic carotid stenosis. The trial was conducted at 100 centers in 14 countries.	Similar to NASCET. Patients with any degree of carotid stenosis were eligible for ECST. 501 patients had stenosis ≥70% and 684 patients were in the moderate stenosis category. Method of measurement of stenosis was different than in NASCET. The ECST method resulted in higher degrees of stenosis compared with NASCET. Very few exclusion criteria.	Results were similar to NASCET with regard to high-grade (≥70%) stenosis. Two-year risk of ipsilateral stroke was 7% for CEA compared with 19.9% for medical therapy. ECST showed negative benefit with CEA in patients with moderate stenosis (50–69%). There was no benefit with CEA for stenosis <50%.	(1) When stenosis was remeasured using NASCET criteria, CEA reduced 5-year stroke and death risk by 5.7%, a modest reduction similar to the results seen in NASCET. (2) ECST defined follow-up stroke as a deficit persisting more than 7 days and did not include retinal TIAs. (3) Medical management has improved since this trial was conducted.

Abbreviations: CEA, carotid endarterectomy; TIA, transient ischemic attack.
Source: Tummala RP, Souslian FG. Extracranial arterial occlusive disease. In: Deshaies E, Eddleman C, Boulos A, eds. Handbook of Neuroendovascular Surgery. 1st ed. New York, NY:Thieme; 2011:330–331. Table 17.2

Major CAS Trials

	Purpose	Eligibility	Results	Criticism
Stent-Protected Angioplasty versus Carotid Endarterectomy Trial (SPACE)13	Prospective, randomized trial, designed to establish noninferiority of CAS compared with CEA for symptomatic extracranial carotid stenosis in low surgical risk patients.	Inclusion criteria—patients from 35 different centers throughout Europe with symptomatic severe carotid stenosis (≥70% on duplex ultrasound, ≥50% by NASCET criteria, ≥70% by ECST criteria). 1183 patients were randomized within 6 months of a TIA or stroke to receive either CAS or CEA. High-risk surgical candidates were excluded from the study. Primary endpoint was stroke or death, with follow-up at 30 days and at 2 years following treatment.	The 30-day post-treatment results failed to support noninferiority of CAS compared with CEA. The rate of ipsilateral stroke or death was 6.34% in the CEA group and 6.84% in the CAS group, which was not statistically significant. The 2-year post-treatment results showed that the rates of ipsilateral stroke between the two modalities are similar (8.8% in the CEA group and 9.5% in the CAS group, p = 0.62).	(1) Enrollment was halted well short of intended enrollment of 1900 patients. Interim analysis suggested that 2500 patients would be needed to demonstrate significance. The trial did not have funds to meet this goal and was terminated early. (2) Use of embolic protection devices was not required and was used in 27% of the CAS cases.
Endarterectomy versus Angioplasty in Patients with Symptomatic Severe Carotid Stenosis (EVA-3S)14	Prospective, randomized, assessor-blinded trial designed to compare CEA versus CAS in patients with symptomatic extracranial carotid stenosis.	527 patients with symptomatic severe carotid artery stenosis (≥60% on angiography or duplex ultrasound and MRA) from 30 different centers in France were randomized within 4 months of stroke. Primary endpoint was stroke or death within 30 days following treatment. The trial was stopped prematurely after it was estimated that at least 4000 patients would have to be enrolled to test the non-inferiority of carotid stenting. As in the SPACE trial, high-risk surgical candidates were excluded from this trial.	30-day rate of death or any stroke was 3.9% in the CEA group versus 9.6% in the CAS group (significant). 6-month rate of death or stroke was 6.1% for CEA and 11.7% for CAS. 30-day rate of disabling stroke was 1.3% for CEA and 3.4% for CAS (not significant).	(1) The inexperience of the operators performing CAS in this trial has been cited as one factor for the high complication rate for CAS. The complication rate for CAS was much higher than described in previously published papers. (2) Embolic protection devices were recommended after half the trial duration was completed. (3) Dual antiplatelet therapy was used in fewer than 50% of the CAS patients. (4) Rates of MI were not assessed.

(Continued)

(Continued) Major CAS Trials

	Purpose	Eligibility	Results	Criticism
Stenting and Angioplasty with Protection in Patients at High Risk for Endarterectomy (SAPPHIRE)15	A prospective observational randomized trial that included 29 centers throughout North America. This study compared high-risk surgical patients who were symptomatic with ≥50% carotid stenosis (with duplex ultrasound or angiography) to high-risk surgical patients who were asymptomatic with ≥80% stenosis. Primary endpoints were major adverse events that included stroke, death, and MI (unlike EVA-3S and SPACE).	Only high-risk surgical candidates were included in the study. They defined high-risk as having one or more of the co-morbidities listed in Table 15.3.	This trial demonstrated that CAS was not inferior to CEA in high-risk patients. The 30-day rates of death, stroke, or MI were 5.8% for CAS and 12.6% for CEA. At 6 months, combined major adverse events rate was 12.2% with CAS and 20.1% in the CEA group. There was a signifi cant decrease in cranial nerve injuries with CAS.	(1) Almost 29% of patients in both treatment groups had recurrent arterial stenosis, which favors carotid stenting. This is because repeat surgery is associated with a higher complication rate. (2) Many patients were lost to follow-up at 3 years. (3) The inclusion of MI as an endpoint was not part of the NASCET or ECST trials.

(Continued)

(Continued) Major CAS Trials

	Purpose	Eligibility	Results	Criticism
Carotid Revascularization Endarterectomy versus Stenting Trial (CREST)16	CREST was a randomized, multicenter, prospective trial that compared CEA to CAS in 2502 patients with symptomatic and asymptomatic carotid stenosis. The trial was conducted at 117 centers in the US and Canada.	Symptomatic: transient ischemic attack (TIA), amaurosis fugax (AF), or non-disabling stroke within the past 180 days, and who have an ipsilateral carotid stenosis ≥50% by angiography or ≥70% by ultrasound or ≥70% by CTA or MRA. Asymptomatic subjects: Patients who have carotid stenosis ≥60% by angiography or ≥70% by ultrasound or ≥80% by CTA or MRA are eligible for this study. (Subjects with symptoms beyond 180 days are considered asymptomatic.) Outcome: Mortality, stroke, or myocardial infarction at 30 days postoperatively; ipsilateral stroke at 30 days postoperatively.	For 2502 patients (median follow-up 2.5 years), there was no significant difference in the estimated 4-year rates of the primary endpoint between the CAS group and the CEA group (7.2% and 6.8%, respectively; hazard ratio with CAS, 1.11; 95% confidence interval, 0.81 to 1.51; p = 0.51). There was no differential treatment effect with regard to the primary endpoint according to symptomatic status (p = 0.84) or sex (p = 0.34). The 4-year rate of stroke or death was 6.4% with CAS and 4.7% with CEA (hazard ratio, 1.50; p = 0.03); the rates among symptomatic patients were 8.0% and 6.4% (hazard ratio, 1.37; p = 0.14), and the rates among asymptomatic patients were 4.5% and 2.7% (hazard ratio, 1.86; p = 0.07), respectively. Periprocedural rates of individual components of the endpoints differed between the CAS group and the CEA group: for death (0.7% versus 0.3%, p = 0.18), for stroke (4.1% versus 2.3%, p = 0.01), and for myocardial infarction (1.1% versus 2.3%, p = 0.03). After this period, the incidences of ipsilateral stroke with CAS and with CEA were similarly low (2.0% and 2.4%, respectively; p = 0.85).	N/A

Source: Tummala RP, Souslian FG. Extracranial arterial occlusive disease. In: Deshaies E, Eddleman C, Boulos A, eds. Handbook of Neuroendovascular Surgery. 1st ed. New York, NY:Thieme; 2011:332–334. Table 17.3

Unruptured Aneurysm Natural History

Natural History Rupture Risks of Unruptured Intracranial Aneurysms (UIAs) in the International Study of Unruptured Intracranial Aneurysms (ISUIA Parts 1 and 2), Stratified by Aneurysm Diameter3,4

ISUIA Part 1 (7.5-Year Risks)	N	< 10 mm		10–24 mm	≥ 25 mm
All group 1*	446	0.4%		~ 6%	~ 12%
All group 2*	438	~ 4%		~ 5%	
ISUIA Part 2 (5-Year Risks)	**N**	**< 7 mm**	**7–12 mm**	**13–24 mm**	**≥ 25 mm**
Anterior circulation (excludes cavernous carotid artery)	1037	Group 1: 0% Group 2: 1.5%	2.6%	14.5%	40%
Posterior circulation (includes aneurysms at posterior communicating artery)	445	Group 1: 2.5% Group 2: 3.4%	14.5%	18.4%	50%

*Groups 1 and 2 refer respectively to UIAs without and with prior history of SAH from another aneurysm in the same patient.
Source: Awad IA, Dey M, Brorson J, Lee S-K. Incidental aneurysms. In: Spetzler R, Kalani M, Nakaji P, eds. 2nd ed. Neurovascular Surgery. New York, NY:Thieme; 2015:749. Table 62.1

Subarachnoid Hemorrhage Grading

WFNS SAH grade

WFNS grade	GCS score[a]	Major focal deficit[b]
0[c]		
1	15	–
2	13–14	–
3	13–14	+
4	7–12	+ or –
5	3–6	+ or –

[a]GCS = Glasgow Coma Scale
[b]aphasia, hemiparesis or hemiplegia (+ = present, – = absent)
[c]intact aneurysm
Source: Greenberg MS. Introduction and general information, grading, medical management, special conditions. In: Handbook of Neurosurgery. 8th ed. New York, NY: Thieme; 2016:1163. Table 77.4

Hunt and Hess criteria

Grade	Criteria	Mortality (%)
1	Asymptomatic or minimal headache with slight nuchal rigidity	11
2	Moderate to severe headache, nuchal rigidity, no neurological deficit other than cranial nerve palsy	26
3	Drowsy, confused, mild focal deficit	37
4	Stupor, moderate to severe hemiparesis	71
5	Deep coma, decerebrate rigidity	100

Source: Cohen M, Jethwa P, Prestigiacomo CJ, Gandhi CD. Subarachnoid hemorrhage: workup and diagnosis. In: Spetzler R, Kalani M, Nakaji P, eds. 2nd ed. Neurovascular Surgery. New York, NY:Thieme; 2015:41. Table 6.2

Modified grading system of Fisher (correlation between the amount of blood on CT and the risk of vasospasm)

Modified Fisher scale group	Blood on CT[a]	Symptomatic vasospasm
	No SAH or IVH	
1	focal or diffuse thin SAH, no IVH	24%
2	focal or diffuse thin SAH, with IVH	33%
3	focal or diffuse thick SAH, no IVH	33%
4	focal or diffuse thick SAH, with IVH	40%

[a]measurements made in the greatest longitudinal & transverse dimension on a printed EMI CT scan (no scaling to actual thickness) performed within 5 d of SAH in 47 patients; falx never contributed more than 1 mm thickness to interhemispheric blood
Source: Greenberg MS. Critical care of aneurysm patients. In: Handbook of Neurosurgery. 8th ed. New York, NY: Thieme; 2016:1180. Table 78.2

Spetzler-Martin AVM Grading

Spetzler-Martin AVM grading system

Graded feature	Points
Size[a]	
small (< 3 cm)	1
medium (3–6 cm)	2
large (> 6 cm)	3
Eloquence of adjacent brain	
non-eloquent[b]	0
eloquent[b]	1
Pattern of venous drainage[c]	
superficial only	0
deep	1

[a]largest diameter of nidus on non-magnified angiogram (is related to and therefore implicitly includes other factors relating to difficulty of AVM excision, e.g. number of feeding arteries, degree of steal, etc.)
[b]eloquent brain: sensorimotor, language and visual cortex; hypothalamus and thalamus; internal capsule; brain stem; cerebellar peduncles; deep cerebellar nuclei
[c]considered superficial if all drainage is through cortical venous system; considered deep if any or all is through deep veins (e.g. internal cerebral vein, basal vein, or pre-central cerebellar vein)
Source: Greenberg MS. Vascular malformations. In: Handbook of Neurosurgery. 8th ed. New York, NY: Thieme; 2016:1243. Table 82.6

Dural Arteriovenous Malformation Grading

Commonly Used Classification Schemes for Dural Arteriovenous Fistulas

	Djindjian21	Cognard17	Borden22
Type I	Drainage into sinus or meningeal vein	Normal anterograde flow into a dural sinus	Venous drainage directly into dural venous sinus or meningeal vein
Type II	Initial drainage into sinus with reflux into other sinuses or cortical veins	a: Drainage into a sinus with retrograde flow within the sinus b: Drainage into a sinus with CVR a+b: Drainage into a sinus with retrograde flow within the sinus and cortical vein (s)	Venous drainage into dural sinus or meningeal vein with CVR
Type III	Initial drainage into cortical vein	Direct drainage into a cortical vein without venous ectasia	Venous drainage directly into subarachnoid veins
Type IV	Initial drainage into cortical vein with giant venous pouch	Direct drainage into a cortical vein with ectasia > 5 mm and 3× larger than the diameter of the draining vein	
Type V		Direct drainage into spinal perimedullary veins	

Abbreviation: CVR, cortical venous reflux.
Source: Mendes GAC, Puglia P Jr., Frudit ME, Mendes Pereira Caldas JG. Endovascular management of intracranial fistulas. In: Spetzler R, Kalani M, Nakaji P, eds. 2nd ed. Neurovascular Surgery. New York, NY:Thieme; 2015:934. Table 77.1

Spine Arteriovenous Malformation Grading

Classification of spinal vascular malformations based on the scheme developed by Spetzler et al

Classification	Description
Extradural AVFs	Uncommon, direct anastomosis between radicular artery and epidural venous plexus; high-flow lesions that may cause symptoms from mass effect from engorgement
Intradural dorsal AVFs	Most common, similar to Di Chiro type I spinal AVM, direct anastomosis between a radicular artery and a dural vein; commonly in thoracic spinal cord
Intradural ventral AVFs	Midline lesions with direct anastomosis between ASA and coronal venous plexus; type A are small, slow-flow lesions; types B and C are larger, higher-flow lesions

(Continued)

(Continued) Classification of spinal vascular malformations based on the scheme developed by Spetzler et al

Classification	Description
Extradural–intradural AVMs	Rare lesions, analogous to Di Chiro type III juvenile AVMs
Intramedullary AVMs	Seated within the spinal cord parenchyma; receive arterial input from the ASA and the PSA; high-pressure, high-flow lesions associated with aneurysm formation; analogous to Di Chiro type II lesions
Conus medullaris AVMs	Complex nidus with multiple shunts from ASA, PSA, and radicular arteries

Abbreviations: ASA, anterior spinal artery; AVF, arteriovenous fistula; AVM, arteriovenous malformation; PSA, posterior spinal artery.
Source: Wemhoff MP, Tsimpas A, Ashley WW Jr. Emergent presentation and management of spinal dural arteriovenous fistulas and vascular lesions. In: Loftus C, ed. Neurosurgical Emergencies. 3rd ed. New York, NY: Thieme; 2017:274. Table 29.1

Tumor

Karnofsky Scale

Karnofsky performance status scale (modified)

Score	Criteria	General category
100	normal: no complaints, no evidence of disease	Able to carry on normal activity and work. No special care is needed
90	able to carry on normal activity: minor signs or symptoms	
80	normal activity with effort: some signs or symptoms	
70	cares for self: unable to carry on normal activity or to do active work	Unable to work. Able to live at home, care for most personal needs. Variable assistance is required
60	requires occasional assistance: cares for most of needs	
50	requires considerable assistance and frequent care	
40	disabled: requires special care and assistance	Unable to care for self. Requires equivalent of institutional or hospital care. Disease may be rapidly progressing
30	severely disabled: hospitalized; death not imminent	
20	very sick: hospitalized; active supportive care needed	
10	moribund: fatal processes are progressing rapidly	
0	dead	

Source: Greenberg MS. Outcome assessment. In: Handbook of Neurosurgery. 8th ed. New York, NY: Thieme; 2016:1358. Table 88.1

House-Brackmann Facial Nerve Grading

House-Brackmann Facial Nerve Grading Classification

Grade	Description
I	Normal function
II	Mild dysfunction: slight weakness on testing, can close eye, normal tone and symmetry at rest
III	Moderate gross dysfunction: at rest, normal tone and symmetry Synkinesis: not severe Movement: moderate weakness but active movement still observed Eye: can close with maximum effort
IV	Moderately severe: obvious weakness/asymmetry with movement At rest, normal tone and symmetry Eye closure incomplete
V	Severe: barely observed movement maximal effort Asymmetry at rest Eye closure incomplete
VI	Total paralysis: no movement, asymmetry at rest

Source: Di Ieva A, Lee J, Cusimano M. Otorhinolaryngology and Principles of Neurotology in Skull Base Surgery. In: Handbook of Skull Base Surgery. 1st ed. Thieme; 2016:201. Table 8.2

Decision Making for 1–4 Brain Mets

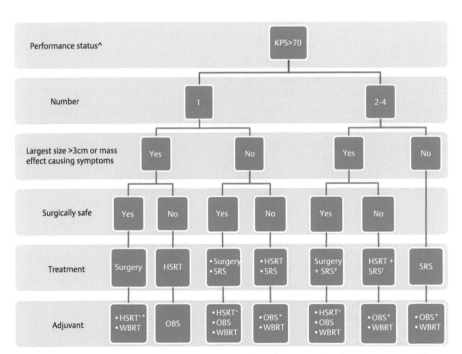

Source: Myrehaug S, Lo SS, Jabbari S, Ma L, Das S, Karotki A, Chang EL, Sahgal A. Stereotactic radiosurgery for the management of one to four brain metastases. In: Lunsford L, Sheehan J, eds. Intracranial Stereotactic Radiosurgery. 2nd ed. Thieme; 2015:240. Figure 28.2

Dose Tolerance for SRS

Reasonable organ-at-risk (OAR) dose-tolerance parameters for intracranial single fraction SRS

OAR	Volume parameter	Dose	Clinical end point	Note
Brain	5–10 cc	12 Gy	Radionecrosis	Tolerance and clinical sensitivity dependent on location and eloquence
Brainstem	Dmax	12.5 Gy	Brainstem radionecrosis	For brainstem metastasis, 15 Gy to lesions < 2 cm in volume is practiced
Optic pathway	Dmax	10–12 Gy	Radiation-induced visual injury	Refers to optic nerve and chiasm
Cochlea	Marginal (Dmax) dose	12–14 Gy Mean dose < 4–6 Gy	Sensorineural hearing loss	Cochlear nucleus may also be important but further data required

Abbreviation: Dmax = maximum point dose to structure.
Source: Jabbari S, Ma L, Lee YK, Lo SS, Chang EL, Grimm J, Altenau L, White D, Udani V, Goetsch SJ, Larson D, Sahgal A. Critical structures and tolerance of the central nervous system. In: Lunsford L, Sheehan J, eds. Intracranial Stereotactic Radiosurgery. 2nd ed. Thieme; 2015:56. Table 7.3

Pediatrics

ETV Success Score

ETV Success Score

Category	Description	Value	Score
Age	< 1 month	0%	___%
	1 to < 6 months	10%	
	6 months to < 1 year	30%	
	1 to > 10 years	40%	
	≥ 10 years	50%	
Etiology	post infectious	0%	___%
	myelomeningocele post IVH non-tectal brain tumor	20%	
	aqueductal stenosis tectal tumor other	30%	

(Continued)

(*Continued*) ETV Success Score

Category	Description	Value	Score
Shunt history	previous shunt	0%	__%
	no previous shunt	10%	
		Total (range 0–90%)	__%

Source: Greenberg MS. Treatment of hydrocephalus. In: Handbook of Neurosurgery. 8th ed. New York, NY: Thieme; 2016:416. Table 25.1

Craniosynostosis

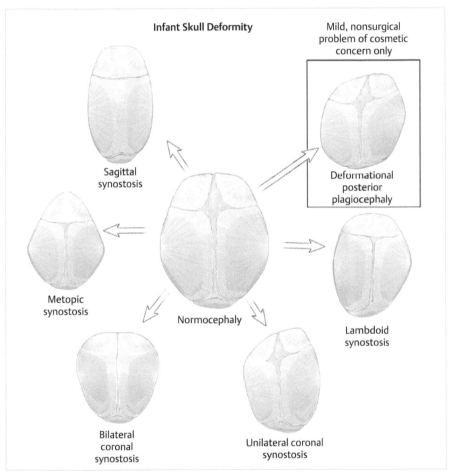

Source: Baird LC, Proctor MR. Craniosynostosis. In: Albright A, Pollack I, Adelson P, eds. Principles and Practice of Pediatric Neurosurgery. 3rd ed. Thieme; 2014:238. Figure 19.2

Peripheral Nerve

Peripheral Nerve Injury Classification

Grading of peripheral nerve injuries

Sunderland grade	Seddon grade	Pathological features	Clinical outcome
I	Neuropraxia	Conduction block, myelin loss	Excellent
II	Axonotmesis	Axon loss	Very good
III		Grade II and endoneurium loss	Variable
IV		Grade III and perineurium loss	Poor/no recovery
V	Neurotmesis	Nerve trunk disruption	No recovery

Source: Addas BMJ. Nerve injuries: anatomy, pathophysiology, and classification. In: Socolovsky M, Rasulic L, Midha R, et al., eds. Manual of Peripheral Nerve Surgery. From the Basics to Complex Procedures. 1st ed. Thieme; 2017:19. Table 3.2

EMG and Lesion Severity Correlation

Clinical correlation: correlating electrophysiological findings with nerve lesions

Grade injury	Neurapraxia	Axonotmesis	Neurotmesis
	I	II–IV	V
NCS	Conduction block with decreased amplitude that is restored within a few weeks	First day: proximal CMAP amplitude reduced. After 4 days, distal CMAP amplitude reduced	Absent proximal CMAP. After 4 days, absent distal CMAP
EMG	No spontaneous activity Normal MUP Recruitment decreased of MU that is restored within a few weeks	First day: recruitment decreased. After 3 weeks: spontaneous activity, abnormal MUP If reinnervation: polyphasic and prolonged MUP If recovery: fewer denervation signs and increased recruitment	First day: absent MUP with no spontaneous activity. After 3 weeks: spontaneous activity, absent MUP. Reinnervation signs only if reconstructive surgery successful; otherwise spontaneous activity disappears by fibrosis

Abbreviations: CMAP, compound motor action potential; EMG, electromyography; MU, motor unit; MUP, motor unit potentials; NCS, nerve conduction studies.
Source: Rodríguez Aceves CA, Domínguez Páez M, Fernández Sánchez VE. Electrodiagnostic pre-, intra-, and postoperative evaluations. In: Socolovsky M, Rasulic L, Midha R, et al., eds. Manual of Peripheral Nerve Surgery. From the Basics to Complex Procedures. 1st ed. Thieme; 2017:53. Table 6.2

Reinnervation on EMG

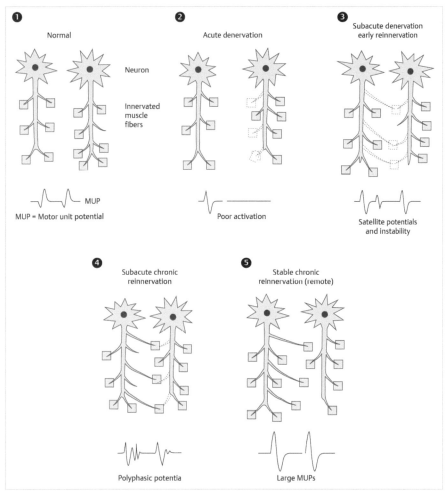

Source: Patel K, Horak HA. Electrodiagnostic testing in spine surgery. In: Baaj A, Mummaneni P, Uribe J, et al., eds. Handbook of Spine Surgery. 2nd ed. Thieme; Figure to follow 2016:67. Figure 10.2

Glossary

ABCs	airway, breathing, circulation
ABG	arterial blood gases
AC	anterior commissure
ACA	anterior cerebral artery
ACAS	Asymptomatic Carotid Atherosclerosis Study
ACDF	anterior cervical diskectomy and fusion
ACE	angiotensin-converting enzyme
ACh	acetylcholine
ACom	anterior communicating artery
ACTH	adrenocorticotropic hormone
ADH	antidiuretic hormone
ADI	atlantodental interval
AFB	acid-fast bacilli
AFib	atrial fibrillation
AFP	α fetal protein
AICA	anterior inferior cerebellar artery
AIDP	acute inflammatory demyelinating polyradiculoneuropathy
AIDS	acquired immunodeficiency syndrome
ALIF	anterior lumbar interbody fusion
ALL	anterior longitudinal ligament
ALS	amyotrophic lateral sclerosis
ANA	antinuclear antibody test
AOS	anterior odontoid screw
AP	anteroposterior
ARDS	acute respiratory distress syndrome
ASA	aspirin
ATV	all-terrain vehicle
AVF	arteriovenous fistula
AVM	arteriovenous malformation
b.i.d.	twice a day
BAER	brainstem auditory evoked response
BBB	blood–brain barrier
BCNU	carmustine
BF	blood flow
Botox	botulism toxin
BP	blood pressure
BUN	blood urea nitrogen
CABG	coronary artery bypass graft
CAD	coronary artery disease
CBC	complete blood count
CBF	cerebral blood flow
CCA	common carotid artery
CCB	calcium channel blocker
CCF	carotid–cavernous fistula
CCNU	lomustine

CEA	carotid endarterectomy
CESI	cervical epidural steroid injection
CHF	congestive heart failure
CJD	Creutzfeldt–Jakob disease
CK	creatine kinase
$CMRO_2$	cerebral metabolic rate of oxygen
CNS	central nervous system
COPD	chronic obstructive pulmonary disease
COWS	cold opposite, warm same
CPA	cerebellopontine angle
CPN	common peroneal nerve
CPP	cerebral perfusion pressure
CRP	C-reactive protein
CRPS	complex regional pain syndrome
CSF	cerebrospinal fluid
CSW	cerebral salt wasting
CT	computed tomography
CTA	computed tomography angiography
CTS	carpal tunnel syndrome
CVA	cerebrovascular accident
CVP	central venous pressure
CXR	chest X-ray
DANG THE RAPIST	diabetes and drugs; amyloid; neoplasm and nutritional (B_{12}); Guillain–Barré syndrome; trauma; hereditary; endocrine, electrolytes, and entrapment; renal and radiation; alcohol and AIDS; porphyria and paraneoplastic syndrome; infectious, immunologic, and ischemic; sarcoid; and toxins
DBM	demineralized bone matrix
DBS	deep brain stimulation
DDAVP	desmopressin acetate
DI	diabetes insipidus
DIC	disseminated intravascular coagulopathy
DISH	diffuse idiopathic skeletal hyperostosis
DM	diabetes mellitus
DNA	deoxyribonucleic acid
DREZ	dorsal root entry zone
DTRs	deep tension reflexes
DVT	deep venous thrombosis
DWI	diffusion-weighted imaging
DXA	dual-energy X-ray absorptiometry
EAM	external acoustic meatus
EBV	Epstein–Barr virus
ECA	external carotid artery
ECG	electrocardiogram
EDH	epidural hemorrhage
EEG	electroencephalogram
ELISA	enzyme-linked immunosorbent assay
EMG	electromyogram
ENT	ear, nose, and throat
ER	emergency room

ESR	erythrocyte sedimentation rate
ET	endotracheal
ETOH	ethanol
EVD	external ventricular drain
FFP	fresh frozen plasma
FMD	fibromuscular dysplasia
FSH	follicle-stimulating hormone
GBM	glioblastoma multiforme
GBS	Guillain–Barré syndrome
GCS	Glasgow Coma Scale
GERD	gastroesophageal reflux disease
GGT	gamma glutamyl transferase
GH	growth hormone
GPi	globus pallidus interna
GTC	generalized tonic-clonic
GTR	gross total resection
GU	genitourinary
Gy	gray (unit of radiation)
HCP	hydrocephalus
HCT	hematocrit
HFS	hemifacial spasm
HHH	hypervolemic-hypertensive-hemodilution
HLA-B27	human leukocyte antigen-B27
HOB	head of bed
HSV	herpes simplex virus
HTN	hypertension
IBS	irritable bowel syndrome
ICA	internal carotid artery
ICP	intracranial pressure
Ig	immunoglobulin
IGF	insulin-like growth factor
IgG	immunoglobulin G
INR	international normalized ratio
IQ	intelligence quotient
IT	intrathecal
IV	intravenous
IVDA	intravenous drug abuser
IVH	intraventricular hemorrhage
JCV	JC virus
KUB	kidney, ureter, and bladder
LD	lumbar drain
LE	lower extremity
LH	luteinizing hormone
LINAC	linear accelerator
LMN	lower motor neuron
LOAF	lumbricals 1 and 2, opponens pollicis, and abductor and flexor pollicis brevis muscles
LOC	loss of consciousness
LP	lumbar puncture
MAEW	moves all extremities well

MAO	monoamine oxidase
MCA	middle cerebral artery
MCV	mean corpuscular volume
MEPS	motor evoked potentials
METS	metastasis
MI	myocardial infarction
MM	myelomeningocele
MRA	magnetic resonance angiography
MRI	magnetic resonance imaging
MRV	magnetic resonance venography
MS	multiple sclerosis
MVD	microvascular decompression
NAP	nerve action potentials
NASCET	North American Symptomatic Carotid Endarterectomy Trial
NCCT	noncontrast computed tomography
NCV	nerve conduction velocity
NF-1	neurofibromatosis type I
NG	nasogastric
NPO	nothing by mouth
NS	normal saline
NSAID	nonsteroidal antiinflammatory drug
NSCCA	non-small cell carcinoma
OCP	oral contraceptive pill
OFC	occipital-frontal circumference
OPCA	olivopontucerebellar atrophy
OPLL	ossified posterior longitudinal ligament
OR	operating room
Osm	osmolarity
PC	posterior commissure
PCA	posterior cerebral artery
PCD	primary ciliary dyskinesia
PCom	posterior communicating artery
PCR	polymerase chain reaction
PD	Parkinson disease
PEG	percutaneous endoscopic gastrostomy tube
PET	positron emission tomography
PGA	polyglycol alcohol
PICA	posterior inferior cerebellar artery
PLIF	posterior lumbar interbody fusion
PLL	posterior longitudinal ligament
PMH	Past medical history
PML	progressive multifocal leukoencephalopathy
PMN	polymorphonuclear neutrophil
PNET	primitive neuroectodermal tumor
PNS	peripheral nervous system
PO	taken orally
POD	postoperative day
PSNP	progressive supranuclear palsy
PT	physical therapy
PT	prothrombin time

PTA	post-traumatic amnesia
PTH	parathyroid hormone
PTT	partial thromboplastin time
PVD	peripheral vascular disease
QHS	every bedtime
rBMP	recombinant bone morphogenetic protein
REZ	root entry zone
RF	radiofrequency
RF	Rheumatoid Factor
RIND	reversible ischemic neurological deficit
RLN	recurrent laryngeal nerve
RPR	rapid plasma reagin
RSD	reflex sympathetic dystrophy
SACE	serum angiotensin-converting enzyme
SAH	subarachnoid hemorrhage
SATCHMO	sarcoid, aneurysm/adenoma (pituitary), teratoma, craniopharyngioma, hypothalamic hamartoma/histiocytosis X, meningioma, optic glioma
SBP	systolic blood pressure
SCD	sequential compression devices
SCI	spinal cord injury
SCIWORA	spinal cord injury without radiographic abnormality
SCM	sternocleidomastoid
SCS	spinal cord stimulation
SCSD	subacute combined systems disease
SDH	subdural hematoma
SEGA	subependymal giant cell astrocytoma
SG	specific gravity
SI	sacroiliac
SIADH	syndrome of inappropriate antidiuretic hormone
SLE	systemic lupus erythematosus
SLR	straight leg raise
SMA	superior mesenteric artery
SNHL	sensorineural healing loss
SOMI	sternal-occipital-mandibular immobilizer
SPECT	single photon emission computed tomography
SQ	subcutaneous
SR	solute ratio
SRS	stereotactic radiosurgery
SSEP	somatosensory evoked potential
SSPE	subacute sclerosing panencephalitis
SSS	superior sagittal sinus
STA	superficial temporal artery
STIR MRI	short T1-inversion recovery magnetic resonance imaging
STN	subthalamic nucleus
t.i.d.	three times daily
TB	tuberculosis
TCL	transverse carpal ligament
TED	thromboembolic deterrent
TENS	transcutaneous electrical nerve stimulation

TIA	transient ischemic attack
TLIF	transforaminal lumbar interbody fusion
TLSO	thoracolumbar spinal orthosis
TM	transverse myelitis
TMJ	temporomandibular joint disorder
t-PA	tissue-plasminogen activator
TSH	thyroid-stimulating hormone
UA	urinalysis
UE	upper extremity
UMN	upper motor neuron
UOP	urine output
V/Q	ventilation-perfusion
VA	vertebral artery
VDRL	Venereal Disease Research Laboratory
VHL	Von Hippel-Lindau disease
VIM	ventral intermediate thalamic nucleus
VIND	vascular, infectious, neoplastic, demyelinating
VMA	vanillylmandelic acid
VP	ventriculoperitoneal
w/u	workup
WBCs	white blood cells
WBRT	whole brain radiation therapy
XRT	radiation therapy

Index

Note: Page numbers set in **bold** or *italic* indicate headings or figures, respectively.